Anti-oxidant and Anti-inflammatory Properties of Natural Compounds

Anti-oxidant and Anti-inflammatory Properties of Natural Compounds

Editor

Othmane Merah

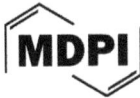

Basel • Beijing • Wuhan • Barcelona • Belgrade • Novi Sad • Cluj • Manchester

Editor
Othmane Merah
University of Toulouse
Toulouse
France

Editorial Office
MDPI AG
Grosspeteranlage 5
4052 Basel, Switzerland

This is a reprint of articles from the Special Issue published online in the open access journal *Cosmetics* (ISSN 2079-9284) (available at: https://www.mdpi.com/journal/cosmetics/special_issues/Antioxidant_Compounds).

For citation purposes, cite each article independently as indicated on the article page online and as indicated below:

Lastname, A.A.; Lastname, B.B. Article Title. *Journal Name* **Year**, *Volume Number*, Page Range.

ISBN 978-3-7258-2045-0 (Hbk)
ISBN 978-3-7258-2046-7 (PDF)
doi.org/10.3390/books978-3-7258-2046-7

© 2024 by the authors. Articles in this book are Open Access and distributed under the Creative Commons Attribution (CC BY) license. The book as a whole is distributed by MDPI under the terms and conditions of the Creative Commons Attribution-NonCommercial-NoDerivs (CC BY-NC-ND) license.

Contents

About the Editor vii

Preface ix

Othmane Merah
Special Issue "Anti-Oxidant and Anti-Inflammatory Properties of Natural Compounds"
Reprinted from: *Cosmetics* **2023**, *10*, 80, doi:10.3390/cosmetics10030080 1

Emna Habachi, Iness Bettaieb Rebey, Sarra Dakhlaoui, Majdi Hammami, Selmi Sawsen, Kamel Msaada, et al.
Arbutus unedo: Innovative Source of Antioxidant, Anti-Inflammatory and Anti-Tyrosinase Phenolics for Novel Cosmeceuticals
Reprinted from: *Cosmetics* **2022**, *9*, 143, doi:10.3390/cosmetics9060143 4

Yoo-Kyung Kim and Dae-Jung Kang
Anti-Pollution Activity, Antioxidant and Anti-Inflammatory Effects of Fermented Extract from *Smilax china* Leaf in Macrophages and Keratinocytes
Reprinted from: *Cosmetics* **2022**, *9*, 120, doi:10.3390/cosmetics9060120 21

Young-Ah Jang, Yong Hur and Jin-Tae Lee
Anti-Inflammatory Activity of the Active Compounds of Sanguisorbae Radix in Macrophages and In Vivo Toxicity Evaluation in Zebrafish
Reprinted from: *Cosmetics* **2019**, *6*, 68, doi:10.3390/cosmetics6040068 30

Kamel Zemour, Amina Labdelli, Ahmed Adda, Abdelkader Dellal, Thierry Talou and Othmane Merah
Phenol Content and Antioxidant and Antiaging Activity of Safflower Seed Oil (*Carthamus Tinctorius* L.)
Reprinted from: *Cosmetics* **2019**, *6*, 55, doi:10.3390/cosmetics6030055 42

Nattawut Whangsomnuek, Lapatrada Mungmai, Kriangsak Mengamphan and Doungporn Amornlerdpison
Efficiency of Skin Whitening Cream Containing *Etlingera elatior* Flower and Leaf Extracts in Volunteers
Reprinted from: *Cosmetics* **2019**, *6*, 39, doi:10.3390/cosmetics6030039 53

Peggy Schlupp, Thomas M. Schmidts, Axel Pössl, Sören Wildenhain, Gianni Lo Franco, Antonio Lo Franco and Bandino Lo Franco
Effects of a Phenol-Enriched Purified Extract from Olive Mill Wastewater on Skin Cells
Reprinted from: *Cosmetics* **2019**, *6*, 30, doi:10.3390/cosmetics6020030 63

Olívia R. Pereira, Gleiciara Santos and Maria João Sousa
Hop By-Products: Pharmacological Activities and Potential Application as Cosmetics
Reprinted from: *Cosmetics* **2022**, *9*, 139, doi:10.3390/cosmetics9060139 76

Asma El Zerey-Belaskri, Nabila Belyagoubi-Benhammou and Hachemi Benhassaini
From Traditional Knowledge to Modern Formulation: Potential and Prospects of *Pistacia atlantica* Desf. Essential and Fixed Oils Uses in Cosmetics
Reprinted from: *Cosmetics* **2022**, *9*, 109, doi:10.3390/cosmetics9060109 92

Agnieszka Kulawik-Pióro and Weronika Joanna Goździcka
Plant and Herbal Extracts as Ingredients of Topical Agents in the Prevention and Treatment Radiodermatitis: A Systematic Literature Review
Reprinted from: *Cosmetics* **2022**, *9*, 63, doi:10.3390/cosmetics9030063 115

Punniamoorthy Thiviya, Ashoka Gamage, Dinushika Piumali, Othmane Merah and Terrence Madhujith
Apiaceae as an Important Source of Antioxidants and Their Applications
Reprinted from: *Cosmetics* **2021**, *8*, 111, doi:10.3390/cosmetics8040111 . . . . **159**

About the Editor

Othmane Merah

Dr. Othmane MERAH is an Associate Professor at the Paul Sabatier University, Toulouse, working as a teacher and researcher in the Laboratory of Agroindustrial Chemistry (Institut National Polytechnique, Toulouse, France). After obtaining an engineer's degree in Agronomic Sciences from the National Agronomic School of Rennes (France) and the University of Blida (Algeria), he completed his PhD at the Institute of Plant Biotechnology (Paris XI University) and the National Institute for Agronomic Research (Montpellier). He completed his Habilitation Diploma for supervising doctoral research at the National Polytechnic Institute of Toulouse. He investigates genetic and morpho-physiological diversity in cereals, oilseed, and aromatic plants. His research program is focused on studying the physiology and genetics of drought tolerance in cereals and oilseed crops under conventional and organic conditions. He is a crop scientist and agronomist with wide experience in large-scale research programs and leading multidisciplinary and international collaboration projects. He is the author of over 150 publications. He is an editorial and/or advisory board member of several international journals. He has attended many international congresses and symposiums. He has participated in the development of three cultivars of brown mustard in Burgundy (France) for the famous "Moutarde de Dijon" condiment. He was the scientific referent for the genetic program of the mustard network in Burgundy. He works on the valorization of bioactive molecules from plants for foods and cosmetics.

Preface

Plants have historically been a source of nutrition for humans, for their health, for the pharmaceutical industry, and also for their well-being and social appearance. This societal demand has become more demanding over the years, as have the naturalness of molecule sources and extraction and processing methods. At present, these requirements are the focus of marketing, environmental protection labels and the recycling of industrial by-products, the circular bioeconomy, and 'green' sources that guarantee the authenticity sought after by consumers. The following Special Issue responds to this demand by attempting to take an overview of acquired knowledge and new research on plant sources around the world.

This Special Issue, entitled 'Anti-oxidant and Anti-inflammatory Properties of Natural Compounds', is a collection of eleven articles, both original research, and reviews, exploring the diversity of plant sources for their antioxidant and anti-inflammatory activities.

The contributions in this Special Issue provide an overview of the diversity of sources of antioxidant and anti-inflammatory molecules around the world. Other works show the interest of certain botanical species in providing us with natural compounds that respond to current concerns about pollution or for the confection of specific cosmetic products. This Special Issue also focuses on the use of plant processing residues. These by-products are wonderful sources of molecules of interest to the cosmetics industry and provide answers to anti-ageing, anti-pollution, anti-stress, anti-inflammatory, and antioxidant needs necessary for an intense and stressful life and well-being. The works published in this printed collection contribute in several ways to the enrichment of our knowledge, either through a consistent effort to summarise the state of the art on what plants can contribute to cosmetics or through case research on a given plant. I have had the honor and pleasure of editing this Special Issue and would like to express my thanks and profound gratitude to the authors who have chosen to contribute to it.

Othmane Merah
Editor

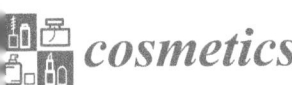

Editorial

Special Issue "Anti-Oxidant and Anti-Inflammatory Properties of Natural Compounds"

Othmane Merah [1,2]

[1] Laboratoire de Chimie Agro-industrielle (LCA), Université de Toulouse, INRAe, INPT, 31030 Toulouse, France; othmane.merah@ensiacet.fr; Tel.: +33-5-3432-3523
[2] Département Génie Biologique, IUT A, Université Paul Sabatier, 32000 Auch, France

Throughout history, humans have utilized plants as conscious or unconscious sources of molecules for food, health and well-being [1,2]. With the evolution of human activity, the stresses generated, and the necessity of resorting to medicinal solutions to manage them, discovering and employing natural products has become crucial. Thus, the use of plants as a source of care and well-being has become increasingly vital.

Thiviya et al. [3] present one of the oldest plant families used for food, traditional medicine and cosmetics. They review the current scientific knowledge of many umbelliferous plants regarding their composition and their biological, anti-inflammatory, anti-ageing and anti-cancer activities; above all, they provide some examples of the research conducted on the application of antioxidants from this family in the cosmetics industry.

Kulawik-Pióro and Goździcka [4] present, in a review, cases of the utilization of herbal extracts in preparations for the prevention and treatment of radiodermatitis. Some of these extracts can be employed as cosmetic supplements. The dominant biological effects of these extracts are related to their antioxidant, anti-inflammatory and antimicrobial activities.

The Atlas pistachio tree, an endemic species of North Africa, is endangered. Nevertheless, El Zerey-Belaskri et al. [5] shed light on the application of Atlas pistachio oils in the development of novel formulations, and as sources of new ingredients and products inspired by indigenous knowledge. This focus may illuminate the plight of this species and generate interest regarding how it might be saved and perhaps exploited as a proven local source of antioxidants and anti-inflammatories.

Oils are often used as ingredients in moisturizing or regenerating creams. Few studies have shown the anti-inflammatory properties of plant oils. The study by Zemour et al. [6] examines the antioxidant and anti-ageing activity of three varieties of safflower grown in three successive years. The results highlight the applicative potential of safflower as a valuable source of oil in cosmetic formulations. The choice of variety and growing conditions have crucial influence on these activities. These results highlight the fascinating potential of safflower oil as a source of phenols, alongside its valuable antioxidant and anti-ageing activity, and its possible application in cosmetics.

Arbutus unedo L., also named the strawberry tree, is known for its fruits, which are consumed in several countries, and for its high content of bioactive molecules, such as polyphenols, flavonoids and monoterpenoids [7]. The effects of extracts from this species, when procured via various methods, are studied by Habachi et al. [8]. As expected, the method of extraction has an impact on the phytochemical composition of the extracts. Moreover, these extracts exhibit a promising whitening effect, with high anti-tyrosinase activities. In addition, their fascinating anti-inflammatory activity and absence of cytotoxicity have been reported.

It is established that air pollution has a substantial effect on human skin, indicating that each pollutant has a distinct toxicological impact on it. This pollution can cause oxidative stress that exceeds the antioxidant capacity of the skin. It can lead to oxidative damage and the premature ageing of the skin, depending on which pollutants the skin is repeatedly

Citation: Merah, O. Special Issue "Anti-Oxidant and Anti-Inflammatory Properties of Natural Compounds". *Cosmetics* **2023**, *10*, 80. https://doi.org/10.3390/cosmetics10030080

Received: 27 April 2023
Accepted: 5 May 2023
Published: 16 May 2023

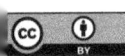

Copyright: © 2023 by the author. Licensee MDPI, Basel, Switzerland. This article is an open access article distributed under the terms and conditions of the Creative Commons Attribution (CC BY) license (https://creativecommons.org/licenses/by/4.0/).

exposed to. The application of naturally occurring antioxidants could help the skin to overcome this repeated aggression. Kim et al. [9] examine the possibility of utilizing the fermented extract of *Smilax china* leaves (FESCL) as an anti-pollution cosmetic material. FESCL significantly diminishes pollutant-induced luciferase activity at a concentration of 1%. This study reveals the applicative potential of FESCL as an anti-pollutant material in cosmetic formulations.

It has been previously proved that *Etlingera elatior* leaf extracts possess strong antioxidant activity and whitening and anti-aging properties, which make it an excellent source for cosmeceuticals. This is investigated in the study of Whangsomnuek et al. [10], which evaluates the efficiency of whitening cream containing both the flower and leaf extracts of E. *elatior* in human volunteers and the degree of skin irritation experienced. The results show that the application of creams formulated with the flower and leaf extracts of E. elatior significantly diminishes the quantity of melanin in the skin compared to non-treated skin This finding indicates that the formulate cream is safe and effective for skin whitening.

The dried roots of *Sanguisorba officinalis* L., also called Sanguisorbae Radix (SR), are known to possess several properties often employed in traditional Chinese medicine. In a study by Jang et al. [11], the antioxidant compounds procured from an acetone extract of SR are isolated, and their anti-inflammatory effects and toxicity are studied in vivo. The various compounds isolated from the SR extract are able to inhibit nitric oxide, tumor necrosis factor alpha and prostaglandin production in a dose-dependent manner. This result demonstrates the potential of compounds extracted from Sanguisorbae Radix, and particularly quercetin, to provide non-toxic and anti-inflammatory biomaterial for the skin.

The economic problems of countries, current geostrategic conflicts, and humanitarian crises around the world are limiting the use of land for non-food purposes. The more efficient utilization of directly produced plant material, or unused or processed residues, appears to be an invaluable source of antioxidant molecules. Thus, in their review, Pereira et al. [12] detail the phytochemicals and biological and pharmacological activities of hops, and their potential application in skin care products. They also highlight the current interest in exploiting the rejected parts of hops and the by-products of the brewing industry, which possess applicative potential in the cosmetic industry.

Olive oil is known to be rich in polyunsaturated fatty acids and possess medicinal properties. The residues remaining after pressing are a precious source of polyphenols, which have many positive health effects. The work of Schlupp et al. [13] evaluates the cell viability, cell proliferation, anti-inflammatory and antioxidant properties of a phenol-enriched olive mill wastewater (OMWW) extract and its effect on an immortal keratinocyte cell line. It was discovered that this phenol-enriched extract exhibits excellent antimicrobial activity, and minimizes the formation of reactive oxygen species and the release of interleukin 8 in HaCaT cells. It also inhibits the growth of A375 melanoma nodules in the skin model. This study reveals that olive mill wastewater is a promising ingredient for dermal applications, and is able to improve skin health and have a positive impact on skin ageing.

These studies and reviews highlight the potential significance of plants as a source of invaluable compounds for application in the cosmetics industry, both by utilizing plant organs or the by-products of industrial processes.

Conflicts of Interest: The author declares no conflict of interest.

References

1. Sayed Ahmad, B.; Talou, T.; Saad, Z.; Hijazi, H.; Merah, O. The Apiaceae: Ethnomedicinal family as source for industrial uses. *Ind. Crop. Prod.* **2017**, *109*, 661–671. [CrossRef]
2. Thiviya, P.; Gamage, A.; Gama-Arachchige, N.S.; Merah, O.; Madhujith, T. Seaweeds as a Source of Functional Proteins. *Phycology* **2022**, *2*, 216–243. [CrossRef]
3. Thiviya, P.; Gamage, A.; Piumali, D.; Merah, O.; Madhujith, T. Apiaceae as an Important Source of Antioxidants and Their Applications. *Cosmetics* **2021**, *8*, 111. [CrossRef]
4. Kulawik-Pióro, A.; Goździcka, W.J. Plant and Herbal Extracts as Ingredients of Topical Agents in the Prevention and Treatment Radiodermatitis: A Systematic Literature Review. *Cosmetics* **2022**, *9*, 63. [CrossRef]

5. El Zerey-Belaskri, A.; Belyagoubi-Benhammou, N.; Benhassaini, H. From Traditional Knowledge to Modern Formulation: Potential and Prospects of *Pistacia atlantica* Desf. Essential and Fixed Oils Uses in Cosmetics. *Cosmetics* **2022**, *9*, 109. [CrossRef]
6. Zemour, K.; Labdelli, A.; Adda, A.; Dellal, A.; Talou, T.; Merah, O. Phenol Content and Antioxidant and Antiaging Activity of Safflower Seed Oil (*Carthamus Tinctorius* L.). *Cosmetics* **2019**, *6*, 55. [CrossRef]
7. Bajoub, A.; Ennahli, N.; Ouaabou, R.; Chaji, S.; Hafida, H.; Soulaymani, A.; Idlimam, A.; Merah, O.; Lahlali, R.; Ennahli, S. Investigation into Solar Drying of Moroccan Strawberry Tree (*Arbutus unedo* L.) Fruit: Effects on Drying Kinetics and Phenolic Composition. *Appl. Sci.* **2023**, *13*, 769. [CrossRef]
8. Habachi, E.; Rebey, I.B.; Dakhlaoui, S.; Hammami, M.; Sawsen, S.; Msaada, K.; Merah, O.; Bourgou, S. *Arbutus unedo*: Innovative Source of Antioxidant, Anti-Inflammatory and Anti-Tyrosinase Phenolics for Novel Cosmeceuticals. *Cosmetics* **2022**, *9*, 143. [CrossRef]
9. Kim, Y.-K.; Kang, D.-J. Anti-Pollution Activity, Antioxidant and Anti-Inflammatory Effects of Fermented Extract from *Smilax china* Leaf in Macrophages and Keratinocytes. *Cosmetics* **2022**, *9*, 120. [CrossRef]
10. Whangsomnuek, N.; Mungmai, L.; Mengamphan, K.; Amornlerdpison, D. Efficiency of Skin Whitening Cream Containing *Etlingera elatior* Flower and Leaf Extracts in Volunteers. *Cosmetics* **2019**, *6*, 39. [CrossRef]
11. Jang, Y.-A.; Hur, Y.; Lee, J.-T. Anti-Inflammatory Activity of the Active Compounds of Sanguisorbae Radix In Macrophages and in Vivo Toxicity Evaluation in Zebrafish. *Cosmetics* **2019**, *6*, 68. [CrossRef]
12. Pereira, O.R.; Santos, G.; Sousa, M.J. Hop By-Products: Pharmacological Activities and Potential Application as Cosmetics. *Cosmetics* **2022**, *9*, 139. [CrossRef]
13. Schlupp, P.; Schmidts, T.M.; Pössl, A.; Wildenhain, S.; Lo Franco, G.; Lo Franco, A.; Lo Franco, B. Effects of a Phenol-Enriched Purified Extract from Olive Mill Wastewater on Skin Cells. *Cosmetics* **2019**, *6*, 30. [CrossRef]

Disclaimer/Publisher's Note: The statements, opinions and data contained in all publications are solely those of the individual author(s) and contributor(s) and not of MDPI and/or the editor(s). MDPI and/or the editor(s) disclaim responsibility for any injury to people or property resulting from any ideas, methods, instructions or products referred to in the content.

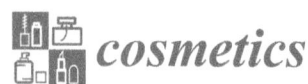

Article

Arbutus unedo: Innovative Source of Antioxidant, Anti-Inflammatory and Anti-Tyrosinase Phenolics for Novel Cosmeceuticals

Emna Habachi [1], Iness Bettaieb Rebey [1], Sarra Dakhlaoui [1], Majdi Hammami [1], Selmi Sawsen [1], Kamel Msaada [1], Othmane Merah and Soumaya Bourgou [1,*]

[1] Laboratory of Medicinal and Aromatic Plants, Biotechnology Center of Borj-Cedria, BP 901, Hammam-Lif 2050, Tunisia
[2] Laboratoire de Chimie Agro-Industrielle (LCA), Université de Toulouse, INRA, INPT, 31030 Toulouse, France
[3] Département Génie Biologique, IUT A, Université Paul Sabatier, 32000 Auch, France
* Correspondence: bourgousoumaya@yahoo.com

Citation: Habachi, E.; Rebey, I.B.; Dakhlaoui, S.; Hammami, M.; Sawsen, S.; Msaada, K.; Merah, O.; Bourgou, S. *Arbutus unedo*: Innovative Source of Antioxidant, Anti-Inflammatory and Anti-Tyrosinase Phenolics for Novel Cosmeceuticals. *Cosmetics* **2022**, *9*, 143. https://doi.org/10.3390/cosmetics9060143

Academic Editors: Adeyemi Oladapo Aremu and Antonio Vassallo

Received: 13 November 2022
Accepted: 14 December 2022
Published: 16 December 2022

Publisher's Note: MDPI stays neutral with regard to jurisdictional claims in published maps and institutional affiliations.

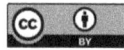

Copyright: © 2022 by the authors. Licensee MDPI, Basel, Switzerland. This article is an open access article distributed under the terms and conditions of the Creative Commons Attribution (CC BY) license (https:// creativecommons.org/licenses/by/ 4.0/).

Abstract: Phenolic compounds are valuable cosmetic ingredients. They display skin protective potential and play an important role in preserving cosmetic formulations due to their ability to neutralize free radicals. Considering this fact, the current study aims to obtain a phenolic-enriched fraction from *Arbutus unedo* for topical application in cosmeceutical products. The chemical composition and the antioxidant, anti-inflammatory, and anti-tyrosinase activities of different extracts from the plant were investigated and compared. Samples were obtained by maceration, reflux, and ultrasound using water and ethanol. The findings indicated that the extraction methods impacted the phytochemical composition of the extracts. The high-performance liquid chromatography with diode-array detection (HPLC–DAD) analysis showed a wide range of phenolic compounds, comprising phenolic acids and flavonoids. Among the extracts, the water reflux had significant levels of both total polyphenols, flavonoids, and tannins and possessed the most important content on hyperoside. It displayed the most significant antioxidant activities with high antiradical and reducing power, as well as strong total antioxidant activity. It possesses a promising whitening effect with high anti-tyrosinase activities. Furthermore, it shows no cytotoxicity and moderate anti-inflammatory activity. Finally, due to its high yield efficiency and activities, water reflux was selected to formulate a cosmeceutical oil-in-water nanoemulsion that displayed optimal pH and stability.

Keywords: *Arbutus unedo*; phytocosmetics; phenolic compounds; antioxidants; anti-inflammatory; anti-tyrosinase; cosmetic formulation; nanoemulsion

1. Introduction

Skin aging is characterized by a progressive loss of physiological properties and regenerative potential due to intrinsic (genetic factors and hormones) and extrinsic factors caused by the environment [1]. The most harmful of the external factors is UV radiation, known as photoaging, which induces the production of reactive oxygen species (ROS) that can result in oxidative stress and induces aging skin [2], contributing to wrinkle, roughness, dryness, elasticity loss, and pigmentation [3]. Nowadays, cosmetics incorporating natural active compounds are gaining great interest compared to synthetic ingredients [4] due to their capacity to limit the intrinsic aging processes of the skin and to counteract extrinsic processes [5]. Plants' anti-aging effects are mainly attributed to their antioxidant metabolites. Topical antioxidants can protect the skin from free radical damage, and daily use can influence the biological functions of the skin and reverse photodamage, helping skin reparations [6]. Moreover, plant secondary metabolites can modulate the activity of enzymes involved in skin aging. Tyrosinase is an enzyme often a target for the cosmetic sector. It is a copper-containing enzyme that catalyzes melanin biosynthesis in human skin. Melanin provides protection against environmental parameters, in particular, UV radiation. However, the hyperpigmentation induced by excessive melanin production may lead to skin disorders such as age spots and melasma and post-inflammatory hyperpigmentation leading to flaw and premature aging appearance [7]. Therefore, targeting tyrosinase activity could be a recommended approach to treating disordered pigmentation problems and developing cosmetic products. [7]. However, synthetic ingredients used in cosmetics and medical preparations are not widely accepted by consumers due to their adverse side effects. Kojic acid is a well-known tyrosinase inhibitor but exhibits cellular toxicity [8]. Therefore, further research is required to identify safe and effective natural tyrosinase inhibitors.

Antioxidants inhibit or quench free radicals and slow the oxidation of oxidizable biomolecules like fats, proteins, and DNA. Antioxidants consist of enzymatic and non-enzymatic forms. Enzymatic antioxidants include the primary enzymes catalase, superoxide dismutase, and glutathione peroxidase. The secondary enzymes consist of glutathione reductase and glucose-6-phosphate dehydrogenase. Non-enzymatic antioxidants are vitamin C, vitamin E, plant phenolic compounds, carotenoids, and glutathione [9].

Phenolics are metabolites with variable phenolic structures and one or more hydroxyl groups and aromatic rings in free or glycosylated form. They are well-known for their precious health advantages and are components of various cosmetic and pharmaceutical applications depending on their bioactivities. Polyphenols have an important role as cardioprotective and neuroprotective, antidiabetic, and anticancer substances. They have antioxidant and anti-inflammatory activities that prevent UV-induced ROS generation in fibroblasts and keratinocytes and the production of pro-inflammatory mediators. [10]. They can restore the proper function of the skin (e.g., DNA repair and viability of human keratinocytes and dermal fibroblasts) after UVA and UVB-caused damages [10–13]. All these precious benefits make phenolics prime candidates for anti-aging therapies as antioxidants. Furthermore, antioxidant testing is a complex topic due to the lack of a standardized test. Two general categories, namely those associated with lipid peroxidation and electron or radical scavenging tests, are widely used for various antioxidant analyses. The former includes the β-carotene bleach test, the lipid peroxidation test with TCA-TBA solution, and the latter includes the ABTS (2, 2′-azino-bis3-ethylbenzthiazoline-6-sulfonic acid) radical cation decolorization test, DPPH (1, 1-Diphenyl-2-picryl-hydrazyl) radical scavenging test, ferric reducing antioxidant power test, superoxide anion scavenging activity test, ferrous ion chelation test, etc. The choice of a suitable test is, therefore, crucial to examine the antioxidant activity of biological extracts [14].

Arbutus unedo, also called the strawberry tree, belongs to the Ericaceae family. It grows in the Canary Islands, north-eastern Africa, western Asia, and Europe. This species has been traditionally used as food by using fruits to make marmalades, liquor, jams, and jellies. In traditional medicine, the leaves are used for their astringent, diuretic, urinary antiseptic, antidiarrheal and purgative properties and are useful in the treatment of diabetes, rheumatism and inflammation, and skin diseases [15].

Several pharmacological studies pointed to biological properties such as antitumor, antimicrobial, spasmolytic, antioxidant, and neuroprotective. Phytochemical reports underlined the presence of tannins, flavonoids, phenolic glycosides, irroids, tocopherol, anthocyanins, carotenoids, terpenoids, and fatty acids [16]. It has been shown that genetic variability and environmental factors, as well as extraction techniques, may greatly affect the phytochemical content of *A. unedo* and, thus, its biological capacity [17]. Thus, the selection of extraction method is crucial, depending on the sample matrix and the targeted compound to be recovered. Although *Arbutus* from the European region has been studied, mainly from Portugal, Croatia, and Italy [16–19], there is a scarcity of the phytochemistry and bioactivities of *Arbutus unedo* from Tunisia. Therefore, the objective of this study was to examine the effect of different extraction methods (maceration, reflux, and ultrasound extraction) on the pharmacological potentials of *Arbutus unedo*, including its antioxidant, anti-inflammatory, and anti-tyrosinase activities. A topical emulsion containing a selected phenolics-enriched extract associated with the highest activities was further developed. Its stability via physicochemical means was evaluated.

2. Materials and Methods

2.1. Plant Material

Leaves of *Arbutus unedo* were collected from Ain draham (North Tunisia). A specimen was deposited at the Center of Biotechnology of Borj Cedria (voucher number AU002020.10). The air-dried leaves were finely ground with an A10 knife mill (Ika-Werk, Staufen, Germany) and stored in the dark.

2.2. Extraction Procedure

Plant material was subjected to different extraction procedures, reflux: 30 g of *Arbutus unedo* leaves powder was extracted using 300 mL of boiling water under reflux for 30 min, static maceration: 10 g of powder was separately extracted by solvents for 12 h at room temperature, ultrasound: ten grams of powdered were deposited in capped glass vials, mixed with 100 mL solvents and immersed into the ultrasonic bath (SONOREX DIGIPLUS, BANDELIN, Berlin, Germany) (180 W, 40 kHz frequency) for 30 min. For maceration and ultrasound extractions, water, ethanol, and ethanol: water (50:50) were used as solvents. After filtering through the Whatman No.1 filter paper, solvents were removed.

2.3. Total Phenolics Evaluation

The number of total polyphenols in *A. unedo* extracts was carried out by spectrophotometric analysis using the Folin-Ciocalteu method [20]. A sample of 125 µL of the extract was mixed with 500 µL of distilled water and 125 µL of Folin–Ciocalteu reagent. The mixture was stirred before the supply of 1.25 mL of 7% Na_2CO_3, and distilled water was added to reach a final volume of 3 mL, and the mix was thoroughly shaken. The mixture was incubated in the dark for 90 min. The absorbance was measured at 760 nm. The standard used was gallic acid at different concentrations to establish a calibration curve. The polyphenol contents were expressed as micrograms of gallic acid equivalents per gram of dry matter (mg GAE/g DW).

2.4. Total Flavonoids Measurement

The total flavonoid content of extracts was performed according to the protocol described by Bourgou et al. [20]. Each sample (250 mL) was mixed with 75 mL of the solution of $NaNO_2$ (5%; w/v), and then 150 mL $AlCl_3 \times 6H_2O$ (10%; w/v) was added. This mixture was supplied with 500 mL of NaOH (1 M), and the final volume was adjusted to 2.5 mL with distilled water. The mixture was then carefully stirred. Absorbance was assessed at 510 nm. Flavonoid contents were expressed as mg catechin equivalent per gram of dry residue (mg CE/g DW) using the calibration curve of (+)-catechin, with concentrations ranging from 0 to 500 µg/mL.

2.5. Evaluation of Total Condensed Tannins

Total tannin contents were performed according to Sun et al. [21]. H_2SO_4 solution (1.5 mL) was added to a 50 µL aliquot of extract. The extract solvent was used as a blank, and the absorbance was measured at 500 nm. Total condensed tannins were expressed as mg catechin/g DW. A calibration curve of catechin with a 50 to 400 µg/mL concentration range was used for this purpose.

2.6. Identification of Phenolic Compounds

The system of high-performance liquid chromatography (consisting of a vacuum degasser, an autosampler, and a binary pump with a maximum pressure of 400 bar; Agilent 1260, Agilent Technologies, Waldronn, Germany) with a 4.6 × 100 mm reversed-phase C18 analytical column with a particle size of 3.5 µm (Zorbax Eclipse XDB C18, Agilent Technologies GmbH, Böblingen Germany) was used to analyze phenolic compounds in

A. unedo extracts. The diode array detector was configured over a scan range of 200–400 nm. The temperature of the column was 25 °C. Two microliters of the sample were injected. The mobile phase was composed of a mixture of methanol (solvent A) and milli-Q water with 0.1% formic acid (solvent B). The identification of phenolic compounds was performed by comparing their retention times with those of the standards. Gallic, caffeic, *p*-coumaric and ellagic acids were used as phenolic acid standards, while the flavonoid standards were arbutin, catechin, epigallocatechin, rutin, and hyperoside. The detected phenolic compounds were determined using the calibration curves of the corresponding standard solutions. The content of each compound was expressed in micrograms per gram of residue (µg/g DR).

2.7. Antioxidant Activity

2.7.1. Total Antioxidant Activity (TAA)

The total antioxidant capacity of *A. unedo* extracts was carried out, according to Bourgou et al. [20]. The extract was homogenized with 1 mL of reagent solution (0.6 N sulfuric acid, 28 mM sodium phosphate, and 4 mM ammonium molybdate) and incubated at 95 °C for 90 min. The mixtures were cooled to room temperature, and the absorbance was read at 695 nm. The activity was expressed as mg gallic acid equivalent per gram dry weight (mg GAE/g DW).

2.7.2. ABTS Radical Scavenging Assay

2,2′-Azino-bis(3-ethylbenzothiazoline-6-sulphonic acid (ABTS) assays were carried out by mixing 950 µL of the diluted ABTS solution and 50 µL of extract increasing concentrations. After incubation for 6 min, absorbance was measured at 734 nm. ABTS scavenging ability was expressed as IC_{50} value (the extract's concentration resulting in 50% inhibition of absorbance).

2.7.3. DPPH Radical Scavenging Assay

DPPH quenching ability of extracts were evaluated according to Bourgou et al. [20]. Samples were added to a 0.2 mM solution of DPPH. After 30 min of incubation at room temperature, the absorbance was read against a blank at 517 nm. The results were given as half-maximal inhibitory concentration (IC_{50}) and presented in µg/mL.

2.7.4. Iron Reducing Power

The sample extract was supplied with sodium phosphate buffer (0.2 M, pH 6.6) and potassium ferricyanide (10 g/L) [20]. The mixture was then incubated at 50 °C for 20 min. Trichloroacetic acid (100 g/L) was then added. After centrifugation, the upper layer was mixed with deionized water and ferric chloride (0.01 g/L). The generated blue-green color was measured at 700 nm.

2.7.5. Chelating Effect

The chelating activity was evaluated according to Zhao and others [22]. Different concentrations of the sample were added to $FeCl_2 \times 4H_2O$ solution (2 mM) and incubated at room temperature for 5 min. Then, the reaction was initiated by adding ferrozine (5 mM), and the absorbance of the solution was then measured spectrophotometrically at 562 nm. Results were expressed as IC_{50}.

2.8. Cell Culture

RAW 264.7 murine macrophage cells (American Type Culture Collection, Manassas, VA, USA) were cultured at 37 °C in a humidified atmosphere of 5% carbon dioxide; the RPMI medium supplemented with 10% of fetal bovine serum (*v*/*v*), 100 µg/mL of streptomycin and 100 U/mL of penicillin.

2.9. Cell Viability Assay

Cell viability was assessed using a Resazurin assay [23]. RAW 264.7 (2×10^5 cells/mL) cells were cultured in 24-well and incubated for 24 h. RAW 264.7 cells were treated with *A. unedo* extracts at different concentrations. Indeed, the extracts were dissolved in DMSO and then diluted with the culture medium into different concentrations to make the final DMSO concentration at less than 0.1% (v/v) in order to avoid solvent toxicity. After 24 h of treatment, the fluorescence was measured using an automated 96-well Fluoroskan Ascent FlTM plate reader (Thermo-Labsystems) at an excitation wavelength of 530 nm and an emission wavelength of 590 nm.

2.10. Anti-Inflammatory Activity

The anti-inflammatory activity of the studied *A. unedo* extracts was evaluated on the murine macrophage RAW 264.7 cell line by measuring NO generated by the cells using the Griess reagent. Cells were plated in 24-well plates at a 2×10^5 cells/mL and incubated for 24 h. Then the cells were treated with Lipopolysaccharide (LPS) (1 µg/mL) in the absence or presence of various concentrations of samples. After a 24 h LPS stimulation, the cell-free supernatants were collected, and nitric oxide (NO) levels were assessed using Griess's reagent. The absorbance was evaluated at 540 nm, and the final nitrite concentration was determined using a sodium nitrite standard curve (0–50 µM).

2.11. Tyrosinase Inhibition Assay

The mushroom tyrosinase activity of *A. unedo* extracts was measured according to Momtaz et al. [24]. L-DOPA and tyrosine have been used as substrates, while kojic acid and arbutin as standard inhibitors. The reaction mixture contained 70 µL of extract (dissolved in dimethyl sulfoxide (DMSO) and further diluted in potassium phosphate buffer (50 mM, pH 6.5) and 30 µL of tyrosinase (333 units/mL in phosphate buffer, pH 6.5). After 5 min of incubation at room temperature, the substrate was added. Absorbance was read at 492 nm. The IC_{50} value was determined as the concentration of tyrosinase inhibitor to inhibit 50% of its activity under the assay conditions.

2.12. Development of Formulation

Oil-in-water (O/W) emulsion was elaborated using the formulation given in Table 1 in two phases (aqueous and oily) according to Khairi et al. with modification [25]. The oily phase was heated to 70 °C using a heating plate with constant stirring until a homogeneous mixture obtaining. The aqueous phase was heated at the same temperature in a beaker until complete melting. Subsequently, the water phase, and the oil phase were placed in a 100 mL glass vessel and homogenized using an Ultraturrax homogenizer at 15.000 rpm. The freshly prepared cosmetic emulsion was then subjected to the following studies.

Table 1. Composition of the O/W formulation containing *A. unedo* phenolic extract.

Components	% (w/w)
Aqueous phase	
Glycerin	1
A. unedo extract	1
Xanthan gum	0.1
Phenoxyethanol	0.1
Distilled water	75.3
Oily phase	
Almond oil	15
Glyceryl monostearate	7.5

2.13. Encapsulation Efficiency Measurement

The percentage of phenolic compounds held within the emulsion was assessed following the Regan and Mulvihill method [26]. About 3 g of the emulsion was mixed with

3 g of phosphate buffer solution (pH 7) and centrifuged at 4500 rpm for 30 min. Then, the lower phase was collected. The percentage of encapsulated compounds (E) was identified by using Equation:

$$E\ (\%) = (1 - C2/C1) \times 100$$

where C2 is the concentration of phenolic compounds found in the aqueous phase after centrifugation, and C1 is the initial concentration of phenolic compounds in the inner aqueous phase [26,27].

2.14. Preliminary Stability Tests

2.14.1. Centrifugation Test

Analytical centrifugation was performed (3000 rpm) for 30 min at room temperature. The appearance and homogeneity characteristics were assessed by macroscopic analyses.

2.14.2. Thermal Stress

Consecutive storage was done for eight days at 4 °C and 40 °C in a drying and heating oven [28].

2.14.3. pH Analysis

The determination of pH was measured by a pH meter at 22 ± 2 °C.

2.14.4. Particle Size and Zeta Potential Evaluation

Measurement of the mean droplet diameter and zeta potential was performed by Zetasizer® (Zetasizer Nano-ZS/Malvern Instruments, Worcester, UK). Laser Diffraction Particle Size Analyzer (LS13320, Beckman Coulter, Inc., Brea, CA, USA) after formulations dilution with distilled water 200-fold.

2.15. Statistical Analysis

An analysis of variance (ANOVA) was performed to compare the effect of methods of extraction on the measured traits, and Duncan's test means comparison was used to determine significant differences among means of measured traits.

3. Results and Discussion

3.1. Yield of Arbutus unedo Leaves Extracts

Many researchers are currently focusing on replacing harmful solvents with environmentally friendly substitutes. The use of green and sustainable solvents such as ethanol and water, combined with the use of low environmental impact technologies, is a promising holistic approach to the development of "green" extraction processes. Ethanol is recognized as a green solvent and offers greater industrial safety. On the other hand, water has a low environmental impact and is inexpensive in terms of production, transport, and disposal. On the other hand, the possibility of modifying the physico-chemical properties of water by varying the conditions (temperature, pressure, etc.) has increased the interest in its use as an extraction solvent. In this study, ethanol and water were used in order to evaluate and optimize the extracting ability of phenolic compounds from the leaves of *Arbutus unedo*, as well as their influence on the biological activities of this specie, by varying the extraction process. The extraction of phenolic compounds by "green" non-toxic solvents was carried out by two conventional (or classic) methods, maceration and reflux extraction, and an unconventional (or innovative) namely extraction by sonication (Table 2).

Yield results are significantly different and vary markedly depending on the solvent and extraction technique (Table 2). Generally, *Arbutus unedo* seems rich in polar compounds. In fact, the best performance was observed using the reflux extraction technique and water as solvent (38%), followed by extraction with 50% ethanol by maceration and sonication with yields of 35% and 30%, respectively. Cold water extraction and sonication have also shown high yields (28% and 29%). Absolute ethanol, especially by maceration, proved to be the least efficient with the lowest yields (5%). The variation in yields agrees with data from the literature, which indicates that the yield depends on the extraction solvent's nature and polarity [29]. Our results suggest that the yield increases with increasing solvent polarity.

Table 2. Mean values of Yield, total phenolic, tannin, and flavonoid contents of *A. unedo* leaves extracts from different extraction methods (mean ± standard deviation, n = 3).

	Yield (%)	Total Phenolics (mg GAE/g DW)	Total Flavonoids (mg CE/g DW)	Total Tannins (mg CE/g DW)
Reflux water	38	73 ± 0.7 [a]	51 ± 1.9 [a]	54 ± 3.8 [a]
Maceration water	28	79 ± 3.6 [a]	22 ± 0.9 [c]	29 ± 2.6 [c]
Maceration ethanol	5	32 ± 1.0 [d]	11 ± 0.4 [e]	17 ± 1.3 [d]
Maceration ethanol 50%	35	67 ± 2.7 [b]	18 ± 1.6 [d]	34 ± 1.1 [bc]
Ultrasound water	29	48 ± 1.5 [c]	19 ± 0.3 [cd]	30 ± 1.4 [c]
Ultrasound ethanol	20	76 ± 2.1 [a]	21 ± 0.4 [cd]	38 ± 2.6 [b]
Ultrasound ethanol 50%	30	74 ± 1.2 [a]	27 ± 1.3 [b]	32 ± 1.0 [bc]

For each column, different letters indicate significant differences between extracts using Duncan's test at a 0.05 probability level.

Regardless of the extraction method, we observed that the yields using 50% ethanol were much higher than those using pure ethanol, which indicated that the extracting power of ethanol is improved by adding water following the increase in its polarity. Moreover, our results are consistent with several works in the literature indicating the efficiency of water in extracting soluble compounds from *Arbutus unedo* leaves. In effect, Oliveira et al. [30] reported a significant yield difference as a function of the polarity of the solvent used, varying from 2.8% using petroleum ether to 32.4% using boiling water. These authors showed an average yield of 15% using ethanol. Similarly, Malheiro et al. [18] worked on 19 *Arbutus* ecotypes Portuguese and noticed hot water extraction yields ranging from 27% to 61%. However, Orak et al. [31] noticed that ethanol and water showed yields close to 40% and 39%.

3.2. Effect of Solvent and Extraction Method on Total Phenolics, Flavonoids, and Tannins Contents

The choice of solvent is crucial in the extraction process as it determines the selectivity and then impacts the chemical composition and functional properties of the final extract. This choice usually depends on the solubility of the target compound. Since solubilization involves electrostatic repulsions and attractions between the solvent and the solute, a polar solvent would be the best for the solubilization and extraction of polar molecules, while a less polar solvent would be suitable for less polar compounds.

3.2.1. Total Phenolic Contents

The impact of solvents and extraction methods on polyphenol content has been extensively studied. Despite the fact that aqueous alcoholic solvents are generally considered the most suitable for phenolic extraction, no universal extraction method is adequate for every phenolic [31]. Table 2 provides a summary of the total contents of phenolics, flavonoids, and tannins in *A. unedo* leaves. According to these results, the maximum total phenolic content was noted in water extract obtained by maceration (79 mg GAE/g DW) as well as ethanol, ethanol 50% ultrasound extracts, and reflux water (76, 74 and 73 mg GAE/g DW, respectively) and the lowest in ethanol extract by maceration (32 mg GAE/g DW). In this case, Oliveira et al. [30] reported a higher amount of total polyphenol in Portuguese *A. unedo* leaves (172.21 and 192.66 mg EAG/g DW, respectively, for aqueous and ethanolic extracts). Tenuta et al. [16] examined four methods for bioactive component extraction from fresh and dried leaves of *A. unedo* and observed a significant impact of solvents and extraction techniques on the content of phytochemicals. Indeed, ethanol 60% by maceration was better than decoction to extract polyphenols from dried leaves with a content of 329 mg/g. These differences observed in plant extracts are probably due to geographical factors, extraction method, and maturity level of the plant at the time of harvest effects [31]. Besides, the contents of total polyphenols are known to be considerably influenced by various extrinsic and intrinsic factors, particularly environmental factors.

Furthermore, we noticed in our study that the extraction technique greatly influenced the phenolic contents of *A. unedo* leaves. In fact, ultrasonic extraction using ethanol 50% seems to enhance the phenolic contents extraction compared to extraction by maceration using this solvent (Table 2), while water use shows a negative effect in ultrasonic extraction. It has been reported that, for some plant materials, excessive extraction time in the water would lead to the degradation of some target compounds, resulting in reduced concentrations [32].

3.2.2. Total Flavonoids

The results in Table 2 show variability in the flavonoid content of *A. unedo* leaves by varying the extraction process and type of solvent. Reflux extraction was the most efficient method to extract flavonoids from *A. unedo* leaves, displaying the highest total concentration of 51 mg CE/g DW (Table 2).

Considering the extraction solvent, we notice that compared to ethanol, water is much more effective in extracting flavonoids with high levels ranging from 19 to 51 mg CE/g DW where reflux extraction showed the highest content. This indicates that heating improves the extractive power of water. The beneficial effect of increasing the temperature would be linked to an increase in the transfer of matter, inducing an increase in the diffusion of molecules [32]. The ethanolic extracts showed lower but interesting flavonoid contents. Indeed, pure ethanol used in ultrasonic extraction has a content of 27 mg CE/g DW followed by 50% ethanol using the same process (21 mg CE/g DW). While the lowest content was found with the maceration extract with 100% ethanol (11 mg EC/g DW). The richness of the aqueous extract of *A. unedo* on flavonoids compared to ethanol extracts is confirmed by the work of Jurica et al. [33], who showed that the leaves' aqueous extract has lower levels of total polyphenols than the methanolic extract but was richer in flavonoids. Moreover, compared to data from the literature, the Tunisian *Arbutus* was richer in flavonoid content than *Arbutus* from Algeria and Portugal [34,35]. Flavonoids have the ability to act as antioxidants in biological systems.

3.2.3. Condensed Tannins

Tannins can be widely found in plants and have several health benefits. As shown in Table 2, *Arbutus unedo* leaves were rich in condensed tannins. Indeed, regardless of the solvent involved and the extraction process adopted, water reflux had the highest content (54 mg CE/g DW). Thus, extraction using hot water leads to obtaining an *Arbutus* extract rich in tannins. As for polyphenols and total flavonoids, ultrasound improves tannin extraction using ethanol as a solvent. Indeed, the ultrasound extraction with pure ethanol and 50% ethanol were richer in tannins (38 and 32 mg CE/g DW, respectively) compared to pure ethanol by maceration (17 mg CE/g DW).

The various results suggest that using water as a solvent at a high temperature ensures the extraction of the maximum level of tannins.

3.3. Phytochemicals Identification

Although the total contents of bioactive molecules are valuable data regarding the phytochemical profile of a plant, they do not allow the separate quantification of the main bioactive compounds. For this reason, a detailed assessment of the phenolic compounds in the seven different extracts was performed by HPLC-DAD analysis, and the results are displayed in Table 3. The main compounds in the extracts of *Arbutus unedo* leaves were flavonoids and phenolic acids. The obtained data highlighted the richness of extracts on hyperoside (quercetin 3-*O*-galactoside) with amounts ranging from 30 to 56 mg/g DR. The highest content was observed in reflux water (56 mg/g DR) and ultrasound ethanol (55 mg/g DR). As previously reported in the literature, hyperoside was the most predominant phenolic compound in Croatian *Arbutus unedo* leaves [19].

Table 3. Identification and quantification (mg/g DR) of the main polyphenols present in *A. unedo* extracts (mean ± standard deviation, *n* = 3).

	Phenolic Acids					Flavonoids			
	Gallic Acid	Caffeic Acid	*p*-Coumaric Acid	Ellagic Acid	Arbutin	Catechin	Epigallocatechin	Rutin	Hyperoside
Reflux water	0.42 ± 0.1 [b]	0.07 ± 0.00 [e]	0.39 ± 0.00 [d]	1.27 ± 0.05 [bc]	1.2 ± 0.2 [bc]	ND	0.96 ± 0.2 [a]	ND	56.06 ± 1.8 [a]
Maceration water	0.18 ± 0.0 [c]	0.05 ± 0.00 [e]	0.27 ± 0.04 [d]	0.83 ± 0.1 [d]	2.78 ± 1.2 [a]	0.58 ± 0.1 [b]	0.19 ± 0.04 [b]	1.55 ± 0.4 [c]	31.32 ± 3.1 [b]
Maceration ethanol	0.09 ± 0.0 [c]	0.27 ± 0.1 [d]	0.59 ± 0.01 [c]	1.26 ± 0.2 [bc]	2.26 ± 0.7 [a]	ND	0.77 ± 0.1 [a]	2.07 ± 0.3 [b]	34.24 ± 6.1 [b]
Maceration ethanol 50%	0.08 ± 0.0 [c]	0.31 ± 0.08 [bc]	0.28 ± 0.03 [d]	1.06 ± 0.01 [cd]	1.87 ± 0.4 [ab]	1.22 ± 0.6 [a]	0.34 ± 0.1 [b]	2.14 ± 0.01 [ab]	33.97 ± 4.5 [b]
Ultrasound water	1.83 ± 0.6 [c]	0.38 ± 0.02 [b]	1.45 ± 0.9 [a]	1.51 a ± 0.45	0.73 ± 0.02 [c]	0.58 ± 0.03 [b]	0.18 ± 0.07 [b]	ND	30.03 ± 5.5 [b]
Ultrasound ethanol	0.18 ± 0.05 [c]	0.28 ± 0.1 [d]	0.96 ± 0.2 [b]	1.50 ± 0.1 [ab]	0.85 ± 0.1 [c]	ND	0.16 ± 0.04 [b]	2.66 ± 0.7 [a]	55.05 ± 2.1 [a]
Ultrasound ethanol 50%	0.12 ± 0.05 [c]	0.59 ± 0.2 [a]	0.02 ± 0.01 [e]	1.36 ± 0.1 [ab]	2.16 ± 0.1 [ab]	1.22 ± 0.6 [a]	0.34 ± 0.1 [b]	2.56 ± 0.2 [ab]	41.88 ± 6.6 [b]

ND: not detected. For each column, different letters indicate significant differences between extracts using Duncan's test at 0.05 probability level.

Moreover, samples contained interesting amounts of arbutin. The highest quantity was obtained in water maceration extract (3 mg/g DR) followed by ethanol maceration and ethanol 50% ultrasound by about 2 mg/g DR. This hydroquinone-β-D-glucopyranoside is common in the leaves of several plant species, particularly in the Ericaceae. [36]. Jurica et al. [33] compared the effectiveness of different solvents (methanol, methanol 50%, ethyl acetate, and dichloromethane) and techniques for arbutin extraction from *A. unedo* leaves and reported that ultrasound-assisted extraction with methanol was the most suitable extraction procedure for the recovery for arbutin. The arbutin content in *A. unedo* leaves has been reported to vary according to the origin due to the effect of climate and soil characteristics, ranging from 0.6 mg/g to 12.4 mg/g [36,37].

Other flavonoids detected in our study were rutin, catechin, and epigallocatechin (Table 3). Among the phenolic acids, ellagic acid was the most abundant; the highest quantities were recovered in water and ethanol ultrasound extracts (1.5 mg/g DR). Our results agree with several studies which have established that the main phenolic compounds present in *A. unedo* leaves are catechin, epicatechin, catechin gallate, quercetin, gallic acid, ellagic acid and *p*-hydroxybenzoic acid [34,38–40].

3.4. Effect of Solvent and Extraction Method on Antioxidant Activities

To understand the mechanism of action of the antioxidants present in the extracts of *Arbutus unedo* leaves, four different methods were used, and the results are depicted in Table 4.

Table 4. Mean values of Antioxidant activity of *A. unedo* leaves extracts from different extraction methods.

	TAA (mg GAE/g DW)	DPPH IC$_{50}$ (µg/mL)	ABTS IC$_{50}$ (µg/mL)	Reducing Power EC$_{50}$ (µg/mL)	Chelating Power EC$_{50}$ (mg/mL)
Reflux water	194 ± 5.2 [a]	7 ± 1.1 [d]	58 ± 3.2 [e]	82 ± 5.2 [c]	40 ± 3.1 [a]
Maceration water	86 ± 3.2 [b]	17 ± 1.5 [a]	66 ± 5.5 [d]	112 ± 7.4 [a]	33 ± 4.2 [b]
Maceration ethanol	32 ± 2.1 [e]	9 ± 1.0 [c]	114 ± 7.2 [a]	83 ± 4.4 [c]	NA
Maceration ethanol 50%	52 ± 2.1 [d]	10 ± 1.1 [b]	68 ± 4.1 [d]	64 ± 3.2 [d]	NA
Ultrasound water	63 ± 3.2 [c]	9 ± 1.0 [c]	101 ± 4.3 [b]	97 ± 4.3 [b]	34 ± 4.4 [b]
Ultrasound ethanol	65 ± 4.2 [c]	9 ± 0.7 [c]	102 ± 5.1 [b]	60 ± 3.7 [d]	NA
Ultrasound ethanol 50%	59 ± 2.2 [cd]	6 ± 1.1 [d]	94 ± 4.4 [c]	62 ± 3.2 [d]	NA

NA: not active. For each column, different letters indicate significant differences between extracts at 0.05 probability level using Duncan's test).

The results showed that the nature of the solvent and the extraction technique influence the total antioxidant activity of *A. unedo* (Table 4). Water was found to be the most powerful for extracting antioxidant compounds. In particular, water reflux extraction exhibited a very high value of 194 mg GAE/g DW. Water cold and ultrasound extractions also showed interesting activities (86 mg GAE/g DW and 63 mg GAE/g DW, respectively), while ethanol and ethanol 50% maceration presented the lowest activity, around 32 and

52 mg EAG/g DW. We noted that the ultrasound technique improves the activity in ethanol extracts (TAA = 65 and 59 mg GAE/g DW in ethanol and ethanolic 50%, respectively).

Moreover, the results showed that the significant total antioxidant activity of water reflux extract was positively correlated to its richness in flavonoids and tannins. Indeed, this extract showed the highest levels of these compounds, which suggests that flavonoids and total tannins participated actively in the antioxidant activity of *Arbutus unedo* extracts.

The scavenging activity measured by the DPPH assay showed that the different extracts from *A. unedo* exhibited high capacity with low IC_{50} values that do not exceed 17 µg/mL (Table 4). The ethanolic extract (50%) obtained by sonication and water reflux extract showed the highest trapping power of the DPPH (6 and 7 µg/mL, respectively). It should be noted that apart from the cold aqueous extract, the antiradical capacities obtained are higher than the synthetic antioxidant standard BHT (IC_{50} value is equal to 11.5 µg/mL).

Besides, the results relating to the antiradical activity against the ABTS radical are in line with those of antiradical activity against the DPPH radical (Table 4) and indicate that water reflux extract exhibits the best activity displaying a low IC_{50} (58 µg/mL). However, this capacity becomes lower when the solvent used is ethanol. Ethanol 50% (IC_{50} = 68 µg/mL), ethanolic extracts presented moderate antiradical activity since the IC_{50} varies from 94 to 114 µg/mL. Our results agree with other reports, which underlined a significant antiradical potential of *Arbutus* extracts. Moderate scavenging activity has been reported for the Portuguese and Turkish *A. unedo*, with IC_{50} values ranging from 73 to 487.2 µg/mL [30,31,41]. Indeed, the high antiradical potential of the various extracts, especially that of the water extract by reflux, could be due to their richness in flavonoids, in particular, hyperoxide present with levels varying from 28 to 37 mg/g DW (Table 3). The antioxidant activity of hyperoxide has been described as being related to the hydroxyl groups of the A and B rings and the glycosides bound to the C ring [42]. Liu et al. [43] found that hyperoxide could effectively protect PC12 cells from ROS-induced cytotoxicity, including hydrogen peroxide and tert-butyl hydroperoxide, without being damaging. Flavonoids are known to be powerful scavenger agents and effective hydrogen donors, acting as primary antioxidants and stabilizing radicals. In addition, *A. unedo* leaf extracts are rich in *p*-coumaric acid. This last one is one of the most active free radical scavenging hydroxycinnamic acids [44]. Finally, the antiradical activity of the *Arbutus* could also be due to the presence of arbutin. Indeed, this flavonoid has been reported as a powerful radical scavenger [45].

According to the results illustrated in Table 4, we noticed that the reducing powers of *A. unedo* leave extracts were significantly different and varied markedly depending on the solvent and extraction technique. Hence, the ethanolic extracts, as well as that of the water reflux method, presented the lowest values of the EC_{50} (varying from 60 and 83 µg/mL), therefore, the strongest reducing activities of the iron. Indeed, we noted that the pure ethanol extract of the ultrasound is distinguished by the best-reducing power of iron (EC_{50} = 60 µg/mL). As for the previous tests, the water reflux extract showed a very high reducing power with an EC_{50} of 83 µg/mL. On the contrary, lower activity was observed in the aqueous extract obtained by maceration, of which the EC_{50} value is equal to 112 µg/mL. Our results reveal that the Tunisian *Arbutus* exhibits an important reducing power. The lower reducing activity was noted by Malheiro et al. [18] in aqueous extract leaves of 19 Portuguese *A. unedo* genotypes. These authors explained that the antioxidant power of the *Arbutus* would be due to its richness in reducing phenolic compounds.

Concerning the chelating power of iron which was measured by the inhibition of the formation of ferrozine-Fe^2 complex, our study revealed a low chelating capacity of ferrous iron; the aqueous extracts showed moderate activity displaying EC_{50} values ranging from 33 to 40 mg/mL (Table 4).

Our results revealed a strong antioxidant potential of the Tunisian *A. unedo*. In particular, the aqueous extraction under reflux was distinguished by a very high power to trap free radicals as well as a high total and reduced antioxidant activities.

3.5. Effect of Solvent and Extraction Method on Anti-Tyrosinase Activity

A. unedo leaves extracts were analyzed for tyrosinase inhibition activity. Tyrosinase is a copper enzyme that plays a main role by catalyzing the first two steps in melanogenesis. Firstly, it converts L-tyrosine into L-DOPA by hydroxylation, and secondly, this compound is converted into o-dopaquinone by oxidation which polymerizes spontaneously to form melanin, which is the key molecule for skin color [46]. Melanin overproduction can produce hyperpigmentation disorders, such as lentigo, melasma, and hyperpigmentation. As a consequence, tyrosinase inhibitors are promising potential skin-whitening agents [5]. There are well-known tyrosinase inhibitors such as hydroquinone; nevertheless, their adverse effects are a serious concern, which leads to the search for natural compounds that have tyrosinase inhibitory effects [47].

The inhibition of tyrosinase by *A. unedo* extracts was assessed on its two catalysis functions, i.e., monophenolase (the inhibition of L-tyrosine hydroxylation to L-DOPA) and diphenolase (L-DOPA oxidation to dopaquinone) activities. Interestingly and considering monophenolase inhibition, all the extracts were able to inhibit tyrosinase activity efficiently, although to a different extent (Table 5). Ethanol and ethanol 50% maceration extracts exhibited the strongest activities (IC_{50} = 90 µg/mL), followed by ethanol 50% ultrasound (IC_{50} = 150 µg/mL) and decoction (IC_{50} = 200 µg/mL), whereas ultrasound ethanol was the less potent inhibitor for monophenolase activity.

Table 5. Mean values of Anti-tyrosinase activities of *A. unedo* extracts.

	Monophenolase Inhibition (IC_{50} in µg/mL)	Diphenolase Inhibition (IC_{50} in µg/mL)
Reflux water	200 ± 2.5 [d]	2500 ± 9.5 [a]
Maceration water	340 ± 5 [b]	1600 ± 10.0 [c]
Maceration ethanol	90 ± 2.0 [f]	450 ± 5.0 [f]
Maceration ethanol 50%	90 ± 1.0 [f]	500 ± 5.0 [e]
Ultrasound water	290 ± 6.5 [c]	2000 ± 8.0 [b]
Ultrasound ethanol	390 ± 4.5 [a]	900 ± 7.5 [d]
Ultrasound ethanol 50%	150 ± 2.5 [e]	400 ± 5.0 [f]
Arbutin	100 ± 3.5 [f]	NA
Kojic acid	4.7 ± 0.1 [g]	0.018 ± 0.00 [g]

NA: not active. In each column, the same letters mean non-significant differences using Duncan's test at 0.05 probability level.

Some extracts displayed moderate diphenolase activity. Ethanol 50% obtained by ultrasound and maceration as well as ethanol maceration showed the highest activities with IC_{50} values of 400, 450, and 500 µg/mL, respectively. The other extracts were rather ineffective (IC_{50} > 1 mg/mL). These results confirm previous observations on moderate diphenolase *A. unedo* activity. Recently, Deniz et al. [48], have investigated the enzyme inhibitory activity of 92 herbal ethanol extracts and showed that *A. unedo* ethanol 80% leaves extract by maceration showed 32% diphenolase inhibition at 666 µg/mL.

These data pointed out the high potency of *A. unedo* monophenolase activity and revealed strong lightening capacity. This remarkable activity is likely to result from high arbutin content in the different extracts (Table 3), which act as the major tyrosinase-modulating compound. In our study, this phenolic exhibited high monophenolase activity (IC_{50} = 100 µg/mL, Table 5) while it was inactive in diphenolase activity. Recently, the effect of α-arbutin on the monophenolase and diphenolase activities of tyrosinase was analyzed and reported that this compound inhibits monophenolase activity and activates diphenolase activity [49]. In addition, it has been shown that arbutin is also safe and can potentially prevent melanin formation without cytotoxicity [50]. Data on the antioxidant capacity of arbutin are emerging, and these antioxidant properties are proposed to contribute to the skin-lightening effect of the molecule.

There are several other compounds present in extracts from *A. unedo* plants with tyrosinase-modulating properties. Accordingly, Huang et al. [51] explained that ellagic acid inhibited tyrosinase activity in a reversible manner and was a mixed tyrosinase inhibitor. Moreover, catechins and *p*-coumaric acid were reported to inhibit tyrosinase by acting as alternative substrates [52].

3.6. Effect of Solvent and Extraction Method on Cytotoxic and Anti-Inflammatory Activities

Due to the significant side effect profiles of drugs, the use of natural compounds for preventing or reducing inflammation has recently received a lot of attention. The cytotoxicity of *A. unedo* extracts was studied using the resazurin assay. RAW 264.7 cells were treated with different concentrations of extracts (25–300 µg/mL), as shown in Figure 1. Independently of technique, both water and ethanol of *A. unedo* extracts exhibited no cytotoxic effect for the tested concentrations up to 300 µg/mL since cell viability exceeded 80%. Interestingly, *A. unedo* extracts, especially water reflux and ethanol extract by maceration at 50 µg/mL, caused an increase in cell viability by 11% compared to the control. Based on this, concentrations ranging from 25 to 150 µg/mL were selected for further studies.

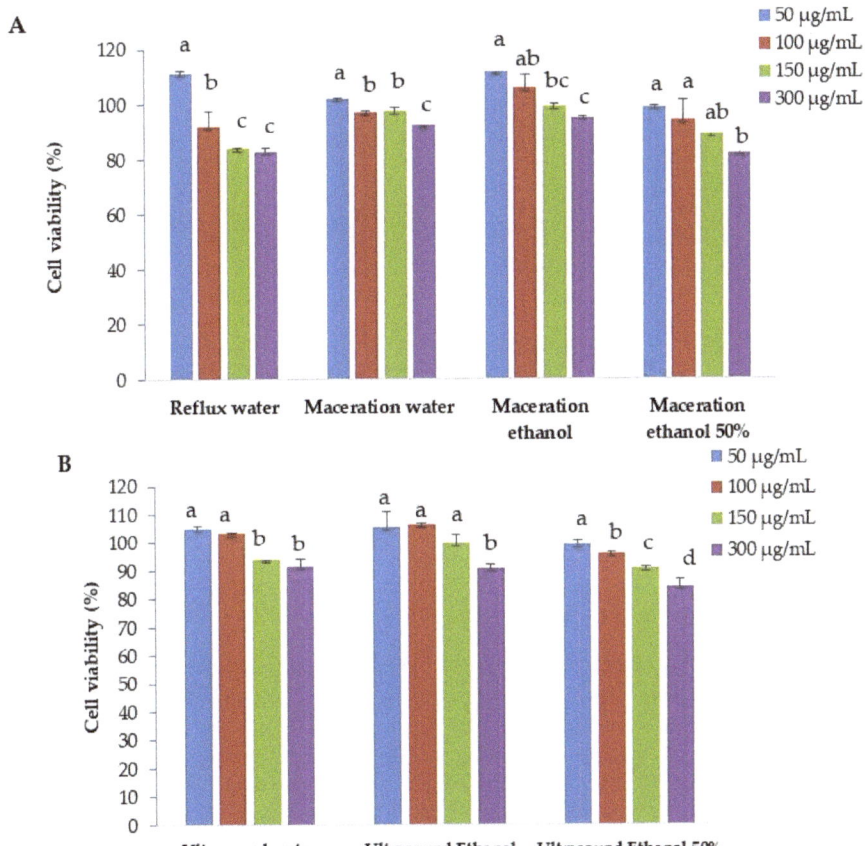

Figure 1. Cell viability (%) evaluation using resazurin assay for *Arbutus unedo* extracts obtained by reflux and maceration (**A**) and ultrasound (**B**) extraction on RAW 264.7 cells. Cells were incubated, for 24 h, with 50–300 µg/mL extract. The percent cell viability was determined by comparison to the untreated control. Data were displayed as mean ± SD calculated from triplicate results. For each extraction method, different letters between extract concentrations mean significant differences using Duncan's test at a 0.05 probability level.

Nitric oxide (NO) is a strong mediator in numerous cellular processes, such as the regulation of neurotransmission, vasodilatation, inhibition of platelet adherence, host defense mechanisms, and inflammation [53]. LPS can activate macrophage cells to initiate proinflammatory mediators, including TNF-α, IL-6, and NO. Therefore, the utilization of NO inhibitors constitutes a substantial therapeutic advance in the treatment of inflammatory diseases. Noncytotoxic *A. unedo* extracts concentrations were examined to explore their potential to inhibit NO production in LPS-treated RAW 264.7 macrophages. Extracts showed anti-inflammatory activity in a concentration-dependent manner (Figure 2). The most active extracts were ethanol maceration and water extract obtained by ultrasound with percentage NO production inhibition of 37 and 35%, respectively, at a high dose of 150 µg/mL. Some studies highlighted the potential activity of *A. unedo* extracts as anti-inflammatory candidates. Tenuta et al. [16] showed that *A. unedo* ethanolic and hydroalcoholic macerations were able to reduce nitrite production in HFF1 cells stimulated with interleukin-2β.

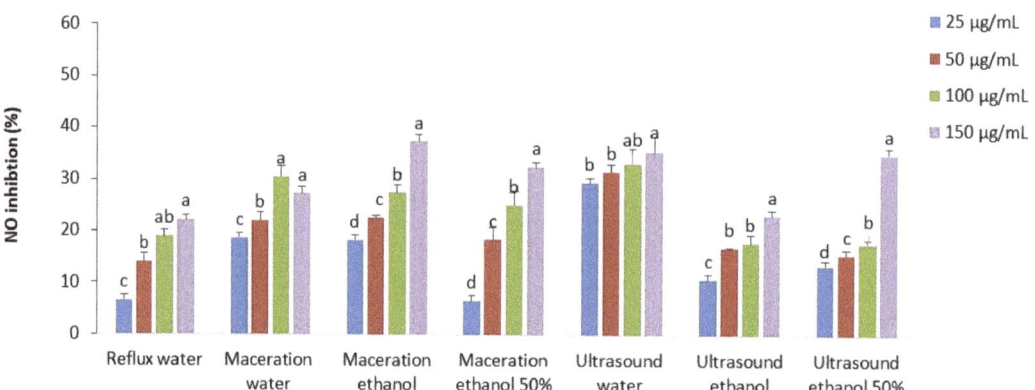

Figure 2. Anti-inflammatory activity of *A. unedo* extracts from different extraction methods (mean ± SD, n = 3 replicates). Cells were incubated with 25–150 µg/mL extract and Lipopolysaccharide (LPS). After a 24 h LPS stimulation, the cell-free supernatants were collected and assayed for nitric oxide (NO) levels. For the same extraction method, different letters (a, b, c, d) mean significant differences between extract concentrations using the Duncan test at the probability level of $p < 0.05$.

Mariotto et al. [54] reported that treatment with an aqueous extract of *A. unedo* decreased acute lung inflammation in an animal model. Among *A. unedo* phenolics, arbutin suppressed LPS-induced production of NO and expression of inducible NO synthase (iNOS) and cyclooxygenase-2 (COX-2) in LPS stimulated BV2 microglial cells in a dose-dependent manner and without causing cellular toxicity [55].

3.7. Characterization of Emulsion Containing A. unedo Extract

After evaluating the phytochemical composition and the activities of the seven *A. unedo* extracts, it was found that the reflux water has the best performance with satisfactory compositional characteristics that allowed its use in the elaboration of a cosmetic emulsion based on a high phenolic compounds content and elevated antioxidant and anti-tyrosinase activities. Thus, a formulation that contained 1% of the selected *A. unedo* extract was developed.

Initially, the formulation loading phenolic-enriched *A. unedo* extract was light yellow and homogeneous, while the base formulation was white homogeneous. This color difference is caused by the color of the extract influencing the color of the end product.

On the other hand, total polyphenols retention evaluation showed a satisfactory level of phenolics retention (60.32%) in the nanoemulsion.

Stability tests are crucial because of their predictive nature. The centrifugation test was carried out to obtain information on possible instability processes. Formulations were centrifuged 24 h after preparation at 3000 rpm for 30 min. The emulsion loading phenolic-enriched *A. unedo* extract showed no change in its initial characteristics and stability. The emulsion was described as stable, as no cremation, flocculation, or phase separation was observed during the available time. Similar behavior was observed in the thermal stress test in which the cream did not show changes during the whole process.

Regarding pH analysis, the emulsion loading phenolic-enriched *A. unedo* extract initially presented a pH value of about 6.9 (Table 6). The value for the emulsion subjected to thermal stress for eight days was 6.5. Both values are compatible with skin [56]. Therefore, these emulsions were considered suitable for use.

Table 6. Mean droplet diameter (Z-average), zeta potential (ZP), and pH values of preliminary stability tests of nanoemulsions containing phenolic-enriched *A. unedo* extract (A-NE) and blank nanoemulsion (NE).

	Z-Average (d.nm)		Zeta Potential (mV)		pH	
	T0	T8	T0	T8	T0	T8
A-NE	197 ± 1.05 [b]	243 ± 0.8 [b]	−56 ± 2 [a]	−64 ± 1.0 [a]	6.9 [b]	6.5 [b]
NE	216.± 0.8 [a]	286 ± 0.5 [a]	−59 ± 1,2 [a]	−70 ± 1.8 [a]	7.6 [a]	7.9 [a]

Mean followed by the same letter at each column are not significantly different using Duncan test at the $p < 0.05$ probability level. Each value represents the mean of three replicates.

Zeta potential and particle size measurement are commonly employed methods to assess the stability of emulsions. Initially, the emulsion possesses 197 nm. After thermal stress for eight days, the sample showed a slight increase in the mean droplet size to 243 nm, as shown in Table 6. However, the radius of the droplets was still within the range of 20–500 nm, which corresponds to the size of a nanoemulsion [57]. The stability of the emulsion is strongly related to the droplet size distribution. Generally, the smaller the droplet size, the more stable the W/O nanoemulsions and the longer their shelf life. The small droplet size of nanoemulsions stabilizes them against gravitational separation and flocculation. Large droplet size can promote Ostwald ripening, which increases droplet size leading to coalescence and creaming [58]. The zeta potential value obtained for the nanoemulsion on day zero was −56 ± 2 mV. Alternatively, the value presented for the nanoemulsion subjected to thermal stress for eight days was −64 ± 1 mV (Table 6). Both values reflect the stability of the emulsion even when subjected to changes in temperature. The zeta potential shows the force of repulsion between adjacent equally charged droplets and consequently proves the important role of the droplets' surface layer in the stabilization process. High values of zeta potential (>|30| mV) indicate resistance to particle aggregation and, therefore, greater stability [59].

4. Conclusions

This study investigated the skin anti-aging activity of *A. unedo* from Tunisia to assess the opportunity of exploiting this plant species as a source of bioactive compounds with numerous applications. Various extraction techniques were compared for the recovery of phenolic compounds from *A. unedo*. Among the different extracts, the reflux water extract was rich in total polyphenols, recovered the highest amounts of flavonoids and tannins, and showed the highest antioxidant activity. Additionally, it showed anti-inflammatory and anti-tyrosinase activities with no cytotoxic effect. Furthermore, the reflux water extract gave the highest yield (38%), which would be advantageous for the cosmetic industry due to its cost-effectiveness. Consequently, in the present study, a cosmetic emulsion containing the reflux extract was developed with high polyphenol content. It is worth noting that in future studies, we will assess the stability of the formulation incorporating the *A. unedo* extract at different times (several weeks) and temperatures.

Author Contributions: Conceptualization, S.B. and O.M.; writing, S.B., E.H. and I.B.R.; methodology, S.B. and M.H.; investigation, E.H., S.D., S.S. and M.H.; formal analysis, S.B. and M.H.; data curation, S.B., E.H. and K.M.; resources, S.B.; writing—review editing, O.M. All authors have read and agreed to the published version of the manuscript.

Funding: This research was supported by the 20PEJC Project "La biodiversité végétale au service des produits de santé naturels: étude des propriétés pharmacologiques d'extraits végétaux et developpement d'une crème anti-taches pour l'industrie cosmétique" funded by the Tunisian Ministry of Higher Education and Scientific Research (LR19CBBC06).

Institutional Review Board Statement: Not applicable.

Informed Consent Statement: Not applicable.

Conflicts of Interest: The authors declare no conflict of interest.

Abbreviations

ABTS: 2,2′-Azino-bis(3-ethylbenzothiazoline-6-sulphonic acid; A-NE: *A. unedo* extract phenolic-enriched nanoemulsion; COX-2: cyclooxygenase-2; DPPH: 2,2-diphenyl-1-picrylhydrazyl; DMSO: dimethyl sulfoxide; HPLC–DAD: high-performance liquid chromatography coupled to a diode-array detector; IL-6: interleukine 6; iNOS: NO synthase; LPS: lipopolysaccharides; NE: blank nanoemulsion; NO: Nitric oxide; O/W: oil in water; ROS: reactive oxygen species; SD: standard deviation; TAA: Total antioxidant activity; TNFα: Tumor Necrosis Factor; Z-average: Mean droplet diameter; ZP: zeta potential.

References

1. Domaszewska-Szostek, A.; Puzianowska-Kuźnicka, M.; Kuryłowicz, A. Flavonoids in Skin Senescence Prevention and Treatment. *Int. J. Mol. Sci.* **2021**, *22*, 6814. [CrossRef] [PubMed]
2. Lohani, A.; Morganti, P. Age-Defying and Photoprotective Potential of Geranium/Calendula Essential Oil Encapsulated Vesicular Cream on Biochemical Parameters against UVB Radiation Induced Skin Aging in Rat. *Cosmetics* **2022**, *9*, 43. [CrossRef]
3. Farage, M.A.; Miller, K.W.; Elsner, P.; Maibach, H.I. Intrinsic and extrinsic factors in skin ageing: A review. *Int. J. Cosmet. Sci.* **2008**, *30*, 87–95. [CrossRef] [PubMed]
4. Guan, Y.; Chu, Q.; Fu, L.; Ye, J. Determination of antioxidants in cosmetics by micellar electrokinetic capillary chromatography with electrochemical detection. *J. Chromatogr. A* **2005**, *1074*, 201–204. [CrossRef] [PubMed]
5. Chiocchio, I.; Mandrone, M.; Sanna, C.; Maxia, A.; Tacchini, M.; Poli, F. Screening of a hundred plant extracts as tyrosinase and elastase inhibitors, two enzymatic targets of cosmetic interest. *Ind. Crop. Prod.* **2018**, *122*, 498–505. [CrossRef]
6. Michalak, M. Plant-Derived Antioxidants: Significance in Skin Health and the Ageing Process. *Int. J. Mol. Sci.* **2022**, *23*, 585. [CrossRef] [PubMed]
7. Şöhretoğlu, D.; Sari, S.; Barut, B.; Özel, A. Tyrosinase inhibition by some flavonoids: Inhibitory activity, mechanism by in vitro and in silico studies. *Bioorganic Chem.* **2018**, *81*, 168–174. [CrossRef]
8. Saeedi, M.; Eslamifar, M.; Khezri, K. Kojic acid applications in cosmetic and pharmaceutical preparations. *Biomed. Pharmacother.* **2018**, *110*, 582–593. [CrossRef]
9. Nimse, S.B.; Pal, D. Free radicals, natural antioxidants, and their reaction mechanisms. *RSC Adv.* **2015**, *5*, 27986–28006. [CrossRef]
10. Widyarini, S.; Spinks, N.; Husband, A.J.; Reeve, V.E. Isoflavonoid Compounds from Red Clover (*Trifolium pratense*) Protect from Inflammation and Immune Suppression Induced by UV Radiation. *Photochem. Photobiol.* **2001**, *74*, 465–470. [CrossRef]
11. Choi, S.; Youn, J.; Kim, K.; Joo, D.H.; Shin, S.; Lee, J.; Lee, H.K.; An, I.-S.; Kwon, S.; Youn, H.J.; et al. Apigenin inhibits UVA-induced cytotoxicity in vitro and prevents signs of skin aging in vivo. *Int. J. Mol. Med.* **2016**, *38*, 627–634. [CrossRef] [PubMed]
12. Bing-Rong, Z.; Song-Liang, J.; Xiao-E, C.; Xiang-Fei, L.; Bao-Xiang, C.; Jie, G.; Dan, L. Protective effect of the Baicalin against DNA damage induced by ultraviolet B irradiation to mouse epidermis. *Photodermatol. Photoimmunol. Photomed.* **2008**, *24*, 175–182. [CrossRef]
13. El-Mahdy, M.A.; Zhu, Q.; Wang, Q.-E.; Wani, G.; Patnaik, S.; Zhao, Q.; Arafa, E.-S.; Barakat, B.; Mir, S.N.; Wani, A.A. Naringenin Protects HaCaT Human Keratinocytes Against UVB-induced Apoptosis and Enhances the Removal of Cyclobutane Pyrimidine Dimers from the Genome. *Photochem. Photobiol.* **2007**, *84*, 307–316. [CrossRef] [PubMed]
14. Selvakumar, K.; Madhan, R.; Srinivasan, G.; Baskar, V. Antioxidant Assays in Pharmacological Research. *Asian J. Pharm. Tech.* **2011**, *1*, 99–103.
15. Bouzid, A.; Chadli, R.; Bouzid, K. Étude ethnobotanique de la plante médicinale *Arbutus unedo* L. dans la région de Sidi Bel Abbès en Algérie occidentale Ethnobotanical study of the medicinal plant *Arbutus unedo* L. in the region of Sidi Bel Abbes in western Algeria. *Phytothérapie* **2017**, *15*, 373–378. [CrossRef]

16. Tenuta, M.C.; Deguin, B.; Loizzo, M.R.; Dugay, A.; Acquaviva, R.; Malfa, G.A.; Bonesi, M.; Bouzidi, C.; Tundis, R. Contribution of Flavonoids and Iridoids to the Hypoglycaemic, Antioxidant, and Nitric Oxide (NO) Inhibitory Activities of *Arbutus unedo* L. *Antioxidants* **2020**, *9*, 184. [CrossRef]
17. El Haouari, M.; Assem, N.; Changan, S.; Kumar, M.; Daştan, S.D.; Rajkovic, J.; Taheri, Y.; Sharifi-Rad, J. An Insight into Phytochemical, Pharmacological, and Nutritional Properties of *Arbutus unedo* L. from Morocco. *Evid. Based Complement Altern. Med.* **2021**, *2021*, 1–19. [CrossRef] [PubMed]
18. Malheiro, R.; Sá, O.; Pereira, E.; Aguiar, C.; Baptista, P.; Pereira, J.A. *Arbutus unedo* L. leaves as source of phytochemicals with bioactive properties. *Ind. Crop. Prod.* **2012**, *37*, 473–478. [CrossRef]
19. Brčić Karačonji, I.; Jurica, K.; Gašić Uroš, M.; Drami´canin, A.; Teši´c, Ž.; Milojković-Opsenica, D.M. Comparative Study on the Phenolic Fingerprint and Antioxidant Activity of Strawberry Tree (*Arbutus unedo* L.) Leaves and Fruits. *Plants* **2022**, *11*, 25. [CrossRef] [PubMed]
20. Bourgou, S.; Rebey, I.B.; Mkadmini, K.; Isoda, H.; Ksouri, R.; Ksouri, W.M. LC-ESI-TOF-MS and GC-MS profiling of *Artemisia herba-alba* and evaluation of its bioactive properties. *Food Res. Int.* **2017**, *99*, 702–712. [CrossRef]
21. Sun, J.; Chu, Y.-F.; Wu, X.; Liu, R.H. Antioxidant and Antiproliferative Activities of Common Fruits. *J. Agric. Food Chem.* **2002**, *50*, 7449–7454. [CrossRef]
22. Zhao, H.; Dong, J.; Lu, J.; Chen, J.; Li, Y.; Shan, L.; Lin, Y.; Fan, A.W.; Gu, G. Effects of Extraction Solvent Mixtures on Antioxidant Activity Evaluation and Their Extraction Capacity and Selectivity for Free Phenolic Compounds in Barley (*Hordeum vulgare* L.). *J. Agric. Food Chem.* **2006**, *54*, 7277–7286. [CrossRef]
23. O'Brien, J.; Wilson, I.; Orton, T.; Pognan, F. Investigation of the Alamar Blue (resazurin) fluorescent dye for the assessment of mammalian cell cytotoxicity. *Eur. J. Biochem.* **2000**, *267*, 5421–5426. [CrossRef]
24. Momtaz, S.; Mapunya, B.; Houghton, P.; Edgerly, C.; Hussein, A.; Naidoo, S.; Lall, N. Tyrosinase inhibition by extracts and constituents of *Sideroxylon inerme* L. stem bark, used in South Africa for skin lightening. *J. Ethnopharmacol.* **2008**, *119*, 507–512. [CrossRef] [PubMed]
25. Khairi, N.; As'Ad, S.; Djawad, K.; Alam, G. The determination of antioxidants activity and sunblock *Sterculia populifolia* extract-based cream. *Pharm. Biomed. Res.* **2018**, *4*, 2026. [CrossRef]
26. Regan, J.O.; Mulvihill, D.M. Water soluble inner aqueous phase markers as indicators of the encapsulation properties of water-in-oil-in-water emulsions stabilized with sodium caseinate. *Food Hydrocoll.* **2009**, *23*, 2339–2345. [CrossRef]
27. Niknam, S.M.; Escudero, I.; Benito, J.M. Formulation and Preparation of Water-In-Oil-In-Water Emulsions Loaded with a Phenolic-Rich Inner Aqueous Phase by Application of High Energy Emulsification Methods. *Foods* **2020**, *9*, 1411. [CrossRef] [PubMed]
28. Delgado-Arias, S.; Zapata-Valencia, S.; Cano-Agudelo, Y.; Arias, J.C.O.; Vega-Castro, O. Evaluation of the antioxidant and physical properties of an exfoliating cream developed from coffee grounds. *J. Food Process Eng.* **2019**, *43*, e13067. [CrossRef]
29. Wakeel, A.; Jan, S.A.; Ullah, I.; Shinwari, Z.K.; Xu, M. Solvent polarity mediates phytochemical yield and antioxidant capacity of *Isatis tinctoria*. *Peerj* **2019**, *7*, e7857. [CrossRef]
30. Oliveira, I.; Coelho, V.; Baltasar, R.; Pereira, J.A.; Baptista, P. Scavenging capacity of strawberry tree (*Arbutus unedo* L.) leaves on free radicals. *Food Chem. Toxicol.* **2009**, *47*, 1507–1511. [CrossRef]
31. Orak, H.H.; Yagar, H.; Isbilir, S.S.; Demirci, A.; Gümüş, T.; Ekinci, N. Evaluation of antioxidant and antimicrobial potential of strawberry tree (*Arbutus unedo* L.) leaf. *Food Sci. Biotechnol.* **2011**, *20*, 1249–1256. [CrossRef]
32. Bamba, B.S.B.; Shi, J.; Tranchant, C.C.; Xue, S.J.; Forney, C.F.; Lim, L.-T. Influence of Extraction Conditions on Ultrasound-Assisted Recovery of Bioactive Phenolics from Blueberry Pomace and Their Antioxidant Activity. *Molecules* **2018**, *23*, 1685. [CrossRef] [PubMed]
33. Jurica, K.; Brčić Karačonji, I.; Šegan, S.; Milojkovi´c Opsenica, D.; Kremer, D. Quantitative analysis of arbutin and hydroquinone in strawberry tree (*Arbutus unedo* L., Ericaceae) leaves by gas chromatography-mass spectrometry. *Arh. Hig. Rada Toksikol.* **2015**, *66*, 197–202. [CrossRef]
34. Guendouze-Bouchefa, N.; Madani, K.; Chibane, M.; Boulekbache-Makhlouf, L.; Hauchard, D.; Kiendrebeogo, M.; Stévigny, C.; Okusa, P.N.; Duez, P. Phenolic compounds, antioxidant and antibacterial activities of three Ericaceae from Algeria. *Ind. Crop. Prod.* **2015**, *70*, 459–466. [CrossRef]
35. Andrade, D.; Gil, C.; Breitenfeld, L.; Domingues, F.; Duarte, A.P. Bioactive extracts from *Cistus ladanifer* and *Arbutus unedo* L. *Ind. Crop. Prod.* **2009**, *30*, 165–167. [CrossRef]
36. Fiorentino, A.; Castaldi, S.; D'Abrosca, B.; Natale, A.; Carfora, A.; Messere, A.; Monaco, P. Polyphenols from the hydroalcoholic extract of *Arbutus unedo* living in a monospecific Mediterranean woodland. *Biochem. Syst. Ecol.* **2007**, *35*, 809–811. [CrossRef]
37. Pavlović, D.R.; Branković, S.; Kovačević, N.; Kitić, D.; Veljković, S. Comparative study of spasmolytic properties, antioxidant activity and phenolic content of *Arbutus unedo* from Montenegro and Greece. *Phyther. Res.* **2011**, *25*, 749–754. [CrossRef] [PubMed]
38. Maleš, Z.; Plazibat, M.; Vunda´c, V.B.; Zuntar, I. Qualitative and quantitative analysis of flavonoids of the strawberry tree—*Arbutus unedo* L. (Ericaceae). *Acta. Pharm.* **2006**, *56*, 245–250.
39. Jardim, C.E.C.G.; Macedo, D.; Figueira, I.; Dobson, G.; McDougall, G.J.; Stewart, D.; Ferreira, R.B.; Menezes, R.; Santos, C.N. (Poly)phenol metabolites from *Arbutus unedo* leaves protect yeast from oxidative injury by activation of antioxidant and protein clearance pathways. *J. Funct. Foods* **2017**, *32*, 332–346. [CrossRef]

40. Legssyer, A.; Ziyyat, A.; Mekh, H.; Bnouham, M.; Herrenknecht, C.; Roumy, V.; Fourneau, C.; Laurens, A.; Hoerter, J.; Fischmeister, R. Tannins and catechin gallate mediate the vasorelaxant effect of Arbutus unedo on the rat isolated aorta. *Phytotherapy Res.* **2004**, *18*, 889–894. [CrossRef]
41. Mendes, L.; de Freitas, V.; Baptista, P.; Carvalho, M. Comparative antihemolytic and radical scavenging activities of strawberry tree (Arbutus unedo L.) leaf and fruit. *Food Chem. Toxicol.* **2011**, *49*, 2285–2291. [CrossRef] [PubMed]
42. Treml, J.; Šmejkal, K. Flavonoids as Potent Scavengers of Hydroxyl Radicals. *Compr. Rev. Food Sci. Food Saf.* **2016**, *15*, 720–738. [CrossRef]
43. Liu, Z.; Tao, X.; Zhang, C.; Lu, Y.; Wei, D. Protective effects of hyperoside (quercetin-3-o-galactoside) to PC12 cells against cytotoxicity induced by hydrogen peroxide and tert-butyl hydroperoxide. *Biomed. Pharmacother.* **2005**, *59*, 481–490. [CrossRef]
44. Kiliç, I.; Yeşiloğlu, Y. Spectroscopic studies on the antioxidant activity of p-coumaric acid. *Spectrochim. Acta. A. Mol. Biomol. Spectrosc.* **2013**, *115*, 719–724. [CrossRef]
45. Tai, A.; Ohno, A.; Ito, H. Isolation and Characterization of the 2,2′-Azinobis(3-ethylbenzothiazoline-6-sulfonic acid) (ABTS) Radical Cation-Scavenging Reaction Products of Arbutin. *J. Agric. Food. Chem.* **2016**, *64*, 7285–7290. [CrossRef]
46. Pillaiyar, T.; Manickam, M.; Namasivayam, V. Skin whitening agents: Medicinal chemistry perspective of tyrosinase inhibitors. *J. Enzym. Inhib. Med. Chem.* **2017**, *32*, 403–425. [CrossRef]
47. Kooyers, T.; Westerhof, W. Toxicology and health risks of hydroquinone in skin lightening formulations. *J. Eur. Acad. Dermatol. Venereol.* **2006**, *20*, 777–780. [CrossRef]
48. Deniz, F.S.S.; Orhan, I.E.; Duman, H. Profiling cosmeceutical effects of various herbal extracts through elastase, collagenase, tyrosinase inhibitory and antioxidant assays. *Phytochem. Lett.* **2021**, *45*, 171–183. [CrossRef]
49. Qin, L.; Wu, Y.; Liu, Y.; Chen, Y.; Zhang, P. Dual Effects of Alpha-Arbutin on Monophenolase and Diphenolase Activities of Mushroom Tyrosinase. *PLoS ONE* **2014**, *9*, e109398. [CrossRef] [PubMed]
50. Sugimoto, K.; Nishimura, T.; Nomura, K.; Sugimoto, K.; Kuriki, T. Inhibitory effects of α-arbutin on melanin synthesis in cultured human melanoma cells and a three-dimensional human skin model. *Biol. Pharm. Bull.* **2004**, *27*, 510–514. [CrossRef]
51. Huang, Q.; Chai, W.; Ma, Z.; Deng, W.; Wei, Q.; Song, S.; Zou, Z.; Peng, Y. Antityrosinase mechanism of ellagic acid in vitro and its effect on mouse melanoma cells. *J. Food Biochem.* **2019**, *43*, e12996. [CrossRef] [PubMed]
52. Seo, S.-Y.; Sharma, V.K.; Sharma, N. Mushroom Tyrosinase: Recent Prospects. *J. Agric. Food Chem.* **2003**, *51*, 2837–2853. [CrossRef] [PubMed]
53. Oh, J.H.; Lee, T.J.; Park, J.W.; Kwon, T.K. Withaferin A inhibits iNOS expression and nitric oxide production by Akt inactivation and down-regulating LPS-induced activity of NF-kappaB in RAW 264.7 cells. *Eur. J. Pharmacol.* **2008**, *599*, 11–17. [CrossRef] [PubMed]
54. Mariotto, S.; Esposito, E.; di Paola, R.; Ciampa, A.; Mazzon, E.; de Prati, A.C.; Darra, E.; Vincenzi, S.; Cucinotta, G.; Caminiti, R.; et al. Protective effect of Arbutus unedo aqueous extract in carrageenan-induced lung inflammation in mice. *Pharmacol. Res.* **2008**, *57*, 110–124. [CrossRef] [PubMed]
55. Lee, H.-J.; Kim, K.-W. Anti-inflammatory effects of arbutin in lipopolysaccharide-stimulated BV2 microglial cells. *Inflamm. Res.* **2012**, *61*, 817–825. [CrossRef] [PubMed]
56. Hashem, F.; Shaker, D.; Ghorab, M.K.; Nasr, M.; Ismail, A. Formulation, Characterization, and Clinical Evaluation of Microemulsion Containing Clotrimazole for Topical Delivery. *AAPS PharmSciTech* **2011**, *12*, 879–886. [CrossRef]
57. Karami, Z.; Zanjani, M.R.S.; Hamidi, M. Nanoemulsions in CNS drug delivery: Recent developments, impacts and challenges. *Drug Discov. Today* **2019**, *24*, 1104–1115. [CrossRef]
58. Kabri, T.-H.; Arab-Tehrany, E.; Belhaj, N.; Linder, M. Physico-chemical characterization of nano-emulsions in cosmetic matrix enriched on omega-3. *J. Nanobiotechnology* **2011**, *9*, 1–8. [CrossRef]
59. Barreto, S.M.A.G.; Maia, M.S.; Benicá, A.M.; de Assis, H.R.B.S.; Leite-Silva, V.R.; da Rocha-Filho, P.A.; de Negreiros, M.M.F.; Rocha, H.A.D.O.; Ostrosky, E.A.; Lopes, P.S.; et al. Evaluation of in vitro and in vivo safety of the by-product of *Agave sisalana* as a new cosmetic raw material: Development and clinical evaluation of a nanoemulsion to improve skin moisturizing. *Ind. Crop. Prod.* **2017**, *108*, 470–479. [CrossRef]

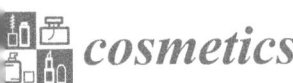

Communication

Anti-Pollution Activity, Antioxidant and Anti-Inflammatory Effects of Fermented Extract from *Smilax china* Leaf in Macrophages and Keratinocytes

Yoo-Kyung Kim and Dae-Jung Kang *

MNHBIO Co., Ltd., 172 Dolma-ro, Bundang-gu, Seongnam-si 13605, Gyeonggi-do, Republic of Korea
* Correspondence: djkang@mnhbio.com; Tel.: +82-31-212-0677

Abstract: Air pollution has considerable effects on the human skin, showing that every single pollutant has a different toxicological impact on it. The oxidative stress that exceeds the skin's antioxidant capacity can lead to oxidative damage and premature skin aging by repeated air pollutant contact. In this study, according to the generalized protocol available to objectively substantiate the 'anti-pollution' claim, we evaluated several biomarkers after pollutants exposure in Raw 264.7 macro-phages and HaCaT keratinocytes to investigate the possibility of anti-pollution cosmetic material of fermented extract from *Smilax china* leaves (FESCL). FESCL decreased pollutants-induced luciferase activity in a dose-dependent manner, and FESCL significantly inhibited XRE-luciferase activity at a concentration of 1%. The IC_{50} value of FESCL showed the same DPPH scavenging activity at 0.0625% as ascorbic acid, and the maximum DPPH scavenging activity (92.44%) at 1%. The maximum permissible non-cytotoxic concentrations of FESCL for a Raw 264.7 cell was determined to be 2%, where PGE_2 production of FESCL was inhibited by 78.20%. These results show the anti-pollution activity of FESCL against the pollutant-stimulated human living skin explants. In conclusion, we confirmed the anti-pollution potential of FESCL as one of the functional materials in cosmetic formulation.

Keywords: anti-pollution; anti-inflammation; antioxidant; fermentation; *Smilax china* leaf; *Lactobacillus* spp.

1. Introduction

Exposure to air pollution has been noted as closely associated with increased morbidity and mortality worldwide. Airborne pollutants are known to penetrate the human body through multiple routes, including direct inhalation and ingestion, as well as dermal contact, and also to cause well-documented acute and long-term effects on human health [1]. Air pollution is composed of a heterogeneous mixture of compounds emitted directly from pollution sources, including gases, low molecular weight hydrocarbons, persistent organic pollutants, (e.g., dioxins), heavy metals, (e.g., lead and mercury), and particulate matter (PM) [1]. Air pollution has considerable effects on the human skin, and it is generally known that every single pollutant has a different toxicological impact on it. Especially being the largest organ of the human body, as well as the boundary between the environment and the organism, the skin unsurprisingly is one of the major targets of air pollutants. Ref. [1] Even though the skin is equipped with an elaborate antioxidant defense system, including enzymatic and non-enzymatic, hydrophilic and lipophilic elements, the oxidative stress that exceeds the skin's antioxidant capacity, can lead to oxidative damage, premature skin aging, and eventually skin cancer by repeated air pollutant contact [2].

Recently, many studies reported potential explanations for outdoor air pollutants' impact on skin damage, focusing their interest, especially on airborne particulate matter (PM) and the ozone [3–5]. PM consists of mixtures of particles of different sizes and compositions and is a major concern in the air of densely populated urban areas [6]. According to previous studies, PM has been known to induce skin oxidative stress, producing reactive oxygen species (ROS), and lead to the secretion of pro-inflammatory cytokines (TNF-α, IL-1β, and IL-8) [7]. Additionally, it was reported that PM could be a relevant risk factor for the development of atopic dermatitis, a chronic inflammatory skin disease, and even exacerbate this condition [8–10]. There has been an increasing interest in anti-pollution products that protect them from various environmental threats.

The genus *Smilax* belongs to the *Liliaceae* family and contains 350 species, and it is known to be widely distributed in the tropical and temperate zones throughout the world, especially in tropical regions of East Asia and South and North America [11]. Many of them have been used as medicinal herbs in East Asian countries. For example, *Smilax china* is commonly used in traditional Chinese medicine for the treatment of diuretics, rheumatic arthritics, detoxication, lumbago, gout, tumors, and inflammatory diseases [12]. Recent pharmacological studies reported that *Smilax china* exhibited anti-inflammatory activity in skin cells [13–16] and significant cytotoxicity against several tumor cell lines [17,18]. In Korea, *Smilax china* L. is called 'Manggae,' and its leaves have been used in wrapping a unique Korean rice cake, called 'Manggae-dduck' of Uiryong-gun. This indigenous 'Manggae' also showed a notable antioxidant activity, similar to foreign *Smilax china* leaf (SCL) [19]. Especially, Li et al. reported that *Smilax china* had positive effects on skin wound healing and skin barrier function by accelerating keratinocyte migration [20].

In this study, according to the generalized protocol available to objectively substantiate the 'anti-pollution' claim, several in vitro tests were investigated. In order to investigate the anti-pollution potential of FESCL as one of the functional materials in the cosmetic formulation, we evaluated several biomarkers after pollutants exposure in Raw 264.7 macrophages and HaCaT keratinocytes. These two cell lines were used according to the generalized protocol available to objectively substantiate the 'anti-pollution' claim.

2. Materials and Methods

2.1. Materials

The dust PM1648a used in this study is urban particulate matter and was purchased from the National Institute of Standards and Technology (NIST; Gaithersburg, MD, USA). It has an average particle size of 5.85 µm. Cadmium chloride (202908), ascorbic acid (A4544), DPPH (D9132), and dexamethasone (D4902) were purchased from Sigma-Aldrich (St. Louis, MO, USA). MRS broth was purchased from Difco™. *Smilax china* leaves (SCL) were collected in 2019 in Uiryong-gun, Korea.

Human keratinocytes (Human adult low calcium high temperature: HaCaT) cells and Raw 264.7 cells used in this experiment were presold by the Korean Cell Line Bank, and DMEM medium containing 1% Penicillin streptomycin (Gibco, Grand Island, NY, USA) and 10% FBS was used. Incubated in a CO_2 incubator adjusted to 37 °C, 5% CO_2.

2.2. Preparation of Standardized SCL Fermented Extracts

SCL was dried at 30–40 °C for 48 h and dried samples were pulverized into a powder having a particle size of 40 mesh using a stainless steel blender (RT-08; MHK., Seoul, Republic of Korea). One kg of pulverized SCL was soaked in 5 L of distilled water for 2 h and then extracted at 100 °C for 2 h. The extract was separated from the insoluble part by filtration with Watman No.1 paper. The extracts were centrifuged at 8000 rpm for 20 min, and the supernatant was concentrated to 1 L under reduced pressure, then it was kept at 4 °C until use. The 1% (w/v) of freeze-dried Lactobacillus bulgaricus (KCTC13554BP) and Lactobacillus reuteri (KCTC14022BP), which were pre-cultured in MRS media, were inoculated in 1 L of SCL concentrated extract. This culture was fermented at 37 °C for 16 h and 10 °C for 6 h, sequentially, resulting in preparing the fermented extract of the SCL sample for this study.

The quantification of quercetin was analyzed by high-performance liquid chromatography (HPLC) (Waters 2690; Waters Co., Milford, MA, USA) using a Capcell pak C18 MG column (Shiseido, Ginza, Japan) (4.6 × 250 mm, 5µm) and a UV detector (Waters 2487;

Waters Co.). Samples were eluted isocratically with 10% (*v/v*) acetonitrile containing 0.1% (*v/v*) potassium dihydrogen phosphate monobasic at a flow rate of 1 mL/min and detected at 340 nm. To avoid variations in activity for different preparations, a sufficient extract was obtained in one batch for use throughout the study. The content of the marker quercetin in FESCL was quantitated using high-performance liquid chromatography and the total flavonoid content was analyzed as the quercetin equivalent (QE) mg/g of FESCL. Results indicated that FESCL possessed 25.3 QE mg of quercetin per 1.0 g (Supplementary Figure S1).

2.3. Cytotoxicity Assay

A WST-1 assay was carried for measuring the FESCL cytotoxicity value, about 5×10^5 viable cells were added to each well of a 96-well tissue culture plate with medium containing 10% FBS (fetal bovine serum), 1% Penicillin/Streptomycin (P/S), and incubated overnight at 37 °C to allow cells to attach to wells of the 96-well cell culture plates. The medium was replaced with fresh serum-free and 1% Penicillin/Streptomycin (P/S). Cell viability was measured using the EZ-Cytox cell viability assay kit (Itsbio. Seoul, Republic of Korea). The cells were incubated for 2 h at 37 °C in a serum-free medium diluted with 1 kit reagent. Next, harvested cells resuspended in the media were carefully moved to an empty 96-well plate, and absorbance was measured using an ELISA at 450 nm. Due to the measure of the cytotoxicity of FESCL in heavy metals exposure, after overnight incubation of the cell culture, the medium containing the serum-free and 1% P/S was replaced and treated with 4 µg/mL of cadmium chloride on each culture plate. The treatment of FESCL (0.0625, 0.125, 0.25, 0.5, and 1%) was suspended in cells and maintained for 24 h to confirm the cytotoxic concentration ranges. The percent cytotoxicity was calculated as follows:

$$Cell\ viability(\%) = \frac{(OD\ value\ of\ treatment - OD\ value\ of\ blank)}{(OD\ value\ of\ control - OD\ value\ of\ blank)} \times 100$$

(*OD*: optical density at 450 nm. Control: only cadmium chloride treatment).

2.4. The DPPH Radical Scavenging Activity

The *DPPH* radical scavenging activity of FESCL was determined according to the method of You et al. [21]. After diluting FESCL by concentrations of 0.125 mL for each fermented extract, 0.125 mL of PM1648a were mixed with 0.625 mL of 0.1 mM *DPPH* in ethanol at 4 °C for 30 min. Then, the absorbance of the sample were measured at 520 nm by a spectrophotometer (UV-1601; Shimadzu, Kyoto, Japan). Radical scavenging activity was expressed as a percentage according to the following formula:

$$DPPH\ radical\ scavenging\ activity(\%) = \left\{1 - \left(\frac{sample}{control}\right)\right\} \times 100$$

2.5. XRE-Luciferase Activity

To assay the activity of XRE and ARE-containing promoters, cells were transfected with XRE-luciferase (XRE-Luc) (Stratagene, La Jolla, CA, USA) or ARE-luciferase (ARE-Luc) reporters (Add gene, MA, USA), and Renilla-luciferase plasmid (1µg) (for normalization) (Promega, Madison, WI, USA) using the DharmaFECT® Duo transfection reagent (Thermo Fisher Scientific, Waltham, MA, USA), according to the manufacturers' protocols [22]. At 24 h post-transfection, FESCL by concentrations and PM1648a were added to the cells for a 48 h treatment. The cells were harvested and luciferase activity was measured using the Dual Luciferase Assay system (Promega) on a LB953 luminometer (Berthold, Germany).

2.6. Measurement of Prostaglandin E_2 (PGE_2) Production

The PGE_2 concentration in the culture medium was measured by the PGE_2 immunoassay (ELISA) kit (Enzo Life Sciences, Farmingdale, NY, USA) following the manufacturer's protocol. In brief, culture supernatants from the Raw 264.7 cells treated with various concentrations of FESCL with or without PM1648a (100 µg/mL) for 24 h were placed in

96-well plates with standard reagents. Wells were incubated with PGE_2 conjugate liquid and monoclonal PGE_2 antibody liquid for 24 h at 4 °C. After 24 h of incubation, wells were washed three times with a wash buffer and incubated with a substrate solution for 1 h at 37 °C. Then, the reactions were blocked by adding a stop solution reagent in each well. The optical density was determined using an automated microplate reader at 405 nm.

2.7. Statistical Analysis

All results are expressed as the mean ± standard deviation (SD) of at least three experiments. Statistical analyses were performed using the Statistical Package for the Social Sciences (SPSS 20.0) software. A paired t-test for the independent samples was used for the statistical analysis of the data. Values of * $p < 0.05$ displayed statistical significance.

3. Results

3.1. Cytotoxicity of FESCL in Heavy Metals Exposure

We investigated the cytotoxic effect of FESCL in a HaCaT cell, and it was observed to reduce viability in a concentration-dependent manner (Figure 1a). The viability of a HaCaT cell was not reduced following treatment with 0.125–1% of FESCL, but the viability was significantly reduced from 2% of FESCL. Based on these results, non-cytotoxic concentrations of FESCL (0.125, 0.25, and 1%) were used in further experiments. In order to evaluate the effect of FESCL on skin cells by heavy metals exposure, we measured the cytotoxicity of the HaCaT cell by treating FESCL in the condition of exposing 4 µg/mL of cadmium chloride. The viability of the HaCaT cell was significantly ($p < 0.05$) increased in a FESCL concentration-dependent manner. Notably, the HaCaT cell showed the highest value in 0.5% of FESCL treatments ($p < 0.05$), compared with the not-treated control (Figure 1b). Taken together, these results indicated that FESCL played potential roles in somewhat protecting skin cells from damage by toxic heavy metals exposure.

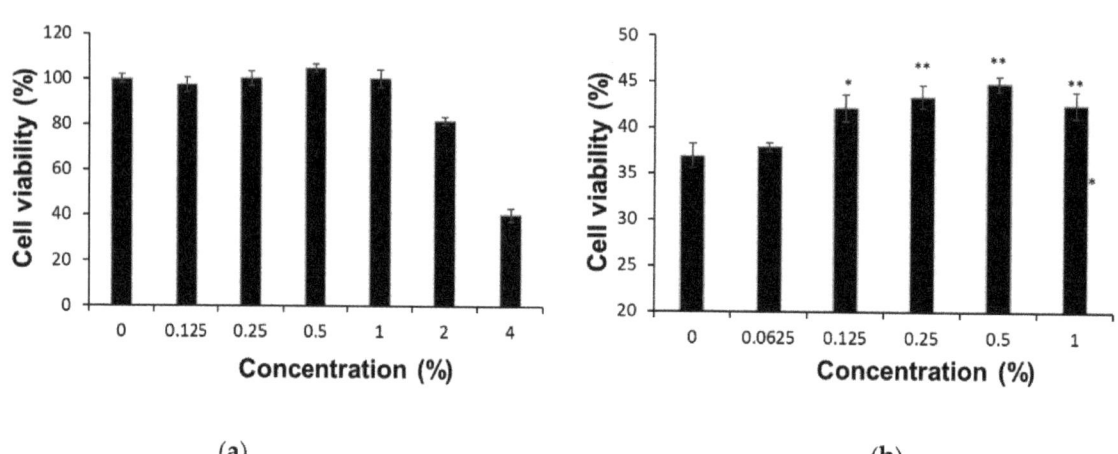

Figure 1. Inhibitory effect of FESCL cell cytotoxicity induced by treatment of Cadmium chloride (4 µg/mL) in HaCaT cells. (**a**) The cell viability of FESCL in HaCaT cells (**b**) The cell viability of FESCL in HaCaT cells with treatment of Cadmium chloride (4 µg/mL). The data are presented as the mean ± SD of three replicates. * $p < 0.05$ and ** $p < 0.01$.

3.2. Inhibitory Effect of FESCL on Air Pollutants

Xenobiotic-responsive elements (XREs) are the domains in the promoter region of some xenobiotic-responsive genes, and these gene expressions can be regulated through the interaction of the XRE and the dimer-containing aryl hydrocarbon receptor (AHR) [23]. The AHR is induced by polycyclic aromatic hydrocarbons (PAHs), and AHR dimerizes with ARNT and binds to xenobiotic-response elements which regulate the expression of cytochrome P450. The oxidation of xenobiotics is important in dermatitis, and even more critical in the detoxification of carcinogens [24]. Accordingly, we evaluated the inhibition effect of FESCL on air pollutant (PM1648a) in the HaCaT cell by an XRE-luciferase activity (Figure 2). The cells were incubated with various concentrations of FESCL (0.25, 0.5, and 1%) and then exposed to the air pollutant (PM1648a-10 μg/mL). As evident in Figure 2, it was confirmed that FESCL decreased pollutant-induced luciferase activity in a dose-dependent manner, and FESCL significantly ($p < 0.001$) inhibited XRE-luciferase activity at a concentration of 1%. The results indicated that air pollutant activated the AHR-signaling pathway, but it appeared that FESCL decreased the activated signaling pathway, hence reducing intracellular XRE promotor activity due to PM1648a, which seems to be due to the cell damage defense activity of FESCL by the PM1648a stimulation.

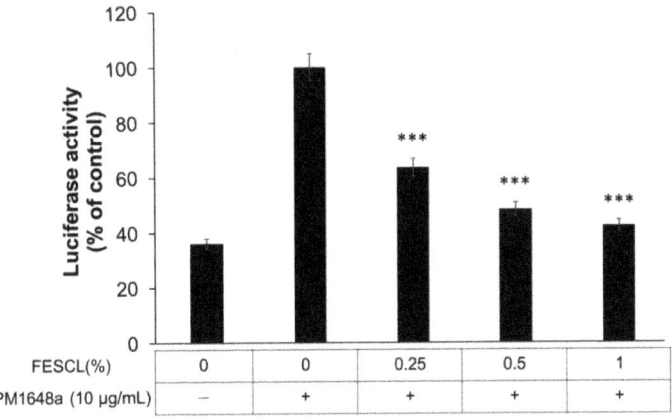

Figure 2. Luciferase activity of FESCL by the treatment of PM1648a (10 μg/mL) in HaCaT cells. The data are presented as the mean ± SD of three replicates. *** $p < 0.001$ vs. the PM1648a treatment control group.

3.3. Free Radical Scavenging Activity of FESCL on Air Pollutants

First, we tested the DPPH radical scavenging activity for PM1648a with ascorbic acid known to have high antioxidant activity as a positive control. As a result, it was confirmed that ascorbic acid exhibited concentration-dependent DPPH radical scavenging activity at a statistically significant level ($p < 0.05$). The entire treatment concentration range of ascorbic acid was from 0.313 to 10 μg/mL, and the IC_{50} of ascorbic acid was 2.87 μg/mL. Then, the DPPH scavenging activity on air pollutant (PM1648a) was performed, respectively, to evaluate the antioxidant activity of FESCL (Figure 3). We also found that FESCL exhibited concentration-dependent DPPH radical scavenging activity at a statistically significant level ($p < 0.05$). The entire treatment concentration range was from 0.015 to 1% of FESCL, and the IC_{50} of FESCL was 0.0618 μg/mL, and the highest DPPH scavenging activity was shown to be 92.44% at 1% concentration of FESCL. This result indicated that FESCL had a noticeable effect on the scavenging free radical and it had high antioxidant activity.

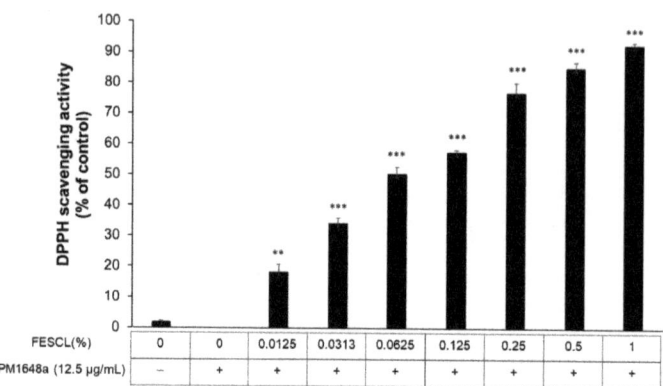

Figure 3. The DPPH radical scavenging activity of various concentrations of FESCL in HaCaT cells by treatment of PM1648a (12.5 μg/mL). All data were reported as the mean ± SD of three replicates. ** $p < 0.01$ and *** $p < 0.001$ vs. the PM1648a treated control group. DPPH; 2,2-diphenyl-1-picrylhydrazyl.

3.4. Anti-Inflammatory Activity of FESCL on Air Pollutants

The production of prostaglandin E_2 (PGE_2) is a representative inflammatory factor in immune cells, and the anti-inflammatory effect can be evaluated through the measurement of PGE_2 production inhibition activity [25]. Therefore, we measured the PGE_2 production inhibition activity of FESCL in Raw cell 264.7. After measuring the cytotoxicity level of fermented extract from SCL for Raw 264.7 cells, the FESCL inhibitory activity on PGE_2 production in the ones exposed to PM 1648a were evaluated. In addition, for the comparison of the positive control group, we tested the inhibition activity of PGE_2 production of 5μM dexamethasone-treated against the PM1648a stimulation and compared the anti-inflammatory effect of FESCL with dexamethasone (Figure 4). The non-cytotoxic concentrations of FESCL for the Raw 264.7 cell were by 2%, and the inhibition rate of PGE_2 production of FESCL was significantly ($p < 0.05$) increased in a concentration-dependent manner (0.125–2%). In particular, it was confirmed that about 78.20% of the PGE_2 production inhibited activity in the 2% concentration treatment group compared to the negative control group. PGE_2 levels in the medium were determined, as described in Materials and Methods. Cell viability by FESCL was also measured by a WST-1 based cell cytotoxicity assay, and there were non-cytotoxic concentrations of FESCL of 2%.

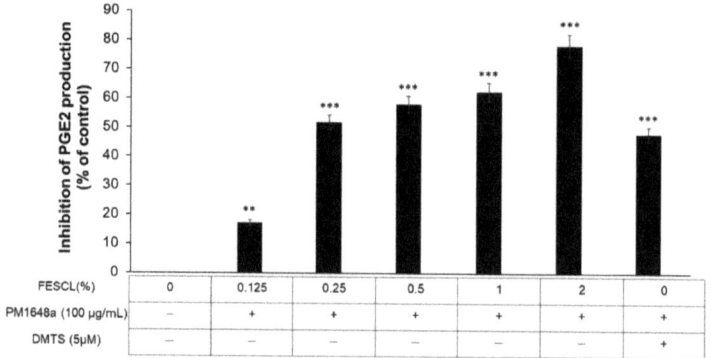

Figure 4. PGE_2 production inhibition activity of various concentrations of FESCL in Raw cell 264.7 by treatment of PM1648a (100 μg/mL). There were non-cytotoxic concentrations of FESCL by 2%. All data were reported as the mean ± SD of three replicates. ** $p < 0.01$ and *** $p < 0.001$ vs. the PM1648a treated control group. DMTS, dexamethasone.

4. Discussion

Cadmium (Cd) is one of the most concerning pollutants possessing high toxicity for both animals and plants. Cadmium is widely dumped into the environment through various anthropogenic activities such as mining, smelting, and the use of fertilizers [26]. Cadmium also affects cellular homeostasis and generates damage via complex mechanisms involving interactions with other metals and oxidative stress induction. Given it is one of the important pollutants which could damage human skin, we investigated a human keratinocyte cell line (HaCaT) as a model to study. In lines of experiments, we could confirm the significant protection activity of FESCL on the Cd exposed keratinocyte. This result was supported by Shi's previous report [27], in which *Smilax glabra* flavonoids extract could also reduce lead-induced cytotoxicity in HEK-293 cells stimulated with Pb.

As well, Urban PM is considered one of the most hazardous pollutants for human health [5], and in this study, the anti-pollution effects of FESCL were investigated by measuring antioxidant activity in the PM1648a-exposed HaCaT cells. As shown in Figures 2 and 3, the XRE-luciferase activity was significantly decreased by the concentration-dependent of FESCL, and the DPPH scavenging activity was significantly higher than the control group. Our results showed similar effect to the previous report related to the ethanol extract of *Smilax china*, but the FESCL appeared to be more effective compared to the ethanol extract of *Smilax china* [19]. According to Seo et al., the ethanol extract of *Smilax china* (IC_{50} = 49.93 µg/mL) showed the highest DPPH radical scavenging activity in four solvents, whereas L-ascorbic acid (33 µg/mL) showed similar results. In contrast, in our study, the IC_{50} value of FESCL was much lower than the IC_{50} value of ascorbic acid (IC_{50} = 0.0618 µg/mL). This means that the content of functional bioactive phytochemicals may be significantly enhanced by microbial fermentation.

Most of the previous studies have reported that *Smilax china* has bioactivities, such as anti-inflammatory, antioxidant, anticancer, and antimicrobial activities. However, these studies were mainly focused on the functionality of bioactive phytochemicals, not by fermentation extract, but the solvent extract of *Smilax china* [14–16]. Since the effects of FESCL on the antioxidant and anti-inflammatory effect had not been investigated yet, our study has great potential for improving skin health.

Since inflammatory reactions in the skin are a kind of defense reaction for protecting skin damage caused by physical irritation, chemicals, bacteria, and pollutants such as fine dust, the inflammatory reaction in the skin-activated macrophages produce inflammatory mediators such as PGE_2, and the inflammatory process could be further deepened [28,29]. We found the anti-inflammatory activity of FESCL by measuring the inhibition activity of PGE_2 production in Raw 264.7 cells. Feng et al. reported that flavonoid-enriched extract of *Smilax china* could affect suppressing inflammation in Raw 264.7 macrophages. Thus, the enhanced anti-inflammation of FESCL may be due to the increased phytochemical-like flavonoids or the synergetic effects of beneficial fermentation by *Lactobacillus*.

Smilax china a member of the *Smilacaceae* family, is widely distributed worldwide in tropical and temperate regions, especially in East Asia [15,19]. Previously, several studies have shown that *Smilax china* has been used in traditional medicine for the treatment of furunculosis, gout, tumors, and inflammation [12,14,27,30–32]. Recently, many studies have been discussing the antioxidant and anti-inflammatory effects of *Smilax china* leaves which has the presence of a significant amount of polyphenols [28,29,33]. The fermentation process itself yields beneficial effects through direct microbial action and the production of metabolites and other complex compounds [34]. During fermentation polyphenol compounds are metabolized and modified by fermenting organisms into other conjugates, glucosides, and/or related forms [34]. There were reports that fermentation positively confers organoleptic characteristics, and improves phenolic constituents and antioxidant activity [28,29]. Notably, FESCL showed high antioxidant and anti-inflammatory activity through a series of experiments using macrophages and keratinocytes after exposurepollutants. Taken together with findings and reports, the potential of FESCL as a functional material for cosmetics was expected to rise dramatically in the future.

5. Conclusions

In this study, we evaluated several biomarkers after pollutant exposure in Raw 264.7 macro-phages and HaCaT keratinocytes to investigate the possibility of anti-pollution cosmetic material of FESCL. FESCL decreased pollutant-induced luciferase activity in a dose-dependent manner, and FESCL significantly inhibited XRE-luciferase activity at a concentration of 1%. The IC_{50} value of FESCL showed the same DPPH scavenging activity at 0.0625% as ascorbic acid, and the maximum DPPH scavenging activity (92.44%) at 1%. The maximum permissible non-cytotoxic concentrations of FESCL for a Raw 264.7 cell was determined to be 2%, where PGE_2 production of FESCL was inhibited by 78.20%. These results show the anti-pollution activity of FESCL against the pollutant-stimulated human living skin explants. In conclusion, we confirmed the anti-pollution potential of FESCL as one of the functional materials in cosmetic formulation.

Supplementary Materials: The following supporting information can be downloaded at: https://www.mdpi.com/article/10.3390/cosmetics9060120/s1, Figure S1: HPLC chromatogram of FESCL and calibration chromatogram of Quercetin as flavonoid marker.

Author Contributions: Conceptualization, Y.-K.K.; methodology, Y.-K.K.; validation, D.-J.K.; formal analysis, Y.-K.K.; writing-original draft preparation, Y.-K.K.; supervision, D.-J.K.; project administration, D.-J.K.; funding acquisition, D.-J.K. All authors have read and agreed to the published version of the manuscript.

Funding: This research received no external funding.

Institutional Review Board Statement: Not applicable.

Informed Consent Statement: Not applicable.

Data Availability Statement: Not applicable.

Acknowledgments: This work was supported by the Technological Innovation R&D Program (S2745843) funded by the Ministry of SMEs and Startups (MSS, Sejong City, Republic of Korea).

Conflicts of Interest: The authors declare no conflict of interest. Author Y.K. Kim has received research grants from MNHBIO Co., Ltd. Author D.J. Kang owns stocks in MNHBIO Co, Ltd.

References

1. Juliano, C.; Magrini, G.A. Cosmetic Functional Ingredients from Botanical Sources for Anti-Pollution Skincare Products. *Cosmetics* **2018**, *5*, 19. [CrossRef]
2. Poljšak, B.; Dahmane, R. Free Radicals and Extrinsic Skin Aging. *Dermatol. Res. Pr.* **2012**, *2012*, 1–4. [CrossRef] [PubMed]
3. Araviiskaia, E.; Berardesca, E.; Bieber, T.; Gontijo, G.; Viera, M.S.; Marrot, L.; Chuberre, B.; Dreno, B. The impact of airborne pollution on skin. *J. Eur. Acad. Dermatol. Venereol.* **2019**, *33*, 1496–1505. [CrossRef]
4. Ali, A.; Khan, H.; Bahadar, R.; Riaz, A.; Bin Asad, M.H.H. The impact of airborne pollution and exposure to solar ultraviolet radiation on skin: Mechanistic and physiological insight. *Environ. Sci. Pollut. Res.* **2020**, *27*, 28730–28736. [CrossRef] [PubMed]
5. Dijkhoff, I.M.; Drasler, B.; Karakocak, B.B.; Petri-Fink, A.; Valacchi, G.; Eeman, M.; Rothen-Rutishauser, B. Impact of airborne particulate matter on skin: A systematic review from epidemiology to in vitro studies. *Part. Fibre Toxicol.* **2020**, *17*, 1–28. [CrossRef]
6. Araujo, J.A. Particulate air pollution, systemic oxidative stress, inflammation, and atherosclerosis. *Air Qual. Atmosphere Health* **2010**, *4*, 79–93. [CrossRef]
7. Kim, K.E.; Cho, D.; Park, H.J. Air pollution and skin diseases: Adverse effects of airborne particulate matter on various skin diseases. *Life Sci.* **2016**, *152*, 126–134. [CrossRef] [PubMed]
8. Kim, J.; Kim, E.-H.; Oh, I.; Jung, K.; Han, Y.; Cheong, H.-K.; Ahn, K. Symptoms of atopic dermatitis are influenced by outdoor air pollution. *J. Allergy Clin. Immunol.* **2013**, *132*, 495–498.e1. [CrossRef] [PubMed]
9. Ahn, K. The role of air pollutants in atopic dermatitis. *J. Allergy Clin. Immunol.* **2014**, *134*, 993–999. [CrossRef]
10. Kim, K. Influences of Environmental Chemicals on Atopic Dermatitis. *Toxicol. Res.* **2015**, *31*, 89–96. [CrossRef]
11. Tian, L.-W.; Zhang, Z.; Long, H.-L.; Zhang, Y.-J. Steroidal Saponins from the Genus Smilax and Their Biological Activities. *Nat. Prod. Bioprospect.* **2017**, *7*, 283–298. [CrossRef] [PubMed]
12. Li, Y.-L.; Gan, G.-P.; Zhang, H.-Z.; Wu, H.-Z.; Li, C.-L.; Huang, Y.-P.; Liu, Y.-W.; Liu, J.-W. A flavonoid glycoside isolated from *Smilax china* L. rhizome in vitro anticancer effects on human cancer cell lines. *J. Ethnopharmacol.* **2007**, *113*, 115–124. [CrossRef] [PubMed]
13. Lü, Y.; Chen, D.; Deng, J.; Tian, L. Effect of *Smilax china* on adjunctive arthritis mouse. *J. Chin. Med. Mater.* **2003**, *26*, 344–346.

14. Shu, X.-S.; Gao, Z.-H.; Yang, X.-L. Anti-inflammatory and anti-nociceptive activities of *Smilax china* L. aqueous extract. *J. Ethnopharmacol.* **2006**, *103*, 327–332. [CrossRef] [PubMed]
15. Khan, I.; Nisar, M.; Ebad, F.; Nadeem, S.; Saeed, M.; Khan, H.; Samiullah; Khuda, F.; Karim, N.; Ahmad, Z. Anti-inflammatory activities of Sieboldogenin from *Smilax china* Linn.: Experimental and computational studies. *J. Ethnopharmacol.* **2009**, *121*, 175–177. [CrossRef] [PubMed]
16. Zhang, Y.; Pan, X.; Ran, S.; Wang, K. Purification, structural elucidation and anti-inflammatory activity in vitro of polysaccharides from *Smilax china* L. *Int. J. Biol. Macromol.* **2019**, *139*, 233–243. [CrossRef] [PubMed]
17. Hu, K.; Yao, X. Protodioscin (NSC-698 796): Its Spectrum of Cytotoxicity Against Sixty Human Cancer Cell Lines in an Anticancer Drug Screen Panel. *Planta Med.* **2002**, *68*, 297–301. [CrossRef] [PubMed]
18. Challinor, V.L.; Parsons, P.G.; Chap, S.; White, E.F.; Blanchfield, J.T.; Lehmann, R.P.; De Voss, J.J. Steroidal saponins from the roots of Smilax sp.: Structure and bioactivity. *Steroids* **2012**, *77*, 504–511. [CrossRef] [PubMed]
19. Seo, H.-K.; Lee, J.-H.; Kim, H.-S.; Lee, C.-K.; Lee, S.-C. Antioxidant and antimicrobial activities of *Smilax china* L. leaf extracts. *Food Sci. Biotechnol.* **2012**, *21*, 1723–1727. [CrossRef]
20. Li, Y.; Won, K.J.; Kim, D.Y.; Bin Kim, H.; Kang, H.M.; Lee, S.Y.; Lee, H.M. Positive Promoting Effects of *Smilax China* Flower Absolute on the Wound Healing/Skin Barrier Repair-Related Responses of HaCaT Human Skin Keratinocytes. *Chem. Biodivers.* **2021**, *18*, e2001051. [CrossRef] [PubMed]
21. You, D.-H.; Park, J.-W.; Yuk, H.-G.; Lee, S.-C. Antioxidant and tyrosinase inhibitory activities of different parts of guava (*Psidium guajava* L.). *Food Sci. Biotechnol.* **2011**, *20*, 1095–1100. [CrossRef]
22. Lee, S.E.; Kwon, K.; Oh, S.W.; Park, S.J.; Yu, E.; Kim, H.; Yang, S.; Park, J.Y.; Chung, W.-J.; Cho, J.Y.; et al. Mechanisms of Resorcinol Antagonism of Benzo[a]pyrene-Induced Damage to Human Keratinocytes. *Biomol. Ther.* **2021**, *29*, 227–233. [CrossRef] [PubMed]
23. Chan, H.Y.; Wang, H.; Tsang, D.S.C.; Chen, Z.-Y.; Leung, L.K. Screening of Chemopreventive Tea Polyphenols Against PAH Genotoxicity in Breast Cancer Cells by a XRE-Luciferase ReporterConstruct. *Nutr. Cancer* **2003**, *46*, 93–100. [CrossRef] [PubMed]
24. Tsay, J.-C.J.; Tchou-Wong, K.-M.; Greenberg, A.K.; Pass, H.; Rom, W.N. Aryl hydrocarbon receptor and lung cancer. *Anticancer. Res.* **2013**, *33*, 1247–1256. [PubMed]
25. Nam, J.-H.; Seo, J.-T.; Kim, Y.-H.; Kim, K.-D.; Yoo, D.-L.; Lee, J.-N.; Hong, S.-Y.; Kim, S.-J.; Sohn, H.-B.; Kim, H.-S.; et al. Inhibitory Effects of Extracts from Arabis glabra on Lipopolysaccharide Induced Nitric Oxide and Prostaglandin E$_2$ Production in RAW264.7 Macrophages. *Korean J. Plant Resour.* **2015**, *28*, 568–573. [CrossRef]
26. Aziz, R.; Rafiq, M.T.; Yang, J.; Liu, D.; Lu, L.; He, Z.; Daud, M.K.; Li, T.; Yang, X. Impact Assessment of Cadmium Toxicity and Its Bioavailability in Human Cell Lines (Caco-2 and HL-7702). *BioMed Res. Int.* **2014**, *2014*, 1–8. [CrossRef] [PubMed]
27. Shi, Y.; Tian, C.; Yu, X.; Fang, Y.; Zhao, X.; Zhang, X.; Xia, D. Protective Effects of Smilax glabra Roxb. Against Lead-Induced Renal Oxidative Stress, Inflammation and Apoptosis in Weaning Rats and HEK-293 Cells. *Front. Pharmacol.* **2020**, *11*, 556248. [CrossRef]
28. Huang, H.-L.; Lu, Z.-Q.; Chen, G.-T.; Zhang, J.-Q.; Wang, W.; Yang, M.; Guo, D.-A. Phenylpropanoid-Substituted Catechins and Epicatechins from *Smilax china*. *Helvetica Chim. Acta* **2007**, *90*, 1751–1757. [CrossRef]
29. Feng, H.; He, Y.; La, L.; Hou, C.; Song, L.; Yang, Q.; Wu, F.; Liu, W.; Hou, L.; Li, Y.; et al. The flavonoid-enriched extract from the root of *Smilax china* L. inhibits inflammatory responses via the TLR-4-mediated signaling pathway. *J. Ethnopharmacol.* **2020**, *256*, 112785. [CrossRef]
30. Chen, L.; Yin, H.; Lan, Z.; Ma, S.; Zhang, C.; Yang, Z.; Li, P.; Lin, B. Anti-hyperuricemic and nephroprotective effects of *Smilax china* L. *J. Ethnopharmacol.* **2011**, *135*, 399–405. [CrossRef]
31. Hirota, B.C.K.; Paula, C.D.S.; de Oliveira, V.B.; da Cunha, J.M.; Schreiber, A.K.; Ocampos, F.M.M.; Barison, A.; Miguel, O.G.; Miguel, M.D. Phytochemical and Antinociceptive, Anti-Inflammatory, and Antioxidant Studies of *Smilax larvata* (Smilacaceae). *Evid.-Based Complement. Altern. Med.* **2016**, *2016*, 1–12. [CrossRef] [PubMed]
32. Adebo, O.A.; Medina-Meza, I.G. Impact of Fermentation on the Phenolic Compounds and Antioxidant Activity of Whole Cereal Grains: A Mini Review. *Molecules* **2020**, *25*, 927. [CrossRef] [PubMed]
33. Shao, B.; Guo, H.-Z.; Cui, Y.-J.; Liu, A.-H.; Yu, H.-L.; Guo, H.; Xu, M.; Guo, D.-A. Simultaneous determination of six major stilbenes and flavonoids in *Smilax china* by high performance liquid chromatography. *J. Pharm. Biomed. Anal.* **2007**, *44*, 737–742. [CrossRef] [PubMed]
34. Huynh, N.T.; Van Camp, J.; Smagghe, G.; Raes, K. Improved Release and Metabolism of Flavonoids by Steered Fermentation Processes: A Review. *Int. J. Mol. Sci.* **2014**, *15*, 19369–19388. [CrossRef] [PubMed]

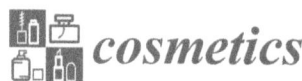

Article

Anti-Inflammatory Activity of the Active Compounds of Sanguisorbae Radix in Macrophages and In Vivo Toxicity Evaluation in Zebrafish

Young-Ah Jang [1], Yong Hur [2] and Jin-Tae Lee [3],*

1   Gennolab Co., Ltd., Gyeongbuk 38540, Korea; yaviol@nate.com
2   Apharm Co., Ltd. 559, Dalseo-daero, Dalseo-gu, Daegu 42709, Korea; coo@drnuell.com
3   Department of Cosmeceutical Science, Daegu Haany University, Gyeongbuk 38540, Korea
*   Correspondence: jtleecosmetics@gmail.com; Tel.: +82-010-5594-8079

Received: 29 October 2019; Accepted: 29 November 2019; Published: 4 December 2019

Abstract: Sanguisorbae Radix (SR) is the root of the *Sanguisorba officinalis* L., a plant native to Asian countries and used in traditional medicine. We isolated the active components of SR and investigated their anti-inflammatory potential. Quercetin (QC), (+)-catechin (CC), and gallic acid (GA) were isolated from acetone extracts of SR. To elucidate the molecular mechanism by which these compounds suppress inflammation, we analyzed the transcriptional up-regulation of inflammatory mediators, such as nuclear factor-kappa B (NF-κB) and its target genes, inducible NOS (iNOS), and cyclooxygenase (COX)-2, in lipopolysaccharide (LPS)-stimulated macrophage RAW264.7 cells. Notably, QC, CC, and GA were found to inhibit the production of nitric oxide, tumor necrosis factor-alpha, and prostaglandin in a dose-dependent manner. Western blot results indicate that the compounds decreased the expression of iNOS and COX-2 proteins. Furthermore, the compounds decreased phosphorylation of IKK, IκB, ERK, p-38, and JNK proteins in LPS-induced cells. The results support the notion that QC, CC, and GA can potently inhibit the inflammatory response, with QC showing the highest anti-inflammatory activity. In in vivo toxicity studies in zebrafish (*Danio rerio*), QC showed no toxicity up to 25 μg/mL. Therefore, QC has non-toxic potential as a skin anti-inflammatory biomaterial.

Keywords: anti-inflammatory biomaterial; macrophages; *Sanguisorba officinalis*; Sanguisorbae Radix

1. Introduction

Inflammation is a response to injury caused by harmful physical or chemical stimuli or microbiological toxins, and occurs in numerous pathologies, such as asthma, arthritis, multiple sclerosis, atherosclerosis, and inflammatory bowel diseases [1,2]. There are three types of mammalian nitric oxide synthase (NOS)—neuronal NOS (nNOS), endothelial NOS (eNOS), and inducible NOS (iNOS). Of these, the iNOS is involved in inflammatory reactions [3]. Nitric oxide (NO) generated by the iNOS isoform is necessary for the innate immune and inflammatory responses of hosts to various pathogens and microorganisms [4,5]. However, excessive production of NO is regarded as a pro-inflammatory mediator that induces inflammation in abnormal physiological situations [6]. Therefore, therapeutic agents that inhibit iNOS may effectively ameliorate these inflammatory conditions. Lipopolysaccharide (LPS)-induced gene products include pro-inflammatory cytokines, such as tumor necrosis factor-alpha (TNF)-α and interleukin-6 (IL-6), and adhesion enzymes, such as iNOS and cyclooxygenase-2 (COX)-2 [7]. COX enzymes are known to produce prostaglandins (PGs) that are involved in many physiological events, such as the progression of inflammation, modulation of the inflammatory response, and transmission of pain [8]. COX-1 is typically expressed in most tissues, which is expected given that COX-1 maintains housekeeping physiological functions.

In contrast, COX-2 is only expressed in some tissues and is transiently induced by growth factors, pro-inflammatory cytokines, tumor promoters, and bacterial toxins [9]. Nuclear factor-kappa B (NF-κB) is a DNA transcription factor that plays a vital role in the expression of various genes involved in the inflammatory response [10–12]. Inactive NF-κB is bound to its inhibitory subunit IκB, and the complexes are sequestered in the cytoplasm. Upon stimulation, IκB proteins are phosphorylated, ubiquitinated, and degraded, allowing NF-κB to translocate to the nucleus, where it can bind to specific DNA sequences located in the promoter regions of target genes, thereby activating gene transcription [13,14]. Recently, many studies demonstrated the role of phytochemicals in anti-inflammatory activity via NF-κB pathway down-regulation [15]. Mitogen-activated protein kinases (MAPKs) have essential functions in the regulation of cell differentiation, cell growth, and cellular responses to cytokines. The MAPK cascades are critical signaling pathways in the immune system and include p38 MAPK, extracellular signal-regulated kinase (ERK), and c-jun N-terminal kinase (JNK) [16]. One of the main functions of MAPK is the activation of transcription factors, some of which increase the expression of pro-inflammatory cytokines [17]. Cytokine-mediated host defense mechanisms induce significant cell and organ injury and play crucial roles in the pathophysiology of sepsis [18].

Sanguisorbae Radix (SR), the dried root of *Sanguisorba officinalis* L., has hemostatic, analgesic, and astringent properties and has been used in traditional Chinese medicine for the treatment of burns, scalds, inflammation, and internal hemorrhage [19–21]. SR is also used to control bloody pus, treat boils, repair damaged tissue, relieve alcohol poisoning, quench one's thirst, and relieve eye pain [22]. Until now, saponin components such as triterpenes and their glycosides (e.g., ziyuglycoside I) and disaccharide (5-O-alpha-D-(3-C-hydroxymethyl)lyxofuranosyl-beta-D-(2-C-hydroxymethyl) arabino furanose) have been reported as the major active compounds of SR that confer these in vitro and in vivo pharmacological effects [22–25]. Although numerous activities of this plant have been reported and published to date, research on the safety of SR has been limited. Zebrafish are economical with regards to maintenance because it requires simpler breeding facilities, and its feed is less expensive than that of other model species. It produces 200–300 embryos with single external fertilization, which makes it suitable for toxicity assessment [26]. Thus, we used the zebrafish (*Danio rerio*) embryo model to investigate the potential anti-inflammatory mechanism of SR against LPS-induced inflammatory response in macrophages, to evaluate the root as a potential safe cosmetic material.

2. Materials and Methods

2.1. Materials and Reagents

RAW264.7 cells were obtained from the Korean Cell Line Bank (KCLB, Seoul, Korea). Dulbecco's Modified Eagle <edium (DMEM), fetal bovine serum (FBS), and penicillin/streptomycin were purchased from Gibco BRL Co. (Grand Island, NY, USA). Lipopolysaccharide (LPS), 3-[4,5-dimethylthiazol-2-yl]-2,5-diphenyl tetrazolium bromide (MTT), acrylamide, and N,N'-bis-methylene-acrylamide were purchased from Sigma-Aldrich Corp. (St, Louis, MO, USA). The iNOS, COX-2, IKK, p-IKK, IκB, p-IκB, ERK, p-ERK, p-38, p-p-38, JNK, p-JNK, and β-actin monoclonal antibodies and the secondary antibody were purchased from Santa Cruz Biotechnology, Inc., (Santa Cruz, CA, USA). Prostaglandin (PGE_2) and TNF-α for ELISA Kits were purchased from R&D Systems Inc. (Minneapolis, MN, USA). Halt™ Protease Inhibitor Cocktail Kits and BSA kits were purchased from Thermo Fisher Scientific (Rockford, IL, USA). GoScript™ Reverse Transcriptase and GoTaq®Flexi DNA Polymerase were purchased from Promega Corporation (Madison, WI, USA).

2.2. Sample Preparation

SR was obtained from Andong City, Kyung-Buk, Korea. The powdered roots of SR were extracted with 70% acetone at 20 °C for 3 days; the solution was filtered using a filter paper (Whatman No. 2, Tokyo, Japan) and the obtained acetone extract was concentrated under reduced pressure. The acetone extract was then dissolved in chloroform in a separatory funnel, and further fractionated by successive solvent extraction with ethyl acetate and n-butanol saturated with H_2O. The n-butanol fraction was fractionated by Diaion HP-20 column chromatography, with stepwise elution of H_2O–MeOH (100:1–1:100) to obtain separated active fractions. To determine the structure of the compounds obtained, ^1H- and ^{13}C-NMR were measured, and the structure of individual substances was determined **Quercetin (1).** Yellow amorphous powder ^1H-NMR (500 MHz, MeOH-d_6): δ 7.79 (1H, d, J = 2.3 Hz, H-2′), 7.69 (1H, dd, J = 2.3, 8.5 Hz, H-6′), 6.99 (1H, d, J = 8.5 Hz, H-5′) 6.55 (1H, d, J = 2.0 Hz, H-6) 6.25 (1H, d, J = 2.0 Hz, H-8). ^{13}C-NMR (125 MHz, MeOH-d_6): δ 175.9 (C-4), 163.9 (C-7), 160.8 (C-5′), 156.2 (C-9), 147.7 (C-4′), 146.8 (C-2), 145.1 (C-3′), 135.8 (C-3), 121.9 (C-1′), 120.0 (C-6′), 115.6 (C-5′), 115.1 (C-2′), 103.1 (C-10), 98.2 (C-6), 93.4 (C-8). **(+)-Catechin (2).** Brown amorphous powder ^1H-NMR (500 MHz, MeOH-d_6): δ 6.84 (1H, dd, J = 8.0, 2.0 Hz, H-6′), 6.76 (1H, dd, J = 2.0 Hz, H-2′), 6.75 (1H, d, J = 8.0 Hz, H-5′), 5.93 (1H, d, J = 2.0 Hz, H-6), 5.86 (1H, d, J = 2.0 Hz, H-8), 4.57 (1H, d, J = 7.5 Hz, H-2), 3.98 (1H, m, H-3), 2.85 (1H, dd, J = 16.0, 5.5 Hz, H-4ax), 2.50 (1H, dd, J = 16.0, 5.5 Hz, H-4eq). ^{13}C-NMR (125 MHz, MeOH-d_6): δ 157.9 (C-7), 157.6 (C-5), 157.0 (C-9), 146.3 (C-3′), 146.3 (C-4′), 132.3 (C-1′), 120.1 (C-6′) 116.1 (C-5′), 115.3 (C-2′), 100.9 (C-10), 96.3 (C-6), 95.9 (C-8), 83.0 (C-2), 68.9 (C-3), 28.6 (C-4). **Gallic acid (3).** White amorphous powder ^1H-NMR (500 MHz, MeOH-d_6): δ 7.15 (2H, s, H-2, 6). ^{13}C-NMR (125 MHz, MeOH-d_6): δ 169.1 (C-7), 145.7 (C-3, 5), 138.7 (C-4), 121.4 (C-1), 109.9(C-2, 6). In this study, three compounds—quercetin (QC), (+)- catechin (CC), and gallic acid (GA)—obtained from SR were used. These compounds were stored in a refrigerator at 4 °C until use.

2.3. MTT Assay

Cells were uniformly dispensed in a 96-well plate (0.18 mL) at a density of 5×10^3 cells/well. QC, CC, and GA were prepared at concentrations of 5, 10, 25, 50, 75, and 100 µg/mL, and 0.02 mL of the solution was added. Then, the cells were cultured in a 5% CO_2 incubator at 37 °C for 24 h. Next, 0.02 mL MTT solution prepared at a concentration of 5 mg/mL was added, and the mixture was cultured for 4 h. Following incubation, the culture solution was removed, and 0.15 mL DMSO was added to each well. After incubation at room temperature for 15 min, absorbance was measured at 540 nm with a Microplate Reader (Winooski, VT, USA). Cell viability was calculated as a percentage of control absorbance.

2.4. Measurement of NO, PGE2, and TNF-α

Cells were plated at a density of 2×10^5 cells/well in a 24-well plate. Cells were induced with LPS (1 µg/mL) and treated with either the control, QC, CC, or GA at concentrations of 10, 25, and 50 µg/mL and cultured. The supernatant was collected, and the inhibitory effect of samples on NO, PGE_2, and TNF-α cytokine production was determined using the Griess reagent enzyme and ELISA kit (Minneapolis, MN, USA), according to the manufacturer's instructions.

2.5. Western Blotting

RAW264.7 cells were uniformly dispensed in a 6-well plate at a density of 1×10^5 cells/well and cultured for 24 h. Then, cells were induced with LPS (1 µg/mL) and treated with the control or QC, CC, or GA at concentrations of 10, 25, and 50 µg/mL and cultured. Protein lysates were obtained by incubating the culture with RIPA lysis buffer (Pierce, IL, USA) for 1 h, followed by centrifugation at 12,000 rpm for 30 min at 4 °C. Then, proteins were quantified by Bradford assay (Hercules, CA, USA) according to the manufacturer's instruction. Equal proteins were electrophoresed using 10% sodium dodecyl sulfate–polyacrylamide gel electrophoresis and transferred to a PVDF membrane (Amersham Pharmacia Biotech, Buckinghamshire, UK) at 60 V for 3 h. After blocking with tris buffer solution containing 5% skim milk for 1 h, the membrane was incubated with dilution of polyclonal antibodies for iNOS, COX-2, IKK, p-IKK, IκB, p-IκB, ERK, p-ERK, p-38, p-p-38, JNK, p-JNK, and β-actin. After extensive washes, the membrane was incubated with the secondary antibody (1:1000 dilution) for 1 h at room temperature. Next, the cells were reacted with Immobilon Western Chemiluminescent

HRP substrate (Millipore, MA, USA) and protein levels were analyzed using EZ-Capture MG (ATTO Corporation, Tokyo, Japan).

2.6. RNA Isolation and RT-PCR

Total RNA was isolated using the TRIsolution™ Santa Cruz Biotechnology, Inc. (Santa Cruz, CA, USA), according to the manufacturer's instructions. One milliliter of Trizol reagent was added to the cells. After the cells were dissolved and kept at room temperature for 5 min, 0.2 mL of chloroform was added and mixed well. The cells were then centrifuged at 12,000× g for 10 min. The isolated RNA was dissolved in distilled water containing diethyl pyrocarbonate and the purity of RNA was measured using the ELISA reader. Then, the concentration of RNA was calculated and used for the experiment. GoScript™ Reverse Transcriptase was used for cDNA synthesis, and PCR was performed using GoTaq®Flexi DNA Polymerase and specific primers. The amplified cDNA was separated by electrophoresis on a 1.5% agarose gel and visualized by the electrophoresis EZ-Capture MG image analyzer.

2.7. Zebrafish Breeding Conditions and Embryo Acquisition

Zebrafish were obtained from the Division of Biomedical & Cosmetics, Mokwon University, Korea, and were used during the breeding period. All experimental protocols were approved and conducted according to the guidelines and regulations of the Animal Ethics Committee of Mokwon University. Wild-type zebrafish were provided by the Zebrafish Center for Disease Modeling, Korea. The rearing condition was kept constant at 28 ± 1 °C with a 16 h/8 h light/dark cycle (Rotifer continuous culture system, GDBC, Korea). They were fed brine shrimp (Ocean Star International, Utah, USA). Female and male fish with at least five spawning experiences were fed adequate feed the day before spawning; 24 h later, irradiation of light was used to produce embryos. The produced embryos were incubated at 28 ± 1 °C for 2 days in pre-manufactured egg water (sea salt solution, Aquarium Systems, France) to avoid exceeding a maximum of 50 eggs in a 100-mm petri dish, and the egg water was replaced periodically. Figure 1 shows the Zebrafish model.

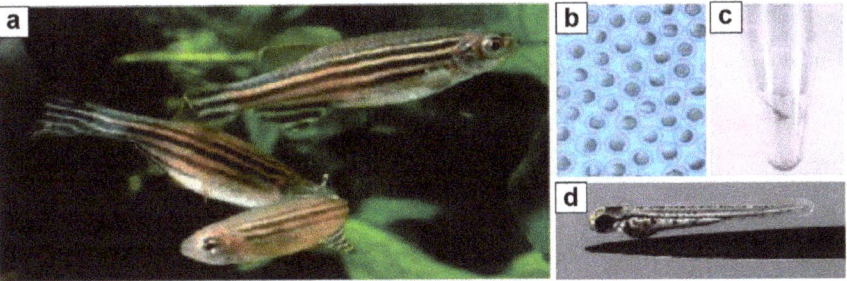

Figure 1. *Danio rerio* animal model. (**a**) *D. rerio* is a small tropical fish of the Cyprinidae family, 4–5 cm in length; (**b**) 6 h of embryonic development, embryos are ~0.7 mm across; (**c**) 1-week-old larva swimming in E. tube; (**d**) embryonic after two days of development, placed on needlepoint.

2.8. Zebra Fish Embryo Toxicity Test

Mature male and female zebrafish were separated in the tank for egg collection. After 24 h, they were put together, and eggs were collected. The culture solution was used as a control. To each well of the 24-well plate, 3 zebrafish eggs were added and treated with different concentrations of QC: 10, 25, and 50 µL/mL. The plate was then placed in the incubator at 28 °C, and the toxicity level of the samples treated with QC was analyzed for coagulation rate and hatching rate at 24, 48, and 72 h after the QC treatment and compared with control.

2.9. Statistical Analysis

Statistical analysis was performed using SPSS 12.0, and differences were considered significant when $p < 0.05, 0.01$ after a t-test using analysis of variance (ANOVA).

3. Results and Discussion

Inflammation is a defensive pathway primarily caused by the action of phagocytic cells, such as macrophages and dendritic cells, which work to protect the body from exogenous pathogens [27]. The innate immune response is part of an appropriate inflammatory reaction that contributes to the development of adaptive immunity. However, excessive and inappropriate inflammatory reactions cause cell necrosis and various chronic diseases [28]. Skin-related diseases are often accompanied by inflammation, which causes aggravation, such as acne and atopy. Studies are being actively conducted to identify natural materials that can alleviate the inflammatory reaction [29]. Herein, we identified three compounds from SR extracts (Figure 2) and then evaluated the toxicity of SR compounds (QC, CC, and GA) at different concentrations against RAW264.7 cells (Figure 3); the cells showed a viability of >85% at all concentrations below 50 µg/mL. Thus, these compounds were considered non-toxic, and further experiments were conducted using a concentration of 50 µg/mL.

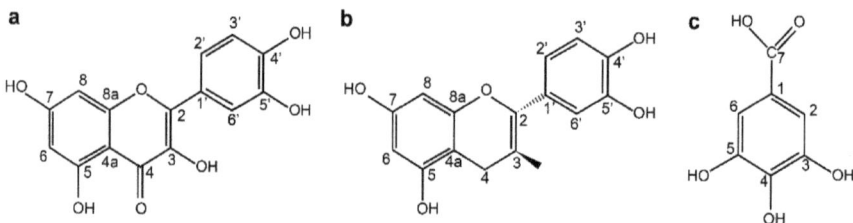

Figure 2. Structure of (**a**) quercetin, (**b**) (+)-catechin, and (**c**) gallic acid isolated from Sanguisorbae Radix.

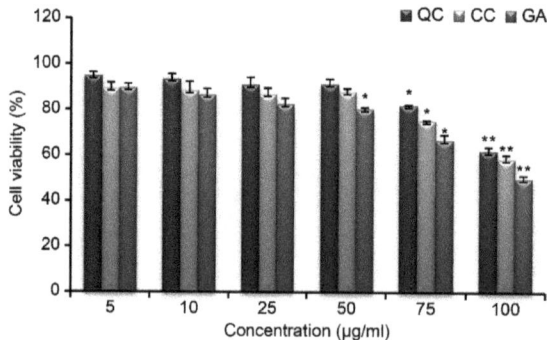

Figure 3. Viability, detected by MTT assay, of RAW264.7 cells after treatment with various concentrations of quercetin (QC), (+)- catechin (CC), and gallic acid (GA), obtained from Sanguisorbae Radix. Data are represented as mean ± standard error ($n = 3$) of three independent experiments. * $p < 0.05$, ** $p < 0.01$, as compared with the control.

Several pro-inflammatory cytokines, such as TNF-α, PGE$_2$, and IL-8, promote systemic inflammation. We measured the production levels of TNF-α and PGE$_2$ using an ELISA Kit and examined the production of NO using the Griess reagent. As shown in Figure 4a,b, SR markedly blocked the production of these inflammatory mediators in LPS-treated RAW264.7 cells. At 50 µg/mL of QC, PGE$_2$ levels decreased by 38.8% and TNF-α levels decreased by 21.9%, which was the highest cytokine inhibition activity observed. TNF-α and PGE$_2$ production were also suppressed by CC and GA treatments in a dose-dependent manner. Additionally, QC was effective at suppressing the release of NO from LPS-induced peritoneal macrophages (Figure 4c).

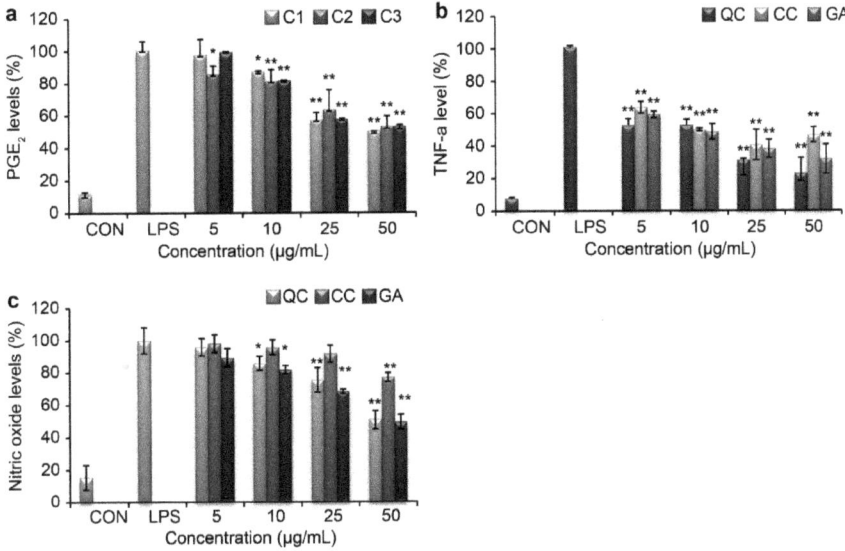

Figure 4. Effect of quercetin (QC), (+)- catechin (CC), and gallic acid (GA) from Sanguisorbae Radix on LPS-induced expression of nitric oxide (NO) in RAW264.7 cells. The cells were incubated for 24 h in DMEM containing 10% FBS, and then simultaneously treated with various concentrations of QC, CC, or GA for 24 h. The supernatant was collected from each well, and (**a**) PGE$_2$ and (**b**) TNF-α levels were determined by ELISA. (**c**) NO level was determined by the Griess reagent. Data are represented as mean ± standard error (n = 3) from three independent experiments. * $p < 0.01$, ** $p < 0.005$.

To investigate the molecular mechanism through which these compounds suppress inflammation, we measured the mRNA and protein expression levels of iNOS and COX-2. LPS stimulation of RAW264.7 cells markedly increased iNOS and COX-2 production compared with that in the negative control. As shown in Figure 5a, the protein expression level of iNOS was found to be 20.7%, 36.2%, and 23.8% upon treatment with 50 μg/mL QC, CC, and GA, respectively. Similarly, the mRNA expression level of iNOS was found to be 40.6%, 53.3%, and 37.3% after treatment with 50 μg/mL of QC, CC, and GA, respectively (Figure 5b). Thus, treatment with the SR compounds markedly inhibited the LPS-mediated induction of iNOS mRNA and protein expression.

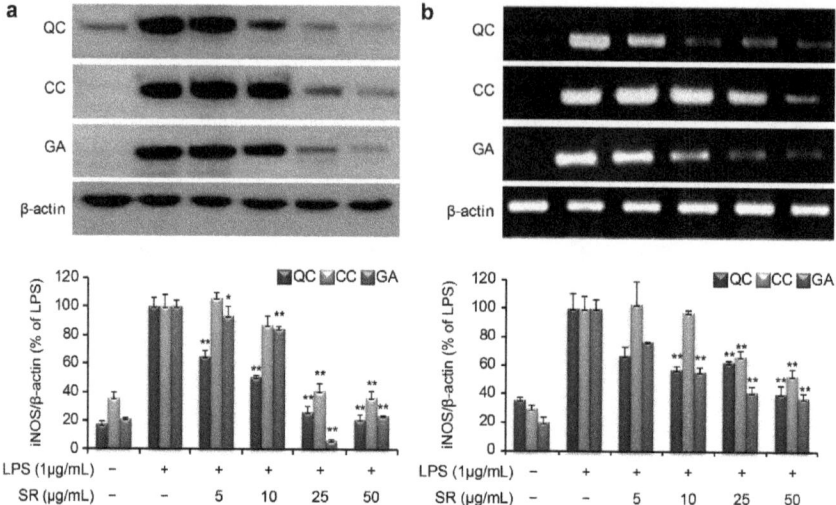

Figure 5. Inhibition of inducible nitric oxide synthase (iNOS) protein (**a**) and mRNA (**b**) expression by quercetin (QC), (+)-catechin (CC), or gallic acid (GA) in LPS-stimulated RAW264.7 cells. Cells were pretreated with the indicated concentrations of QC, CC, or GA 1 h before stimulation with 1 μg/mL LPS and then incubated for 24 h. (**a**) Cell lysates were electrophoresed, and iNOS expression was detected by a specific antibody. (**b**) Total RNA was prepared for reverse transcription polymerase chain reaction analysis of iNOS gene expression. Data are represented as mean ± standard error ($n = 3$) of three independent experiments. * $p < 0.05$, ** $p < 0.01$, compared with control.

Similar to iNOS, the COX-2 mRNA and protein levels were markedly induced by LPS stimulation (Figure 6). However, the protein expression level of COX-2 was reduced to 12.4%, 44.1%, and 23.8% upon simultaneous treatment with 50 μg/mL QC, CC, and GA, respectively (Figure 6a). Consistent with this, the corresponding COX-2 mRNA expression level was reduced to 23.9%, 47.8%, and 35.5% after treatment with 50 μg/mL QC, CC, and GA, respectively (Figure 6b).

Thus, LPS-stimulated macrophages show the rapid induction of genes responsible for production of pro-inflammatory cytokines, such as TNF-α and PGE$_2$, and inflammatory mediators, such as NO. Our data demonstrate that SR markedly inhibited or suppressed these LPS-induced pro-inflammatory effects in RAW264.7 cells at both the mRNA and protein levels.

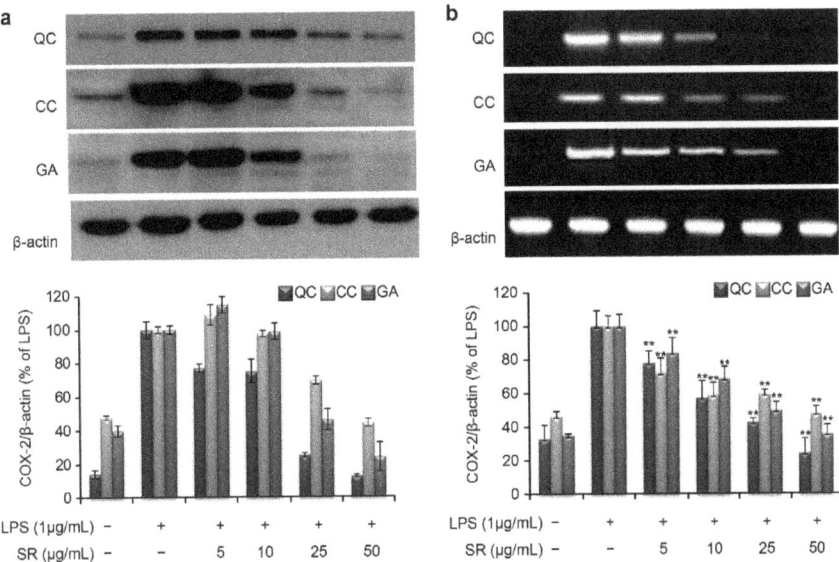

Figure 6. Inhibition of inducible nitric oxide synthase COX-2 protein (**a**) and mRNA (**b**) expression by quercetin (QC), (+)- catechin (CC), or gallic acid (GA) in LPS-stimulated RAW264.7 cells. Cells were pretreated with the indicated concentrations of QC, CC, or GA 1 h before stimulation with 1 µg/mL LPS and then incubated for 24 h. (**a**) Cell lysates were electrophoresed, and COX-2 expression was detected by a specific antibody. (**b**) Total RNA was prepared for reverse transcription polymerase chain reaction analysis of COX-2 gene expression. Data are represented as mean ± standard error ($n = 3$) of three independent experiments. * $p < 0.05$, ** $p < 0.01$, as compared with the control.

A previous study reported that LPS increased activation of NF-κB and regulated the expression of iNOS, COX-2, and other cytokines [30]; thus, NF-κB plays an important role in inflammation. NF-κB binds to inhibitory κBα (IκBα) molecules in the promoter region of an inflammatory response and only becomes active after IκBα is phosphorylated and subsequently degraded; this modification of IκBα occurs at serine 32 and 36 by the IκB kinase (IKK) complex [31]. Thus, we examined the effects of SR on phosphorylation of IκBα and IKK in LPS-induced cells. As a result, treatment with QC, CC, or GA attenuated the phosphorylation of IκBα and IKK in a dose-dependent manner (Figure 7).

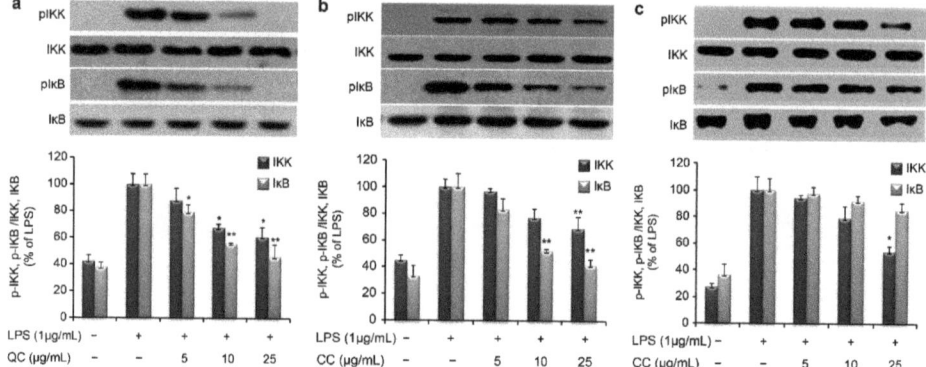

Figure 7. Effect of quercetin (QC), (+)-catechin (CC), and gallic acid (GA) on NF-κB activity in LPS-stimulated RAW264.7 cells. Results are expressed as a ratio of phosphorylated IKK and IκB/non-phosphorylated IKK and IκB. Data are represented as mean ± standard error ($n = 3$) of three independent experiments. * $p < 0.05$, ** $p < 0.01$, compared with control.

The MAPK family consists of ERK, p38, and JNK [32]. In our study, SR effectively suppressed the phosphorylation of ERK, p38, and JNK, which is a critical event in the MAPK signal transduction pathway (Figure 8). These data suggest that SR inhibits the production of inflammation by regulating gene expression involved in the NF-κB and MAPK-mediated inflammatory process.

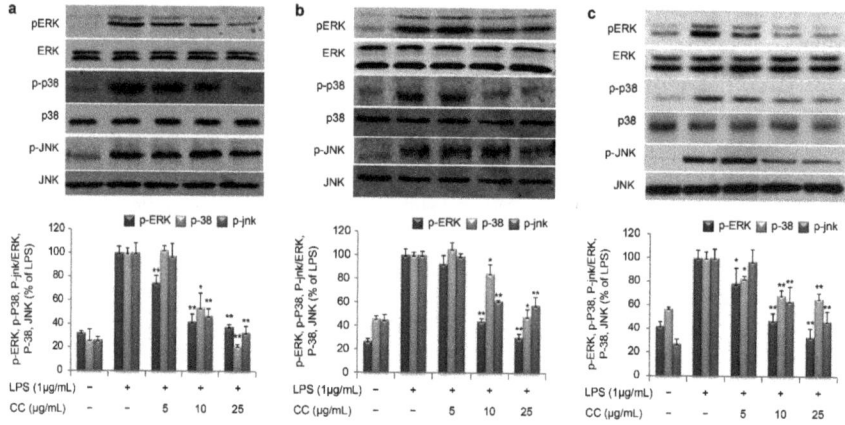

Figure 8. Effect of quercetin (QC), (+)-catechin (CC), and gallic acid (GA) on mitogen-activated protein kinase (MAPK) activity in LPS-stimulated RAW264.7 cells. Results are expressed as a ratio of phosphorylated ERK, p38, and JNK/non-phosphorylated ERK, p38, and JNK. Data are represented as mean ± standard error ($n = 3$) of three independent experiments. * $p < 0.05$, ** $p < 0.01$, compared with control.

To examine the toxicity of QC, zebrafish embryos were treated with 0, 10, 25, and 50 ppm of QC 12 h post-fertilization, and the coagulation rate and hatching rate of embryos were monitored for 72 h (Figure 9a,b). In the control group, the embryos were treated with egg water 24 and 48 h post-fertilization, and the coagulation rate was 0%. In contrast, the coagulation rate of the group treated with 50 ppm QC for 72 h was 33%. The hatching rate of the embryos from the control group after 48 h was 100%, while that of the embryos treated with 10, 25, and 50 ppm of QC was 58%, 41%, and 33%, respectively, indicating a delay in hatching. According to the results, QC qualified as a safe material at a concentration of 50 µg/ml in the safety experiment using the zebrafish model. Nonetheless, the hatching rate was 100% after 72 h in these treatment groups, indicating that the QC extract is safe. Moreover, zebrafish embryos treated with 10 ppm and 25 ppm of QC did not coagulate and underwent normal embryogenesis, similar to that in the control group.

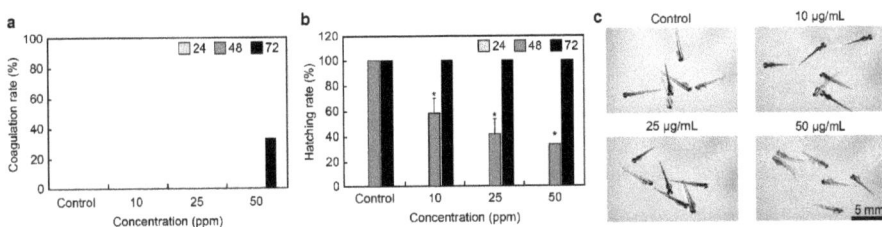

Figure 9. Effect of quercetin (QC) on zebrafish development. (**a**) Embryo coagulation rate, (**b**) hatching rate. (**c**) Representative image of zebrafish treated with control (egg water) or QC at indicated concentrations. Data are represented as mean ± standard error ($n = 3$) of three independent experiments. * $p < 0.05$, compared with control.

Although analysis of the development of zebrafish, when exposed to different concentrations of QC, showed no morphological abnormality at 10 ppm and 25 ppm, yolk swelling and melanin loss were observed at 50 ppm (Figure 9c).

4. Conclusions

In this study, we evaluated the anti-inflammatory effects of SR compounds (QC, CC, and GA) using the RAW264.7 cell line and evaluated their in vivo toxicity using zebrafish. Our results show that QC, CC, or GA was able to suppress iNOS and COX-2 expression, and phosphorylation of p38, JNK, and ERK in LPS-stimulated RAW264.7 cells. Furthermore, the application of QC, CC, or GA effectively suppressed pro-inflammatory cytokines (TNF-α and PGE_2) and NO expression. Of the three compounds, QC showed the highest anti-inflammatory effect. Besides, the toxicity assessment of QC provided evidence that QC is non-toxic at a concentration lower than 25 µg/mL. Therefore, SR has potential applications as a safe anti-inflammatory biomaterial for use in skin-care products.

Author Contributions: Y.-A.J. conceived, designed, and performed the experiments, analyzed the data, and wrote the manuscript. Y.H. reviewed and approved the final manuscript. J.-T.L. designed the manuscript, analyzed the data, and reviewed the final manuscript.

Funding: This research was funded by the Biotherapy Industry Base Construction Project from the Ministry of Trade, Industry, and Energy (MTIE) in 2018, grant number N0001805.

Conflicts of Interest: The authors have no conflicts of interest to declare. The funders of this study had no role in its design or in the collection of data and analysis. The funder did not influence the writing of the manuscript or the decision to publish the results.

References

1. Shim, S.B. Study on Characterizations of Endemic Natural Substances and Efficacy Evaluation of Formulation Using as Cosmetic Ingredients. Ph.D. Thesis, Department of Chemical Engineering, Graduate School, Hanyang University Seoul, Seoul, Korea, 2012; pp. 12–31.
2. Toltl, L.J.; Swystun, L.L.; Pepler, L.; Liaw, P.C. Protective effects of activated protein C in sepsis. *Thromb. Haemost.* **2008**, *100*, 582–592. [CrossRef] [PubMed]
3. Kindt, T.J.; Goldsby, R.A.; Osborne, B.A. *Innate Immunity: Tenney S. Kuby Immunology*, 6th ed.; W. H. Freeman Company: New York, NY, USA, 2007; pp. 52–73.

4. Guzik, T.J.; Korbut, R.; Adamek-Guzik, T. Nitric oxide and superoxide in inflammation and immune regulation. *J. Physiol. Pharmacol.* **2003**, *54*, 469–487. [PubMed]
5. Rankin, J.A. Biological mediators of acute inflammation. *AACN Clin. Issues* **2004**, *15*, 3–17. [CrossRef] [PubMed]
6. MacMicking, J.; Xie, Q.W.; Nathan, C. Nitric oxide and macrophage function. *Annu. Rev. Immunol.* **1997**, *15*, 323–350. [CrossRef] [PubMed]
7. Pfeilschifter, J.; Muhl, H. Immunopharmacology: Anti-inflammatory therapy targeting transcription factors. *Eur. J. Phamacol.* **1999**, *375*, 237–245. [CrossRef]
8. Sharma, J.N.; Al-Omran, A.; Pavathy, S.S. Role of nitric oxide in inflammatory diseases. *Inflammopharmacology* **2007**, *15*, 252–259. [CrossRef]
9. Ahn, K.S.; Aggarwal, B.B. Transcription factor NF-{kappa} B a sensor for smoke and stress signals. *Ann. J. N. Y. Acad. Sci.* **2005**, *1056*, 218–233. [CrossRef]
10. Vane, J.R.; Botting, R.M. Anti-inflammatory drugs and their mechanism of action. *Inflamm. Res.* **1998**, *47*, 78–87. [CrossRef]
11. Prescott, S.M.; Fitzpatrick, F.A. Cyclooxygenase-2 and carcinogenesis. *Biochim. Biophys. Acta Rev. Cancer* **2000**, *1470*, M69–M78. [CrossRef]
12. Tageder, I.; Pfeilschifter, J.; Geisslinger, G. Cyclooxygenase-independent actions of cyclooxygenase inhibitors. *FASEB J.* **2001**, *15*, 2057–2072. [CrossRef]
13. Ghosh, S.; May, M.J.; Kopp, E.B. NF-kappa B and Rel proteins: Evolutionarily conserved mediators of immune responses. *Annu. Rev. Immunol.* **1998**, *16*, 225–260. [CrossRef] [PubMed]
14. Thanos, D.; Maniatis, T. NF-kappa B: A lesson in family values. *Cell* **1995**, *80*, 529–532. [CrossRef]
15. Baldwin, A.S., Jr. The NF-kappa B and I kappa B proteins: New discoveries and insights. *Annu. Rev. Immunol.* **1996**, *14*, 649–681. [CrossRef]
16. Finco, T.S.; Baldwin, A.S. Mechanistic aspects of NF-kappa B regulation the emerging role of phosphorylation and proteolysis. *Immunity* **1995**, *3*, 263–272. [CrossRef]
17. Kundu, J.K.; Surh, Y.J. Breaking the relay in deregulated cellular signal transduction as a rationale for chemo prevention with anti-inflammatory phytochemicals. *Mutat. Res. Fundam. Mol. Mech. Mutagen.* **2005**, *591*, 123–146. [CrossRef]
18. Seger, R.; Krebs, E.G. The MAPK signaling cascade. *FASEB J.* **1995**, *9*, 726–735. [CrossRef]
19. Baldassare, J.J.; Bi, Y.; Bellone, C.J. The role of p38 mitogen-activated protein kinase in iL-1 beta transcription. *J. Immunol.* **1999**, *162*, 5367–5373.
20. Guo, D.L.; Chen, J.F.; Tan, L.; Jin, M.Y.; Ju, F.; Cao, Z.X.; Deng, F.; Wang, L.N.; Gu, Y.G.; Deng, Y. Terpene Glycosides from *Sanguisorba officinalis* and Their Anti-Inflammatory Effects. *Molecules* **2019**, *24*, 2906. [CrossRef]
21. OECD (Organization for Economic Cooperation and Development). Draft Proposal for a New Guideline: Fish Embryo Toxicity (FET) Test. 2006. Available online: http://www.oecd.org/chemicalsafety/testing/36817070.pdf (accessed on 3 October 2019).
22. Kwon, W.J.; Whang, W.K.; Kim, H. Constituents of *Sanguisorba hakusanensis* leaves. *Yathak Hoeji* **1996**, *40*, 262–272.
23. East, J. The effect of certain plant preparations on the fertility of laboratory mammals. *J. Endocrinol.* **1995**, *12*, 273–276. [CrossRef]
24. Hong, J.; Yang, G.; Kim, Y.B.; Eom, S.H.; Lew, J.; Kang, H. Anti-Inflammatory Activity of Cinnamon Water Extract in vivo and in vitro LPS-Induced Models. *BMC Complem. Altern. Med.* **2012**, *12*, 237. [CrossRef]
25. Bogdan, C. Nitric oxide and the immune response. *Nat. Immunol.* **2001**, *2*, 907–916. [CrossRef]
26. Jong, H.P.; Jee, A.H.; Jin, S.K.; Jeon, O.M. Pharmacognostical studies on the "O-I-Pul". *Korean J. Pharmacogn.* **1997**, *28*, 124–130.
27. Park, K.H.; Koh, D.S.; Kim, K.J.; Park, J.; Lim, Y.H. Antiallergic activity of a disaccharide isolated from Sanguisorba officinalis. *Phytother. Res.* **2004**, *18*, 658–662. [CrossRef]
28. Cho, J.Y.; Yoo, E.S.; Cha, B.C.; Park, H.J.; Rhee, M.H.; Han, Y.N. The inhibitory effect of triterpenoid glycosides originating from Sanguisorba officinalis on tissue factor activity and the production of TNF-alpha. *Planta Medica* **2006**, *72*, 1279–1284. [CrossRef]

29. Ban, J.Y.; Nguyen, H.T.; Lee, H.J.; Cho, S.O.; Ju, H.S.; Kim, J.Y.; Bae, K.; Song, K.S.; Seong, Y.H. Neuroprotective properties of gallic acid from Sanguisorbae radix on amyloid beta protein (25–35)-induced toxicity in cultured rat cortical neurons. *Biol. Pharm. Bull.* **2008**, *31*, 149–153. [CrossRef]
30. Kim, Y.H.; Chung, C.B.; Kim, J.G.; Ko, K.I.; Park, S.H.; Kim, J.H.; Eom, S.Y.; Kim, Y.S.; Hwang, Y.I.; Kim, K.H. Anti-wrinkle activity of ziyuglycoside I isolated from a Sanguisorba officinalis root extract and its application as a cosmeceutical ingredient. *Biosci. Biotechnol. Biochem.* **2008**, *72*, 303–311. [CrossRef]
31. Martin, P.; Leibovich, S.J. Inflammatory cells during wound repair: The good, the bad and the ugly. *Trends Cell Biol.* **2005**, *15*, 599–607. [CrossRef]
32. Fan, G.; Zhang, Y.; Jiang, X.; Zhu, Y.; Wang, B.; Su, L.; Cao, W.; Zhang, H.; Gao, X. Anti-Inflammatory Activity of Baicalein in LPS-Stimulated RAW264. 7 Macrophages via Estrogen Receptor and NF-κB-Dependent Pathways. *Inflammation* **2013**, *36*, 1584–1591. [CrossRef]

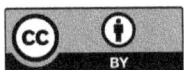

© 2019 by the authors. Licensee MDPI, Basel, Switzerland. This article is an open access article distributed under the terms and conditions of the Creative Commons Attribution (CC BY) license (http://creativecommons.org/licenses/by/4.0/).

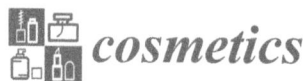

Article

Phenol Content and Antioxidant and Antiaging Activity of Safflower Seed Oil (*Carthamus Tinctorius* L.)

Kamel Zemour [1,2], Amina Labdelli [2,3], Ahmed Adda [2], Abdelkader Dellal [2], Thierry Talou [1] and Othmane Merah [1,4,*]

1. Laboratoire de Chimie Agroindustrielle, LCA, Université de Toulouse, INRA, 31030 Toulouse, France; kamel.zemour@ensiacet.fr (K.Z.); thierry.talou@ensiacet.fr (T.T.)
2. Laboratory of Agro-Biotechnology and Nutrition in Semi-Arid Areas, Ibn Khaldoun University, Tiaret 14000, Algeria; aminalabdelli@yahoo.fr (A.L.); adda2ahmed@yahoo.fr (A.A.); dellal05_aek@yahoo.fr (A.D.)
3. Scientific and Technical Research Centre for Arid Areas (CRSTRA), Biskra 07000, Algeria
4. Université Paul Sabatier, IUT A, Département Génie Biologique, 32000 Auch, France
* Correspondence: othmane.merah@ensiacet.fr; Tel.: +33-5343-23523

Received: 29 August 2019; Accepted: 12 September 2019; Published: 14 September 2019

Abstract: The phenol content of vegetable oil and its antioxidant activity are of primary interest for human health. Oilseed species are considered important sources of these compounds with medicinal effects on a large scale. Total phenol content (TPC) and antioxidant activity (AA) of safflower oil were previously studied. Nevertheless, there is no report on genotypic differences and antiaging activity of safflower oil. The aim of this study was to determine the TPC, diphenyl-picrylhydrazyl (DPPH), and antiaging activity on three respective accessions from Syria, France, and Algeria of seed oil of safflower grown under semi-arid conditions during 3 consecutive years (2015, 2016, and 2017). The results showed that phenol content as well as antioxidant and antiaging activity varied according to both genotype and years. In 2017, the mean value of TPC in oil seed was two times higher than in 2015 and 2016. Moreover, accessions presented different TPC values depending on the year. The highest antioxidant activity was observed among accessions in 2017 compared to 2015 and 2016. As expected, a positive correlation was found between TPC and antioxidant activity. The inhibition in the collagenase assay was between 47% and 72.1% compared to the positive control (83.1%), while inhibition in the elastase assay of TPC ranged from 32.2% to 70.3%, with the positive control being 75.8%. These results highlight the interest of safflower oil as a source of phenols with valuable antioxidant and antiaging activity, and uses for cosmetics.

Keywords: Safflower (*Carthamus tinctorius* L.); oil; phenol; antioxidant activity; anti-collagenase activity; anti-elastase activity; methanolic extract; genotypic variability; year effect

1. Introduction

Safflower, *Carthamus tinctorius* L., an Asteraceae, is cultivated in semi-arid regions mainly for its seed that contains a high level of oil. Safflower oil contains saturated and unsaturated fatty acids coupled by its tocopherol content [1]. Other compounds are also present in safflower oil. Among them, phenolic compounds are in the unsaponifiable phase of oil and are responsible for its stability and important nutritional value. The phenolic compounds have great biological activity mostly due to their antioxidant activity. Moreover, the primary role of antioxidants is to prevent or delay oxidative lipid damage produced in proteins and nucleic acids by reactive oxygen species, including reactive free radicals [2]. In recent years, the food industry has spent time and resources on finding natural antioxidants to replace synthetic compounds in applications and obtain a profit in the growing trend in consumer preferences for natural antioxidants. Koyama et al. [3] confirmed the effects of safflower seed extract and its phenolic constituents on atherosclerosis. Several studies have been carried out to evaluate the phenolic compounds and antioxidant activity of Asteraceae seeds including safflower [4,5], sunflower [6], and artichoke [7]. Moreover, recent research has reported that the root of *Carthamus caeruleus* L. growing wild in Mediterranean regions and especially in Algeria has a potent antioxidant activity [8]. Furthermore, collagen, a major component of skin, plays an important role in its firmness, and elastin fibres lend elasticity and ensure tissue adhesion. Many enzymes are activated when the skin is exposed to UV radiation, indirectly leading to the production of reactive oxygen species (ROS), which generate oxidative stress [9]. The degradation of collagen is caused by enzyme collagenase [10]. Another type of skin degradation is caused by proteolytic enzymes present in the dermis such as elastase. It has been suggested that the degradation of elastin by elastase rises with age and/or repeated UV radiation [11]. Recently, phenolic compounds have been found to inhibit the activity of proteinases, which induce the degradation of skin proteins, such as collagen and elastin. Total phenol content (TPC) and antioxidant activity (AA) of safflower oil were already reported. However, there has been no study on the antiaging activity of oil from safflower.

The aims of the present study were thus to evaluate the total phenol content (TPC) and diphenyl-picrylhydrazyl (DPPH) radical scavenging activity (%) of safflower seed oil (*Carthamus tinctorius* L.) cultivated under semi-arid conditions and to investigate the anti-enzymatic activity of the methanolic extract of safflower oil against callogenase and elastase activity.

2. Materials and Methods

Three accessions of *Carthamus tinctorius* L., namely Alep (Syrie), Gila (France), and Toughourt (Algeria), were used in this study. The morphological characteristics of these accessions are presented in Table 1. Field experiments were conducted at the experimental station of Ibn Khaldoun University of Tiaret (Algeria) (35°20′01″ North, 1°18′48″ East) during 3 successive years: 2015, 2016, and 2017. A complete randomized block design was used with three replicates.

Table 1. Morphological characteristics of the three studied accessions.

Accession	Country	Flower Color	Absence/Presence of Thorns	Precocity
Toughourt	Algeria	y,r	-	Late
Gila	France	w,y,r	+	Early
Alep	Syria	y,r	+	Early

y: Yellow; w: White; r: Red; (+) present; (-) absent.

Table 2 presents rainfall and temperatures during the three plant cycles. The effects of rainfall and temperature on the TPC and antioxidant and antiaging activity of safflower oil were studied across contrasted growing seasons. In 2017, the climatic conditions were characterized by low rainfall amounts and high temperatures (Table 2). Whatever the year, the flowering stage for all genotypes was in July, while maturity took place in August. During maturation, plants were subjected to higher temperatures in 2017 than in the other years (Table 2). Therefore, 2017 could be considered as the hottest year; 2016, in contrast, was the more favorable year, and 2015 was considered intermediate.

Table 2. Rainfall (mm) and temperature (°C, mean, maximum, and minimum values) during the growing season of three safflower accessions during 3 successive years.

Month	Temperature (°C)									Rainfall (mm)		
	2015			2016			2017			2015	2016	2017
	Mean	Max	Min	Mean	Max	Min	Mean	Max	Min			
April	15.3	23.5	7.1	12.8	19.9	5.6	13.0	20.1	6.0	0.0	24.6	6.8
May	19.2	28.3	10.1	16.4	24.3	8.6	19.8	29.0	10.6	12.7	26.7	26
June	21.1	29.3	12.9	21.7	30.4	12.9	25.2	34.0	16.5	7.4	6.5	0.4

Month	Temperature (°C)									Rainfall (mm)		
	2015			2016			2017			2015	2016	2017
	Mean	Max	Min	Mean	Max	Min	Mean	Max	Min			
July	27.0	36.2	17.8	26.7	35.7	17.7	26.8	35.1	18.5	0.0	0.2	1.0
August	27.0	34.6	19.3	25.6	34.7	16.4	27.7	36	19.5	12.0	0	4.8
Mean	21.9	30.4	13.4	20.6	29.0	12.2	22.5	30.4	16.3			
Total										32.1	58.0	39.0

2.1. Oil Extraction

Safflower oil was extracted with the Soxhlet apparatus (NF EN ISO 659) from seeds harvested from the matured heads (browning of leaves and bracts heads), healthy and without impurities. This method consists of oil extraction with an organic solvent (cyclohexane) on 20 g of solid matrix (seed crushed) for 6 h with a ratio of 1:10 w:v. The solvent containing oil was removed using a rotary evaporator at a temperature of 45 °C. The extracted oil was recovered in suitable vials and stored in the dark in a cold room at 4 °C until analysis.

2.2. Polyphenol Extraction

The total phenolic compounds were extracted according to the method described by Ollivier et al. [12] with few modifications. A 0.5-mL aliquot of a methanol/water solution (80/20 *v/v*) was added to 0.5 g of safflower oil in a centrifuge tube. After 10 min of vigorous mixing, the tubes were centrifuged for 15 min at 500 g, and the methanolic phase was recovered. Generally, this operation was repeated two times (three times in total) to ensure a good extraction of TPC, and the volume was brought to 1.5 mL using the methanol/water solution (80/20 *v/v*).

2.3. Total Phenol Content

The total phenol content was determined according to the method described by Merouane et al. [13], using Folin-Ciocalteu reagent and gallic acid as the standard. In brief, 500 µL of Folin-Ciocalteu reagent and 450 µL of distilled water were added to a tube containing 50 µL of extract with vigorous stirring. After 3 min, 400 µL of Na_2CO_3 (75 g·L^{-1}) were added. The tubes were incubated at 25 °C in the dark for 40 min.

The absorbance was determined at 725 nm against a blank that contained methanol instead of the extract. The phenol content of the extract was determined from the gallic acid calibration curve, and the results were expressed in mg of gallic acid equivalent per kg of safflower oil (mg GAE/kg of oil).

2.4. Antioxidant Activity Determination

The antioxidant activity was determined according to the method recommended by Nogala-Kalucka et al. [14]. The method involves the spectrophotometric measurement of the intensity of the color change in solution depending on the amount of DPPH. The reaction was initiated by mixing 1 mL of the methanolic extract with 3 mL methanol, and then adding 1 mL of DPPH (0.012 g/100 mL). Absorbance at a λmax of 517 nm was checked after 15 min. The activity of the extract in scavenging DPPH was calculated as follows:

% DPPH scavenging = [(Absorbance of control − Absorbance of sample)/Absorbance of control] * 100

2.5. Determination of Collagenase and Elastase Inhibition

Collagenase from *Clostridium histolyticum* (Sigma Aldrich, Lyon, France) was used. The activity of collagenase was assessed using N-[3-(2-furyl) acryloyl]-Leu-Gly-Pro-Ala (Sigma Aldrich, Lyon, France) as a substrate following the protocol of Wittenauer et al. [15]. Absorbance decrease was surveyed at 335 nm during 20 min using a microplate reader (BioTek ELX800; BioTek Instruments, Colmar, France). The activity of collagenase in the presence of each genotype for each year was determined in triplicate, and the anti-collagenase activity was expressed as the inhibition percentage relative to the corresponding control (phenol extraction by adding the same volume).

The elastase assay was carried out using porcine pancreatic elastase (Sigma Aldrich, Lyon, France). The elastase activity was evaluated using N-Succ-Ala-Ala-Ala-p-nitroanilide (AAAVPN; Sigma Aldrich) as a substrate [15]. The release of p-nitroaniline was done at 410 nm using a microplate reader (BioTek ELX800; BioTek Instruments). Measurements were performed in triplicate, and the anti-elastase activity was expressed, for each genotype and year, as the inhibition percentage relative to the corresponding control (phenol extraction by adding the same volume of the same solvent).

2.6. Statistical Analyses

Results are presented as the mean ± standard deviation of three replicates for each parameter. A p-value of 0.05 was used to denote significant differences between mean values determined by the analysis of variance (ANOVA) using Statistica 8.0. Two-way ANOVAs were used in order to determine the effect of accession, year, and their interaction. A correlation analysis between antioxidant activity and TPC was also performed.

3. Results

The total phenol content of safflower oil and its antioxidant activity were strongly influenced by the used genotypes and growing conditions (Table 3). Same results were highlighted for both anti-collagenase activity and anti-elastase activity parameters. Significant interaction of year and genotype effects was observed on all measured parameters (Table 3).

Table 3. Effects of accession, year and their interaction on total phenol content, antioxidant and antiaging activity measured in three accessions of safflower grown during three years in Tiaret (semi-arid conditions), Algeria.

Source of Variation	df	Phenol Content	Antioxidant Activity	Anti-Collagenase Activity	Anti-Elastase Activity
Accession	2	7.63 **	53.48 ***	33.84 ***	86.21 ***
Year	2	407.69 ***	744.44 ***	79.6 ***	102.3 ***
Accession Year	4	43.25 ***	281.72 ***	124.2 ***	187.9 ***

** significant at $p < 0.01$; *** significant at $p < 0.001$.

3.1. Total Phenol Content

The highest phenol content was found for 2017 compared with 2015 and 2016. In 2017, the highest content was recorded for the Syrian genotype, while the French accession had the lowest content (Table 4). However, different results were recorded in 2015 and 2016, with the French genotype showing the highest phenol content. Furthermore, the Algerian accession showed intermediate values among the studied genotypes in all years (Table 4).

Table 4. Total polyphenol content and antioxidant activity of the three safflower accessions in 2015, 2016, and 2017.

Year	Accession	Total Phenol Content (mgEAG/kg of oil)	Antioxidant Activity (%)
2015	Syria	140.9 ± 7.0a	20.6 ± 0.6a
	France	199.5 ± 2.9c	33.1 ± 1.0c
	Algeria	168.1 ± 7.1b	24.7 ± 0.7b
	Mean	169.5 ± 16.9	26.15 ± 3.7
2016	Syria	186 ± 4.0a	27.6 ± 0.6a
	France	210.9 ± 0.4b	38.8 ± 0.0c
	Algeria	192.6 ± 4.3a	33 ± 0.8b
	Mean	196.5 ± 7.4	33.13 ± 3.2

Table 4. Cont.

Year	Accession	Total Phenol Content (mgEAG/kg of oil)	Antioxidant Activity (%)
2017	Syria	412.8 ± 1.3b	68.9 ± 0.4b
	France	289.2 ± 8.1a	38.9 ± 1.3a
	Algeria	305.8 ± 17.9a	40.5 ± 0.7a
	Mean	**335.9 ± 38.7**	**49.4 ± 9.7**

In the same column, for each year, means with the same letter were not significantly different at $p < 0.05$.

3.2. Antioxidant Activity

The methanolic extract from safflower oil revealed an antioxidant activity of 20% for all the used genotypes (Table 4). In addition, a similar profile to that of TPC was observed when evaluating antioxidant activity. This activity (%) showed higher values in 2017 compared to 2015 and 2016. In 2017, the highest antioxidant activity was reported for the Syrian accession. In contrary, in 2015 and 2016, this genotype exhibited the lowest antioxidant activity compared to the other genotypes (Table 4). Expectedly, a positive correlation was observed between the total phenol content of safflower oil and its antioxidant activity (Figure 1).

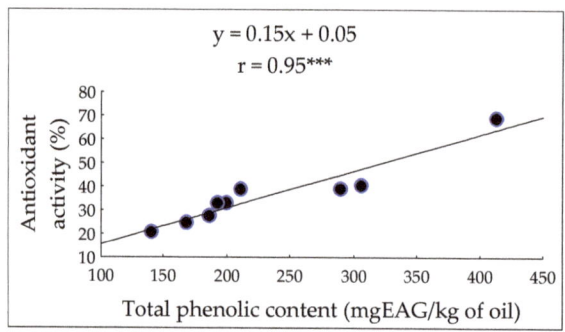

Figure 1. Correlation between total phenol content and antioxidant activity of the three safflower accessions in 2015, 2016, and 2017.

3.3. Antiaging Activity

Antiaging activity was assessed in safflower oil. The results indicated that this oil inhibited collagenase and elastase activity. Moreover, a wide diversity of antiaging activity was observed for all the used genotypes (Table 5).

Separately, a high anti-collagenase activity was found in 2016 and 2015, including a higher value recorded for the Syrian accession. Conversely, in 2017, the French accession shower higher activity compared to the other accessions (Table 5). For the second anti-enzymatic activity, as shown in Table 5, the highest anti-elastase activity was revealed in 2015 and 2017, which was approximately the same as the control. However, in 2016, the inhibition of anti-elastase activity decreased until it reached a minimum value; the lowest value was shown by the Algerian accession, which was half of the control value at 1000 µg/mL (Table 5).

Table 5. Anti-collagenase and anti-elastase activity of the three safflower accessions in 2015, 2016, and 2017.

Year	Accession	Anti-Collagenase Activity		Anti-Elastase Activity	
		IC$_{50}$ (µg/mL)	Inhibition % at 500 µg/mL	IC$_{50}$ (µg/mL)	Inhibition % at 1000 µg/mL
Control	Control	38.7 ± 0.2b	83.1 ± 0.2a	32.3 ± 0.2c	75.8 ± 0.1a
2015	Syria	135.9 ± 0.3a	65.2 ± 0.1b	202.8 ± 0.4a	66.7 ± 0.4b
	France	132.7 ± 0.2a	59.1 ± 0.2c	180.7 ± 0.1b	59.8 ± 0.3c
	Algeria	133.8 ± 0.4a	63.2 ± 0.3b	198.4 ± 0.2a	64.2 ± 0.5b
	Mean	**134.1 ± 0.9**	**62.5 ± 1.8**	**194 ± 6.7**	**63.6 ± 2.0**
2016	Syria	130.1 ± 0.2a	72.1 ± 0.6b	178.6 ± 0.9a	42.4 ± 0.4b
	France	124.6 ± 0.2b	61.6 ± 0.3c	163.7 ± 0.8c	49.1 ± 0.01b
	Algeria	123.4 ± 0.2b	64.9 ± 0.4c	171.4 ± 0.9b	32.2 ± 0.2b
	Mean	**126.03 ± 2.1**	**66.2 ± 3.1**	**171.2 ± 4.3**	**41.2 ± 4.9**
2017	Syria	144.5 ± 0.2a	47.0 ± 0.4b	298.1 ± 1.2a	70.3 ± 0.6ab
	France	134.7 ± 0.2b	52.8 ± 0.3b	254.3 ± 0.9a	63.2 ± 0.4b
	Algeria	136.1 ± 0.2b	49.9 ± 0.8b	274.6 ± 1.1a	67.2 ± 0.8b
	Mean	**138.4 ± 3.1**	**49.9 ± 1.7**	**275.7 ± 12.6**	**66.9 ± 2.0**

In same column, for each year, means with the same letter are not significantly different at $p < 0.05$.

4. Discussion

Polyphenolic compounds are the most important groups of secondary metabolites in medicinal herbs and dietary plants. The results of phenol content observed in safflower oil ranged from 140.9–412.8 mg GAE/kg of oil (Table 4). The high amount of TPC confirmed that safflower oil presents an important source of these components. Similar results were observed in previous studies [4,16–19]. The results showed a high antioxidant activity for all accessions, which ranged from 20.6% to 68.9% (Table 4). This activity has been described by several works [5,19,20]. Shirvani et al. [21] reported that this activity had a rate of 50% at the beginning of safflower seed germination. Kim et al. [21] mentioned that the antioxidant activity of safflower seeds is lower than that of other botanical sections of the safflower plant. In detail, they reported 114.2%, 113.6%, 94.4%, and 86.1% of DPPH radical scavenging activity in petals, leaves, buds, and shoots, respectively.

Interestingly, great importance has been given to anti-inflammatory activity in pharmaceutical and cosmetic uses. Nevertheless, no study has been carried out to date to evaluate the effects of climatic conditions on the antiaging activity of safflower oil. Likewise, and for the first time, the anti-elastase and anti-collagenase properties of the phenol content of safflower oil were assessed in this study to identify a new source of antiaging agent. During the three years, the results suggest that safflower oil has important anti-collagenase activity with 72.1% inhibition at 500 µg/mL, a value corresponding to IC$_{50}$ = 130.1 µg/mL for the Syrian accession. This genotype showed an anti-elastase activity of 70.3% inhibition at 1000 µg/mL, a value corresponding to IC$_{50}$ = 298.1 µg/mL (Table 5). Using essential oils extracted from some medicinal herbs and food plants, Aumeeruddy-Elalfi et al. [22] demonstrated a minimal anti-collagenase activity and anti-elastase activity of 52.2% inhibition at 400 µg/mL and 32.23% inhibition at 800 mg/mL, respectively. A methanolic extract of water-pepper sprout inhibited collagenase activity in a concentration-dependent manner with an IC$_{50}$ value of 156.7 µg/mL [23].

Genotypic variability showed different responses to changes in weather conditions during the three years. Thus, these climatic variations, which were mainly due to variations in temperature and precipitation (Table 2), had significant effects on the studied parameters. Roche et al. [24] reported the effect of climatic conditions on the chemical composition of safflower seeds. In 2017, high temperatures and low rainfall were recorded during the growing season of safflower (Table 2). In the same year, the highest values of TPC (412.8 mg EAG/kg of oil) were reported for the Syrian accession (Table 4). In contrast, a decrease in temperature in 2015 and 2016 (Table 2) induced a decrease in the phenol content and antioxidant activity for all the accessions. Therefore, it appears that these contents are influenced primarily by the increase in mean temperatures. Indeed, heat stress affected the accumulation of phenolic compounds in durum wheat seeds [25]. Another study confirmed that TPC increased significantly with the rise of temperature in sesame [26]. Unexpectedly, the total phenol content in 2016 was higher than 2015 (Table 4). This could be explained by the increase in rainfall, which led to an increase in the phenol content of safflower oil. These results are in accordance with those reported by Palese et al. [27] and in contradiction with those reported by Gucci et al. [28] regarding olive oil.

The influence of the growing conditions during the safflower plant cycle on its antioxidant activity was also investigated. A high antioxidant activity (Table 4) was found for all accessions with the rise of temperatures, confirming results already reported [26]. Taha and Matthäus [16] showed a significant increase in the antioxidant activity of safflower seeds caused by the roasting process. Britz and Kremer [29] reported that heat and drought influenced the tocopherol content in soybean during seed maturation. The content and quality of oil from plant material depends on the nature of the used solvents during its extraction. In our study, cyclohexane, an apolar solvent like hexane, may influence the oil content of safflower [30] and the extracted phenolic of the solid material [31,32]. Terpinc et al. [33] showed the effect of solvent type on the variation of total phenol content and antioxidant activity of different oil cake extracts. A higher percentage of unsaponifiable matter was demonstrated in safflower oil extracted by cyclohexane [34]. The use of a mixture of water and other organic solvents such as methanol in our study remains essential to ensure a perfect extraction of phenolic compounds from safflower seed oil.

The phenylpropanoid biosynthetic pathway is responsible for the synthesis of phenolic compounds [35]. However, biosynthesis stimulation of these compounds is mainly due to the regulation of many genes encoding the main enzymes of the phenylpropanoid pathway according to environmental conditions [36], such as drought stress [37] and high temperature [38,39]. The effect of genotype on phenolic compounds has been previously shown [40]. Moreover, as already seen in safflower and soybean [20,41], we found a positive correlation between TPC and antioxidant activity.

Furthermore, anti-elastase activity increased significantly with the increasing mean temperature recorded in 2017 (Table 5). In contrast, the anti-collagenase activity decreased with increasing temperature. However, the anti-collagenase activity remained higher than 47% inhibition at 500 µg/mL regardless of the temperature.

A great interest in the phenol content and antioxidant activity of the diet was reported among consumers and the scientific community. Phenols, antioxidant activity, and their impact on human health, even if not assessed in our study, have been reported broadly [42–49].

Today, many plants with high antioxidant activity are of interest for pharmaceutical and cosmetic applications. Indeed, a large range of oilseed has been used as skin products and hair cosmetics for a long time in several cultures, including sunflower and olive oil. The application of sunflower seed oil has been shown to preserve the stratum corneum integrity and improve hydration of the adult skin without inducing erythema [50]. Budiyanto et al. [51] reported that olive oil topically applied after UVB exposure can effectively reduce UVB-induced murine skin tumors, possibly via its antioxidant effects in reducing DNA damage by reactive oxygen species, and that the effective component may be labile to UVB. This antioxidant activity presents high potential as a UVB sunscreen agent [10,52]. Argan oil can improve skin elasticity [53] and skin hydration by restoring the barrier function and maintaining the water-holding capacity [54]. Moreover, a natural skin toning cream has been developed from safflower oil [55]. The oil body bound oleosin-rhFGF9 expressed in safflower seed stimulates hair growth and wound healing in mice [56]. Dakhil et al. [57] have reported that safflower oil characteristics can make it a main ingredient in the preparation of topical agents for the treatment of various skin problems. Abdul Karim et al. [52] recommended the possible use of cocoa pod extract as an ingredient in functional cosmetic products, specifically for anti-wrinkles as well as skin whitening or sunscreen products in combination with natural plant extracts to widen the spectrum of protection from sun rays. Furthermore, many studies showed that skin aging and skin wrinkling may be reduced by the action of the antioxidant activity of various botanical extracts [58,59]. Aumeeruddy-Elalfi et al. [22] showed that the inhibitory potential of essential oils extracted from some medicinal plants make them potential candidates for the cosmetic (skin aging) and pharmaceutical industries.

In this study, the excellent anti-collagenase and anti-elastase activity of the phenolic compounds of safflower oil highlight its potential as a natural source of antiaging agents for cosmetic formulations. Besides the phenol content of safflower oil reported in our study, other research has confirmed that safflower oil contains also high proportions of polyunsaturated fatty acids and sterols [24]; the characteristics of all of these compounds could grant safflower oil high importance for pharmaceutical and industrial use.

5. Conclusions

Synthetic antioxidants are often associated with problems of carcinogenticity and toxicity; there is an increasing interest in oilseed as sources of natural antioxidants for cosmetic and pharmaceutical uses. This study focused on the quantitative profiling of methanol extractable (TPC) obtained from safflower seed oil grown in a semi-arid climate, and its antioxidant and antiaging activity. We revealed that safflower seed oil could be an important source of polyphenols with resulting antioxidant and antiaging activity. Genotype, year (climatic conditions), and their interaction significantly affected these properties. This was confirmed by the improvement in total phenol content and DPPH assay, and maintenance of appreciable antiaging activity of safflower oil with increasing temperature and drought. Recently, several studies reported that these compounds have an important role in human health. High levels of phenols as well as antioxidant and antiaging activity were reported for safflower oil seed. Their content and activity depend on both genotype and climatic conditions. Therefore, this highlights the potential interest of this source of valuable compounds for pharmaceutical and cosmetic applications. Moreover, these traits could be managed by modulations according to genotype and climatic conditions.

Author Contributions: Conceptualization, O.M., A.A.; methodology, K.Z., T.T., and A.L.; formal analysis, K.Z., A.L., and O.M., writing—original draft preparation, K.Z., A.L., A.A., A.D., T.T., and O.M.; writing—review and editing, O.M. and A.A.; supervision, O.M.; project administration, O.M., A.D., and A.A.

Funding: This research was supported financially by the Hubert Curien-Tassilli program 16MDU953.

Acknowledgments: This Ph.D. was supported by the Hubert Curien-Tassili program 16MDU953.

Conflicts of Interest: The authors declare no conflict of interest. The funders had no role in the design of the study; in the collection, analyses, or interpretation of data; in the writing of the manuscript; or in the decision to publish the results.

References

1. Mokhtari, N.; Rahimmalek, M.; Talebi, M.; Khorrami, M. Assessment of genetic diversity among and within carthamus species using sequence-related amplified polymorphism (SRAP) markers. *Plant Syst. Evol.* **2013**, *299*, 1285–1294. [CrossRef]
2. Isabelle, M.; Lee, B.L.; Lim, M.T.; Koh, W.P.; Huang, D.; Ong, C.N. Antioxidant activity and profiles of common fruits in Singapore. *Food Chem.* **2010**, *123*, 77–84. [CrossRef]
3. Koyama, N.; Kuribayashi, K.; Seki, T.; Kobayashi, K.; Furuhata, Y.; Suzuki, K.; Arisaka, H.; Nakano, T.; Amino, Y.; Ishii, K. Serotonin derivatives, major safflower (*Carthamus tinctorius* L.) seed antioxidants, inhibit low-density lipoprotein (LDL) oxidation and atherosclerosis in apolipoprotein E-deficient mice. *J. Agric. Food Chem.* **2006**, *54*, 4970–4976. [CrossRef] [PubMed]
4. Ergönül, P.G.; Özbek, Z.A. Identification of bioactive compounds and total phenol contents of cold pressed oils from safflower and camelina seeds. *J. Food Meas. Charac.* **2018**, *12*, 2313–2323. [CrossRef]
5. Xuan, T.D.; Gangqiang, G.; Minh, T.N.; Quy, T.N.; Khanh, T.D. An Overview of chemical profiles, antioxidant and antimicrobial activities of commercial vegetable edible oils marketed in Japan. *Foods* **2018**, *7*, 21. [CrossRef] [PubMed]

6. Karamać, M.; Kosińska, A.; Estrella, I.; Hernández, T.; Dueñas, M. Antioxidant activity of phenolic compounds identified in sunflower seeds. *Eur. Food Res. Technol.* **2012**, *235*, 221–230. [CrossRef]
7. Soumaya, K.; Chaouachi, F.; Ksouri, R.; El Gazzah, M. Polyphenolic composition in different organs of Tunisia populations of *Cynara Cardunculus* L. and their antioxidant activity. *J. Food Nutr. Res.* **2013**, *1*, 1–6. [CrossRef]
8. Baghiani, A.; Boumerfeg, S.; Belkhiri, F.; Khennouf, S.; Charef, N.; Daoud Harzallah, D.; Arrar, L.; Abdel-Wahhab, M.A. Antioxidant and radical scavenging properties of *Carthamus caeruleus* L. extracts grow wild in Algeria flora. *Commun. Sci.* **2010**, *1*, 128–136. [CrossRef]
9. Silva, S.A.M.; Michniak-Kohn, B.; Leonardi, G.R. An overview about oxidation in clinical practice of skin aging. *Anais Brasileiros de Dermatologia* **2017**, *92*, 367–374. [CrossRef]
10. Mukherjee, P.K.; Maity, N.; Nema, N.K.; Sarkar, B.K. Bioactive compounds from natural resources against skin aging. *Phytomedicine* **2011**, *19*, 64–73. [CrossRef]
11. Kacem, R. Phenolic compounds from medicinal plants as natural anti-elastase products for the therapy of pulmonary emphysema. *J. Med. Plant Res.* **2013**, *7*, 3499–3507. [CrossRef]
12. Ollivier, D.; Boubault, E.; Pinatel, C.; Souillol, S.; Guérère, M.; Artaud, J. Analyse de la fraction phénoliques des huiles d'olive vierges. *Ann. Falsif. Exp. Chim. Toxicol.* **2004**, *965*, 169–196.
13. Merouane, A.; Noui, A.; Medjahed, H.; Nedjari Benhadj Ali, K.; Saadi, A. Activité antioxydante des composés phénoliques d'huile d'olive extraite par méthode traditionnelle. *Int. J. Biol. Chem. Sci.* **2014**, *8*, 1865–1870. [CrossRef]
14. Nogala-Kalucka, M.; Rudzinska, M.; Zadernowski, R.; Siger, A.; Krzyzostaniak, I. Phytochemical content and antioxidant properties of seeds of unconventional oil plants. *J. Am. Oil Chem. Soc.* **2010**, *87*, 1481–1487. [CrossRef]
15. Wittenauer, J.; Mäckle, S.; Sußmann, D.; Schweiggert-Weisz, U.; Carle, R. Inhibitory effects of polyphenols from grape pomace extract on collagenase and elastase activity. *Fitoterapia* **2015**, *101*, 179–187. [CrossRef] [PubMed]
16. Taha, E.; Matthäus, B. Effect of roasting temperature on safflower seeds and oil. *J. Food Dairy Sci.* **2018**, *9*, 103–109. [CrossRef]
17. Ben Moumen, A.; Mansouri, F.; Richard, G.; Abid, M.; Fauconnier, M.L.; Sindic, M.; El Amrani, A.; Caid, H.S. Biochemical characterisation of the seed oils of four safflower (*Carthamus tinctorius*) varieties grown in north-eastern of Morocco. *Int. J. Food Sci. Technol.* **2014**, *50*, 804–810. [CrossRef]
18. Yu, S.Y.; Lee, Y.J.; Kim, J.D.; Kang, S.N.; Lee, S.K.; Jang, J.Y.; Lee, H.K.; Lim, J.H.; Lee, O.H. Phenolic composition, antioxidant activity and anti-adipogenic effect of hot water extract from safflower (*Carthamus tinctorius* L.) seed. *Nutrients* **2013**, *5*, 4894–4907. [CrossRef]
19. Sung, J.; Jeong, Y.; Kim, S.; Luitel, B.P.; Ko, H.; Hur, O.; Yoon, M.; Rhee, J.; Baek, H.; Ryu, K. Fatty acid composition and antioxidant activity in safflower germplasm collected from south Asia and Africa. *J. Korean Soc. Int. Agric.* **2016**, *28*, 342–351. [CrossRef]
20. Kim, J.H.; Kim, J.K.; Kang, W.W.; Ha, Y.S.; Choi, S.W.; Moon, K.D. Chemical compositions and DPPH radical scavenger activity in different sections of safflower. *J. Korean Soc. Food Sci. Nutr.* **2003**, *32*, 733–738. [CrossRef]
21. Shirvani, A.; Jafari, M.; Goli, S.A.H.; Soltani Tehrani, N.; Rahimmalek, M. The changes in proximate composition, antioxidant activity and fatty acid profile of germinating safflower (*Carthamus tinctorius*) seed. *J. Agric. Sci. Technol.* **2016**, *18*, 1967–1974.
22. Aumeeruddy-Elalfi, Z.; Lall, N.; Fibrich, B.; Blom Van Staden, A.; Hosenally, M.; Mahomoodally, M.F. Selected essential oils inhibit key physiological enzymes and possess intracellular and extracellular antimelanogenic properties in vitro. *J. Food Drug Anal.* **2018**, *26*, 232–243. [CrossRef] [PubMed]
23. Kawaguchi, T.; Nagata, K. Collagenase inhibition by water-pepper (*Polygonum hydropiper* L.) sprout extract. *J. Herbmed. Pharmacol.* **2019**, *8*, 114–119. [CrossRef]
24. Roche, J.; Mouloungui, Z.; Cerny, M.; Merah, O. Effect of sowing dates on fatty acids and phytosterols patterns of *Carthamus tinctorius* L. *Appl. Sci.* **2019**, *9*, 2839. [CrossRef]
25. De Leonardis, A.M.; Fragasso, M.; Beleggia, R.; Ficco, D.B.M.; De Vita, P.; Mastrangelo, A.M. Effects of heat stress on metabolite accumulation and composition, and nutritional properties of Durum Wheat grain. *Int. J. Mol. Sci.* **2015**, *16*, 30382–30404. [CrossRef] [PubMed]
26. Jannat, B.; Oveisi, M.R.; Sadeghi, N.; Hajimahmoodi, M.; Behzad, M.; Choopankari, E.; Behfar, A.A. Effects of roasting temperature and time on healthy nutraceuticals of antioxidants and total phenolic content in iranian sesame seeds (*Sesamum indicum* L.). *J. Environ. Health Sci. Eng.* **2010**, *7*, 97–102.

27. Palese, A.M.; Nuzzo, V.; Favati, F.; Pietrafesa, A.; Celano, G.; Xiloyannis, C. Effects of water deficit on the vegetative response, yield and oil quality of olive trees (*Olea europaea* L., cv Coratina) grown under intensive cultivation. *Sci. Hort.* **2010**, *125*, 222–229. [CrossRef]
28. Gucci, R.; Caruso, G.; Gennai, C.; Esposto, S.; Urbani, S.; Servili, M. Fruit growth, yield and oil quality changes induced by deficit irrigation at different stages of olive fruit development. *Agric. Water Manag.* **2019**, *212*, 88–98. [CrossRef]
29. Britz, S.J.; Kremer, D.F. Warm temperatures or drought during seed maturation increase free α-tocopherol in seeds of soybean (*Glycine max* [L.] Merr.). *J. Agric. Food Chem.* **2002**, *50*, 6058–6063. [CrossRef]
30. Takadas, F.; Doker, O. Extraction method and solvent effect on safflower seed oil production. *Chem. Proces. Eng. Res.* **2017**, *51*, 9–17.
31. Dobravalskytė, D.; Venskutonis, P.R.; Talou, T.; Zebib, B.; Merah, O.; Ragazinskienė, O. Antioxidant properties of deodorized extracts of *Tussilago farfara* L. *Rec. Nat. Prod.* **2013**, *7*, 201–209.
32. Salem, N.; Msaada, K.; Hamdaoui, G.; Limam, F.; Marzouk, B. Variation in phenolic composition and antioxidant activity during flower development of safflower (*Carthamus tinctorius* L.). *J. Agric. Food Chem.* **2011**, *59*, 4455–4463. [CrossRef] [PubMed]
33. Terpinc, P.; Čeh, B.; Ulrih, N.P.; Abramovič, H. Studies of the correlation between antioxidant properties and the total phenolic content of different oil cake extracts. *Ind. Crops Prod.* **2012**, *39*, 210–217. [CrossRef]
34. Dasari, S.R.; Goud, V.V. Comparative extraction of castor seed oil using polar and non polar solvents. *Int. J. Curr. Eng. Technol.* **2013**, *3*, 121–123.
35. Kallscheuer, N.; Vogt, M.; Marienhagen, J. A novel synthetic pathway enables microbial production of polyphenols independent from the endogenous aromatic amino acid metabolism. *ACS Synth. Biol.* **2017**, *6*, 410–415. [CrossRef] [PubMed]
36. Oh, M.-M.; Trick, H.N.; Rajashekar, C.B. Secondary metabolism and antioxidants are involved in environmental adaptation and stress tolerance in lettuce. *J. Plant Physiol.* **2009**, *166*, 180–191. [CrossRef] [PubMed]
37. Gharibi, S.; Sayed Tabatabaei, B.E.; Saeidi, G.; Talebi, M.; Matkowski, A. The effect of drought stress on polyphenolic compounds and expression of flavonoid biosynthesis related genes in *Achillea pachycephala* Rech.f. *Phytochemistry* **2019**, *162*, 90–98. [CrossRef] [PubMed]
38. Wang, J.; Yuan, B.; Huang, B. Differential heat-induced changes in phenolic acids associated with genotypic variations in heat tolerance for hard fescue. *Crop Sci.* **2019**, *59*, 667–674. [CrossRef]
39. Commisso, M.; Toffali, K.; Strazzer, P.; Stocchero, M.; Ceoldo, S.; Baldan, B.; Levi, M.; Guzzo, F. Impact of phenylpropanoid compounds on heat stress tolerance in carrot cell cultures. *Front. Plant Sci.* **2016**, *7*, 1439. [CrossRef] [PubMed]
40. Gündüz, K.; Özdemir, E. The effects of genotype and growing conditions on antioxidant capacity, phenolic compounds, organic acid and individual sugars of strawberry. *Food Chem.* **2014**, *155*, 298–303. [CrossRef]
41. Zielińska-Dawidziak, M.; Siger, A. Effect of elevated accumulation of iron in ferritin on the antioxidants content in soybean sprouts. *Eur. Food Res. Technol.* **2012**, *234*, 1005–1012. [CrossRef]
42. Reboredo-Rodríguez, P.; Varela-López, A.; Forbes-Hernández, T.Y.; Gasparrini, M.; Afrin, S.; Cianciosi, D.; Zhang, J.; Manna, P.P.; Bompadre, S.; Quiles, J.L.; et al. Phenolic compounds isolated from olive oil as nutraceutical tools for the prevention and management of cancer and cardiovascular diseases. *Int. J. Mol. Sci.* **2018**, *19*, 2305. [CrossRef] [PubMed]
43. Singh, T.; Katiyar, S.K. Green tea polyphenol, (−)-epigallocatechin-3-gallate, induces toxicity in human skin cancer cells by targeting β-catenin signaling. *Toxicol. Appl. Pharmacol.* **2013**, *273*, 418–424. [CrossRef] [PubMed]
44. Kim, H.J.; Bae, Y.C.; Park, R.W.; Choi, S.W.; Cho, S.H.; Choi, Y.S.; Lee, W.J. Bone-protecting effect of safflower seeds in ovariectomized rats. *Calcif. Tissue Int.* **2002**, *71*, 88–94. [CrossRef] [PubMed]
45. Cho, S.H.; Lee, H.R.; Kim, T.H.; Choi, S.W.; Lee, W.J.; Choi, Y. Effects of defatted safflower seed extract and phenolic compounds in diet on plasma and liver lipid in ovariectomized rats fed high-cholesterol diets. *J. Nutr. Sci. Vitaminol.* **2004**, *50*, 32–37. [CrossRef] [PubMed]
46. Singhal, G.; Singh, P.; Bhagyawant, S.S.; Srivastava, N. Anti-nutritional factors in safflower (*Carthamus tinctorius* L.) seeds and their pharmaceutical applications. *Int. J. Rec. Sci. Res.* **2018**, *9*, 28859–28864. [CrossRef]

47. Kim, D.H.; Lee, J.H.; Ahn, E.M.; Lee, Y.H.; Baek, N.I.; Kim, I.H. Phenolic glycosides isolated from safflower (*Carthamus tinctorius* L.) seeds increase the alkaline phosphatase (ALP) activity of humain Osteoblast-like cells. *Food Sci. Biotechnol.* **2006**, *15*, 781–785.
48. Park, G.H.; Hong, S.C.; Jeong, J.B. Anticancer activity of the safflower seeds (*Carthamus tinctorius* L.) through inducing cyclin D1 proteasomal degradation in human colorectal cancer cells. *Korean J. Plant Res.* **2016**, *29*, 297–304. [CrossRef]
49. Kim, E.O.; Oh, J.H.; Lee, S.K.; Lee, J.Y.; Choi, S.W. Antioxidant properties and quantification of phenolic compounds from safflower (*Carthamus tinctorius* L.) seeds. *Food Sci. Biotechnol.* **2007**, *16*, 71–77.
50. Danby, S.G.; AlEnezi, T.; Sultan, A.; Lavender, T.; Chittock, J.; Brown, K.; Cork, M.J. Effect of olive and sunflower seed oil on the adult skin barrier: Implications for neonatal skin care. *Pediatr. Dermatol.* **2013**, *30*, 42–50. [CrossRef]
51. Budiyanto, A.; Ahmed, N.U.; Wu, A.; Bito, T.; Nikaido, O.; Osawa, T.; Ueda, M.; Ichihashi, M. Protective effect of topically applied olive oil against photocarcinogensis following UVB exposure of mice. *Carcinogenesis* **2000**, *21*, 2085–2090. [CrossRef] [PubMed]
52. Abdul Karim, A.; Azlan, A.; Ismail, A.; Hashim, P.; Abd Gani, S.S.; Zainudin, B.H.; Abdullah, N.A. Phenolic composition, antioxidant, anti-wrinkles and tyrosinase inhibitory activities of cocoa pod extract. *BMC Complement. Altern. Med.* **2014**, *14*, 381–393. [CrossRef] [PubMed]
53. Qiraouani Boucetta, K.; Charrouf, Z.; Aguenaou, H.; Derouiche, A.; Bensouda, Y. The effect of dietary and/or cosmetic argan oil on postmenopausal skin elasticity. *Clin. Interv. Aging* **2015**, *10*, 339–349. [CrossRef] [PubMed]
54. Qiraouani Boucetta, K.; Charrouf, Z.; Derouiche, A.; Rahali, Y.; Bensouda, Y. Skin hydration in postmenopausal women: Argan oil benefit with oral and/or topical use. *Przeglad Menopauzalny* **2014**, *13*, 280–288. [CrossRef] [PubMed]
55. Zhaomu, W.; Lijie, D. Current situation and prospects of safflower products development in China. In Proceedings of the 5th International Safflower Conference, Williston, VT, USA, 23–27 July 2001.
56. Cai, J.; Wen, R.; Li, W.; Wang, X.; Tian, H.; Yi, S.; Zhang, L.; Li, X.; Jiang, C.; Li, H. Oil body bound oleosin-rhFGF9 fusion protein expressed in safflower (*Carthamus tinctorius* L.) stimulates hair growth and wound healing in mice. *BMC Biotechnol.* **2018**, *18*, 51–61. [CrossRef] [PubMed]
57. Dakhil, I.A.; Abbas, I.S.; Marie, N.K. Preparation, evaluation, and clinical application of safflower cream as topical nutritive agent. *Asian J. Pharm. Clin. Res.* **2018**, *11*, 495–497. [CrossRef]
58. Garg, C.; Khurana, P.; Garg, M. Molecular mechanisms of skin photoaging and plant inhibitors. *Inter. J. Green Pharm.* **2017**, *11*, 217–232. [CrossRef]
59. Zhang, S.; Duan, E. Fighting against skin aging: The way from bench to bedside. *Cell Transplan.* **2018**, *27*, 729–738. [CrossRef] [PubMed]

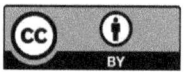

© 2019 by the authors. Licensee MDPI, Basel, Switzerland. This article is an open access article distributed under the terms and conditions of the Creative Commons Attribution (CC BY) license (http://creativecommons.org/licenses/by/4.0/).

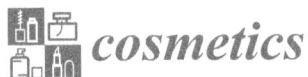

Article

Efficiency of Skin Whitening Cream Containing *Etlingera elatior* Flower and Leaf Extracts in Volunteers

Nattawut Whangsomnuek [1], Lapatrada Mungmai [2], Kriangsak Mengamphan [3,4] and Doungporn Amornlerdpison [3,4,*]

1. Interdisciplinary Agriculture Program, Maejo University, Chiang Mai 50290, Thailand
2. Cosmetic Science, School of Pharmaceutical Sciences, University of Phayao, Phayao 56000, Thailand
3. Center of Excellence in Agricultural Innovation for Graduate Entrepreneur, Maejo University, Chiang Mai 50290, Thailand
4. Faculty of Fisheries Technology and Aquatic Resources, Maejo University, Chiang Mai 50290, Thailand
* Correspondence: doungpornfishtech@gmail.com; Tel.: +66-86-654-6966

Received: 4 June 2019; Accepted: 3 July 2019; Published: 6 July 2019

Abstract: Our previous research demonstrated that *Etlingera elatior* possesses whitening and anti-aging properties and also contains bioactive ingredients for cosmeceuticals. Therefore, this research work aimed to evaluate the efficiency of whitening cream containing both the flower and leaf extracts of *E. elatior* in human volunteers and their degree of skin irritation. Both the flower and leaf extracts were formulated as a cosmetic called "FL1 cream", which was assessed for its physical properties and underwent an accelerated stability test. The FL1 cream was also evaluated for skin irritation and its skin whitening effect among 24 healthy volunteers who used it for four weeks. The FL1 cream demonstrated good physical stability under the various conditions for three months, along with six cycles of heating/cooling. The irritation analysis showed that irritation reactions were absent in all volunteers. The efficiency of FL1 cream in improving the appearance of skin whitening was demonstrated by a significant ($p < 0.05$) and continuous decrease in melanin content compared with the initial value. Additionally, the L^* value was significantly and continuously increased after application of the FL1 cream. The highest melanin reduction was 6.67%. The FL1 cream containing *E. elatior* extracts can be used as a whitening cream in cosmetics.

Keywords: clinical evaluation; *Etlingera elatior*; skin irritation; whitening cream

1. Introduction

Melanin is a pigment that plays an important role in skin protection against UV damage and is involved in pigmentary changes in skin color. It is formed through oxidation and by the amino acid tyrosine through cyclization. Tyrosinase is a melanogenic enzyme that catalyzes the rate-limiting synthetic for melanin production. Melanogenesis initially occurs through hydroxylation of L-tyrosine by tyrosinase converted to L-3,4-dihydroxyphenylalanine (L-DOPA) and by the oxidation of L-DOPA to DOPA-quinone, and eventually to melanin pigments [1,2]. Moreover, in another mechanism, a processes of protein glycosylation, Neu5Acα(2-6)Gal- and possibly sialyl(α2-3)gal-terminated glycans play an important role in melanogenesis and melanosome transfer to keratinocytes [3]. Overproduction and accumulation of melanin results in several skin pigmentation disorders, including solar lentigos (age spots), melasma, freckles, and post-inflammatory hyperpigmentation [4]. Therefore, whitening ingredients that result in inhibited tyrosinase activity, including inhibitory effects on melanogenesis and the melanosome transfer process, are essentially significant for reducing melanin synthesis. Tyrosinase inhibitors are obtained from both natural and synthetic sources, such as hydroquinone, arbutin, kojic acid, L-ascorbic acid, tranexamic acid, ellagic acid, and thiamidol [5]. Lately, Baswan et al. [6–8] reported that cytidine, though not a tyrosinase inhibitor, inhibits melanin synthesis and the melanosome transfer process by interfering with glycosylation processes. In current times, the desire to lighten the complexion has become popular in Asian people seeking beautiful-looking skin. Skin whitening products that propose to lighten the skin's appearance or treat hyper-pigmentation have become highly desirable in the cosmeceutical industries [9]. The use of skin whitening cosmetics has an important role in achieving skin lightening, as well as in diminishing dark spots on the skin [10,11]. Bioactive compounds from plants are gaining popularity for use as cosmetic ingredients in contemporary formulations, as they also contain vitamins, antioxidants, essential oils, proteins, phenolic compounds, and other active compounds [12,13]. Diverse bioactive compounds, including several phenolic compounds, have been reported to contain natural antioxidant compounds, along with having anti-aging, anti-microbial, anti-inflammatory, and tyrosinase-inhibiting actions. Further, these compounds in cosmetic products tend to be safer, biodegradable, more environmentally friendly, and more biologically active when compared with synthetic ingredients [14–16].

Etlingera elatior is a plant in the Zingiberaceae family that is widely cultivated in Southeast Asia as an ornamental flower or is locally consumed as food. The biological activities of *E. elatior* flowers and leaves have been reported over the past few decades. The presence of cosmeceutical properties that are proposed to improve skin appearance, such as antioxidant activity, has been suggested by ferric reducing antioxidant power (FRAP) assay, lipid peroxidation assay, 2, 2-diphenyl-1-picrylhydrazyl (DPPH) radical scavenging, and inhibition of tyrosinase activity, as well as non-toxic properties, as shown by brine shrimp lethality assay [17–20].

In our previous study, *E. elatior* flower and leaf extracts were screened for their amino acid content, phenolic content, and biological activities for cosmetic properties, such as collagenase and tyrosinase inhibition, as well as antioxidant properties, via assay on 2, 2′-azino-bis (3-ethylbenzthiazoline-6-sulfonic acid) (ABTS), DPPH, and superoxide radical scavenging activities. Results indicated that the leaf extract exhibited the strongest antioxidant inhibitor property, higher than those of trolox and gallic acid, and showed the highest phenolic contents of isoquercetin, catechin, and gallic acid, as well as moderate anti-collagenase and amino acid contents. The flower extract showed greater potential to inhibit collagenase activity and more amino acids than the leaf extract, while also showing moderate phenolic compound levels and antioxidant activity. In addition, both the flower and leaf extracts were shown to be capable of suppressing melanogenesis through inhibiting tyrosinase activity [21].

On the basis of the previous study, the research team proposed developing a cosmetic cream for the purpose of skin whitening and with other beneficial properties. The cosmetic cream that was developed contained both the flower and leaf extracts of *E. elatior* together, in a formulation called "FL1 cream". The objective of this study was to evaluate the efficiency of the skin whitening cream containing both the flower and leaf extracts of *E. elatior* in human volunteers and to undertake an irritation test as well.

2. Materials and Methods

2.1. Plant Sample

E. elatior was purchased from a cultivator in the Reso District of Narathiwat Province, Thailand. The flowers and leaves were rinsed several times with distilled water, cut into small pieces, and subsequently shade-dried with a hot-air oven at 50 °C. Dried samples were ground into a fine powder using a high-speed disintegrator machine.

2.2. Plant Extraction

An aqueous solution (1000 mL) including 100 g of powdered flowers or leaves was heated at 50 °C for 8 h, then centrifuged at 4000 rpm for 5 min at ambient temperature and filtered through

Whatman No.1 filter paper. The filtrate extracts were concentrated by a rotary evaporator (KNF RC 900, KNF Neuberger, Trenton, NJ, USA) under vacuum pressure and then lyophilized using a freeze-dryer (Labogene CS 55-4, LaboGene A/S, Allerød, Denmark) to obtain the dried flower and leaf extracts.

2.3. Tyrosinase Inhibition

Tyrosinase inhibition was evaluated using the dopachrome method described by Masuda et al. [22], with some modifications. Solutions of 200 U/mL of tyrosinase from mushrooms and 2.5 mM of L-DOPA (3, 4-dihydroxy-L-phenylalanine) were prepared with 20 mM of phosphate buffer (pH 6.8). The different concentrations and ratios of both flower and leaf extracts, comprising 0.5% and 1% in ratios of 1:1, 1:2, and 1:3 of flower/leaf extracts, were tested. Tyrosinase reactions were performed in a 96-well plate, with each well containing 20 μL of different samples of the extracts, 40 μL of tyrosinase solution, and 140 μL of phosphate buffer. The 96-well plate was allowed to stand for 10 min, and then the reaction was started by adding 40 μL of L-DOPA solution (with phosphate buffer used as a control reaction). The 96-well plate was then incubated at an ambient temperature for 20 min, and the absorbance of tyrosinase activity was measured at 492 nm using a microplate reader (Biochrom EZ read 400) with kojic acid used as a reference substance. Each sample was completed with a blank plate of the sample test, except for the tyrosinase solution. The percentage of tyrosinase inhibition activity was obtained using the following equation:

$$\text{Tyrosinase inhibition (\%)} = [\{(A - B) - (C - D)\} / (A - B)] \times 100.$$

In this equation, A is the absorbance of the control reaction without a sample, B is the absorbance of the blank of the control reaction without a sample, C is the absorbance of the sample test with the presence of sample extracts, and D is the absorbance of the blank of the sample with the presence of sample extracts.

2.4. Formulation of the Whitening Cream

The formulations of FL1 cream containing *E. elatior* flower and leaf extracts are shown in Table 1. The process of preparation for the formulation included the addition of oil phase to the water phase, after which both phases were heated to 80 °C before mixing. Stirring was continued using a mixer homogenizer until the temperature was approximately 50 °C, then sodium hydroxide and preservative were added. Finally, the stirring was continued until the emulsion cooled to an ambient temperature.

Table 1. The formulations of FL1 cream containing *Etlingera elatior* flower and leaf extracts.

Phase	Trade Name	INCI Name	%
A (Oil Phase)	Nikkomulese LH	Glycerin (and) Hydrogenated lecithin (and) Hydroxypropyl methylcellulose stearoxy Ether (and) Squalane (and) Sodium methyl stearoyl taurate	4.00
	DC 350	Dimethicone	3.00
	Squalane	Squalane	5.00
	Cetyl alcohol	Cetyl alcohol	0.30
	Stearyl alcohol	Stearyl alcohol	0.30
B (Water Phase)	Na$_2$EDTA	Disodium EDTA	0.10
	Glycerin	Glycerin	3.00
	Butylene glycol	Butylene glycol	4.00
	Carbopol ultrez 21 polymer	Acrylates/C10-30 alkyl acrylate crosspolymer	0.50
	1Flower/1leaf extract	*Etlingera elatior*	1.00
	DI water	Aqua	q.s. 100
C	NaOH (18% w/v)	Sodium hydroxide (for adjusting pH to 5.5)	0.30
D	Spectrastat BHL	Caprylhydroxamic acid (and) 1,2-hexanediol (and) butylene glycol	2.00

2.5. Stability Testing

The stability was evaluated by the centrifugation method at 4000 rpm and at 20 °C for 30 min to determine the mechanical stress [23]. Accelerated stability testing was also performed in various conditions under room temperature, 4 °C, and 45 °C for three months and six cycles of the heating/cooling method (45 °C, 48 h alternated with 4 °C, 48 h for 1 cycle) [24]. During the stability testing, the physiochemical appearance of the cream, including any change in color or odor, pH, viscosity, phase separation, and precipitation, was investigated.

2.6. Clinical Evaluation in Volunteers

The skin irritation testing and skin whitening efficiency testing on healthy volunteers in this study were approved by the University of Phayao Human Ethics Committee, Thailand (Project identification code: 3/018/61). The efficiency evaluations were performed on 24 healthy volunteers (aged 25–55, $n = 24$). They were investigated for any skin disease and cosmetics allergy history. Before being enrolled in the study, each volunteer received the information protocol that contained the terms and conditions of the clinical testing and signed an informed consent form.

2.7. Skin Irritation Testing

The skin irritation testing was done using a modified Draize model, as described by Bashir and Maibach [25], using Finn chambers®. Skin irritation was performed on the upper outer arm (left-hand side) of volunteers, with each chamber saturated by FL1 cream containing *E. elatior* extracts, 1% w/v of sodium lauryl sulfate (used as a positive reaction), and deionized water (as a negative reaction), before being covered for 48 h. Subsequently, we observed the erythema and edema at 1, 24, and 48 h after removing the patch. Each of the test substances were evaluated based on the primary dermal irritation index (PDII) using the Draize scoring system.

2.8. Efficiency Testing in Human Volunteers

The skin improvement test of the whitening cream was performed with 24 healthy volunteers. They were tested for reduced melanin content after applying the FL1 cream twice a day, morning and evening, on the skin of their left forearm for four weeks. Following Leelapornpisid et al. [24], an untreated area on each volunteer's right forearm was used as a control. Before the study, the volunteers were rested in a suitable room at 20 °C and 50% relative humidity (RH) for 15 min [26]. The study procedures were conducted on Day 0 for the initial value, then on the 1st, 2nd, 3rd, and 4th weeks. The melanin content and CIE-L* value were measured using the skin color probe from DermaLab® Combo (Cortex Technology). Finally, the volunteers were asked to fill out a questionnaire regarding their satisfaction with the whitening cream on Day 30. The ability of the FL1 cream to reduce melanin pigment was obtained using the following equation:

$$\text{Reduction activity (\%)} = [(M_{d0} - M_{dm}) / (M_{d0})] \times 100.$$

In this equation, M_{d0} is the melanin content on the initial day and M_{dm} is the melanin content on the day of measuring.

2.9. Statistical Analysis

The statistical analysis was conducted using the Statistical Package for the Social Sciences (SPSS), version 17.0 for Windows. Viscosity data were analyzed by the use of a one-way analysis of variance (ANOVA) with Tukey's HSD test. A repeated measures ANOVA with pairwise comparisons by the Bonferroni method was used to analyze the skin whitening effect in volunteers. Statistical significance was determined to be at $p < 0.05$.

3. Results and Discussion

3.1. Tyrosinase Inhibition Activity

Tyrosinase is a crucial rate-limiting enzyme in direct melanin synthesis. Therefore, cosmetic products containing tyrosinase inhibitors are becoming more commonly used for their skin whitening properties [27]. In our previous study, flower and leaf at 10 mg/mL showed tyrosinase inhibition activity of 24.37% ± 0.52% and 31.48% ± 1.28%, respectively [21]. This study aimed to develop a cosmetic cream containing both the flower and leaf extracts of *E. elatior* together for the main purpose of skin whitening. Therefore, a suitable concentration and ratio of mixed flower and leaf extracts were investigated. Mushroom tyrosinase was used to determine the role of *E. elatior* in the process of melanogenesis. As shown in Figure 1, the results demonstrated that all concentrations of mixed flower and leaf extracts inhibited tyrosinase activity. In addition, flower and leaf extracts at a concentration of 1% and in a ratio of 1:1 exhibited the highest tyrosinase inhibition activity at 74.61% ± 0.00%. These results indicate that 1% of mixed flower and leaf extracts of *E. elatior* in a ratio of 1:1 is a suitable concentration for use in formulating the cosmetic "FL1". Furthermore, methanol flower and leaf extracts did not show a cytotoxic effect on WRL-68 (human liver) or Vero (African green monkey kidney), or in an *Artemia salina* lethality bioassay [18,20]. Hence, they might be promising for safe use in cosmetic products.

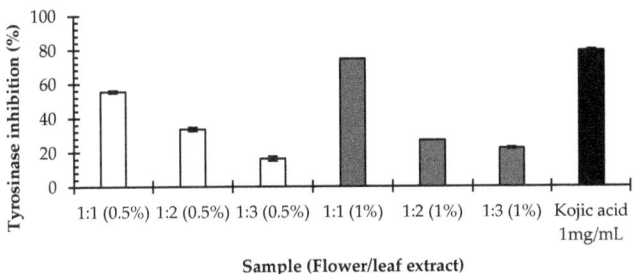

Figure 1. The effect of mixed *E. elatior* flower and leaf extracts on tyrosinase inhibition activity.

3.2. Formulation of the Whitening Cream

In this study, the FL1 cream was evaluated for its physical properties, including pH, color, viscosity (Pa.s), and by centrifugation test, as shown in Table 2. After cosmetic formulation, the physical appearance of the FL1 cream was assessed. The texture was found to be tender, with very good spreadability and a soft feeling on the skin. The FL1 cream was stable and showed no phase separation when centrifuged at 4000 rpm for 30 min.

Table 2. The physical properties of the FL1 cream formulation.

Parameters	pH	Color			Viscosity (Pa.s)	Centrifugation Test
		L^*	a^*	b^*		
FL1 cream	5.5	60.69 ± 0.63	2.47 ± 0.26	20.43 ± 1.08	6.20 ± 0.02	Stable

3.3. Stability Testing

Stability testing under accelerated conditions showed that the pH of the cream kept in all conditions did not change after testing, and separation and precipitation of the FL1 cream were not observed (as shown in Table 3). The viscosity under all conditions compared to the start condition was maintained at room temperature and 4 °C and under heating/cooling cycles was not significantly different ($p > 0.05$). At 45 °C, there was an obvious decrease in viscosity, which may be the effect of heat. Moreover, the physical properties of color under all conditions were also significantly stable ($p > 0.05$), and odor was stable after the stability tests (data not shown). Therefore, FL1 could be stored long term without any change in the pH, color, or viscosity.

Table 3. The stability testing results of FL1 cream after three months and after heating/cooling for six cycles.

Conditions	pH	Viscosity (Pa.s)	Separation and Precipitation	Color		
				L*	a*	b*
Initial	5.5	6.20 ± 0.02 [a]	x	60.69 ± 0.63 [a]	2.47 ± 0.26 [a]	20.43 ± 1.08 [a]
RT	5.5	6.15 ± 0.02 [a]	x	60.18 ± 0.39 [a]	2.40 ± 0.23 [a]	20.07 ± 0.89 [a]
4 °C	5.5	6.17 ± 0.06 [a]	x	60.09 ± 0.34 [a]	2.49 ± 0.23 [a]	19.75 ± 0.84 [a]
45 °C	5.5	6.01 ± 0.03 [b]	x	60.28 ± 0.95 [a]	2.66 ± 0.64 [a]	21.62 ± 0.45 [a]
H/C	5.5	6.15 ± 0.05 [a]	x	60.78 ± 0.51 [a]	2.51 ± 0.41 [a]	20.13 ± 0.24 [a]

Values are expressed as means ± standard deviation. For the viscosity and color values, not sharing the same letter in each column indicates significant difference at $p < 0.05$. RT = Room temperature; H/C = Heating/cooling conditions.

3.4. Irritation Testing

The dermatological test for irritation and allergy effects on human volunteers was performed to ensure the safety of the FL1 cream. The 24 volunteers were tested with FL1 cream, 1% w/v of sodium lauryl sulfate, and deionized water. The results are shown in Table 4. The FL1 cream was non-irritating, with a low Primary Dermal Irritation Index value (PDII < 0.5), whereas sodium lauryl sulfate (SLS), which was used as a positive control, was revealed to be slightly irritating (PDII range from 0.5 to 2.0).

Table 4. The Primary Dermal Irritation Index (PDII) value and skin irritation reaction observed for FL1 cream.

Test Substances	PDII	Classification of Skin Irritation
FL1 cream	0.00	Non-irritating
1% w/v SLS (positive)	0.80	Slightly irritating
DI water (negative)	0.00	Non-irritating

3.5. Skin Whitening Testing

The whitening effect of FL1 cream containing *E. elatior* extracts was evaluated by comparison before the treatment. This was done by measuring the amount of melanin using DermaLab® Combo (Cortex Technology, Hadsund, Denmark) to confirm the efficiency of this product. As shown in Table 5, the results demonstrated that the melanin content in the skin when using FL1 cream was significantly and continuously decreased after one week, until week three of testing ($p < 0.05$). In week four, the melanin content increased, which may be due to the time of testing (March 2019 to April 2019) in Thailand being in the summer season. This period has a corresponding increase in UV exposure, which is one of the causes of melanin synthesis [28,29]; the UV index is shown in Figure 2. Furthermore, the L* value was used for indicating skin lightening after applying the FL1 cream, and it was found that the L* value continuously increased from the 1st to the 3rd week ($p < 0.05$), as did the melanin content. For the untreated areas, the data still showed constant melanin content until week two of testing with no significant difference ($p > 0.05$), but the content increased from the 3rd to the 4th week. However, the L* value of the untreated area was slightly increased until week three and slightly decreased subsequently until week four of testing. In addition, the melanin reduction activity of the FL1 cream reached its highest level of 6.67% after three weeks of testing (Figure 3). There were no significant differences in melanin reduction observed between the FL1-treated and untreated areas of the volunteers during the testing period. These results indicated that *E. elatior* flower and leaf extracts achieved a decent skin whitening effect on human volunteers.

Table 5. The melanin content (%) and L* value after application of the FL1 cream for four weeks.

Test	Parameter	Baseline	Week 1	Week 2	Week 3	Week 4
FL1 cream	Melanin content (%)	36.00 ± 0.33 [a]	35.13 ± 0.38 [b]	33.93 ± 0.53 [c]	33.60 ± 0.44 [c]	35.39 ± 0.55 [ab]
	L* value	37.39 ± 0.40 [a]	38.54 ± 0.47 [b]	39.41 ± 0.47 [c]	41.00 ± 0.65 [d]	39.13 ± 0.70 [bc]
Untreated area	Melanin content (%)	36.44 ± 0.37 [a]	36.15 ± 0.34 [a]	36.01 ± 0.34 [a]	37.13 ± 0.39 [ab]	37.52 ± 0.47 [b]
	L* value	37.57 ± 0.42 [a]	38.07 ± 0.47 [ab]	38.33 ± 0.46 [b]	37.95 ± 0.42 [a]	36.54 ± 0.80 [a]

Values are expressed as means ± standard error. For each parameter of each sample test, not sharing the same letter in each row indicates significant difference at $p < 0.05$.

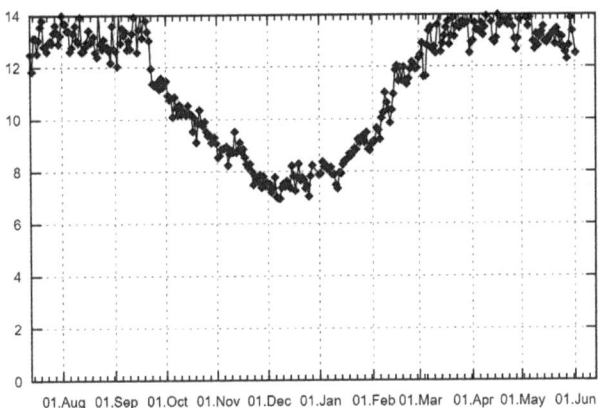

Figure 2. The UV index in Chiang Mai city, Thailand, from August 2018 to June 2019, © weatheronline.co.uk [36].

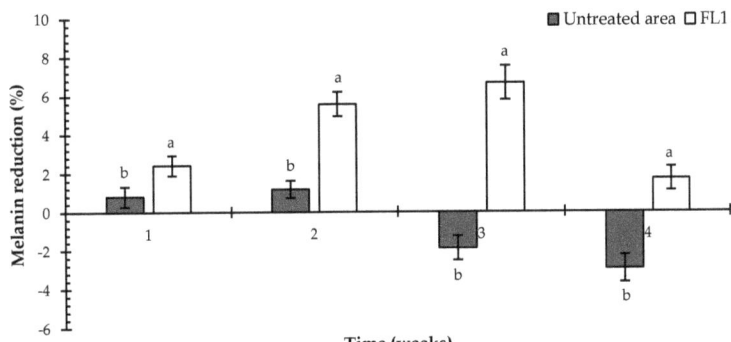

Figure 3. The effect of FL1 cream on melanin reduction. Values are expressed as means ± standard error. For groups in the same week, not sharing the same letter indicates significant difference at $p < 0.05$.

Traditionally, commercial skin whitening agents for suppressing tyrosinase activity have included hydroquinone, arbutin, kojic acid, azelaic acid, ascorbic acid, ellagic acid, and tranexamic acid. These have been widely used in formulations of cosmetic products, with some drawbacks and side effects [27,30]. In the past few decades, research has demonstrated that natural bioactive compounds are increasingly being used in whitening cosmetic formulations. In addition, there are several plant extracts that have been shown to be effective agents to suppress the overproduction of melanin or to regulate melanin synthesis, such as *Cassia fistula* flowers [31], *Asphodelus microcarpus* [32], *Magnolia officinalis* [33], *Dendrobium tosaense* [34], and *Kummerowia striata* [35]. The results of the present study indicated that extracts of *E. elatior* flowers and leaves achieved a decent skin whitening effect on human volunteers; therefore, these extracts act as the active whitening ingredient in FL1 cream.

3.6. Satisfaction Testing

The volunteers were asked to fill in a questionnaire after using the FL1 cream for 30 days. The satisfaction level was determined using a 5-point scale, in which the point value represented the volunteers' feelings about how well the product worked, from very well (5) to very poorly (1). The results revealed that the volunteers' satisfaction with the FL1 cream was high, with responses between "well" and "very well" for all areas measured, as shown in Figure 4. Further, the most satisfying areas of the FL1 cream were the softness of the cream, its spreadability, and overall satisfaction, which had a mean of 4.67, while the lowest was the cream's glossiness, with a mean of 4.33. Additionally, none of the volunteers suffered skin irritation or allergic reactions during the test period.

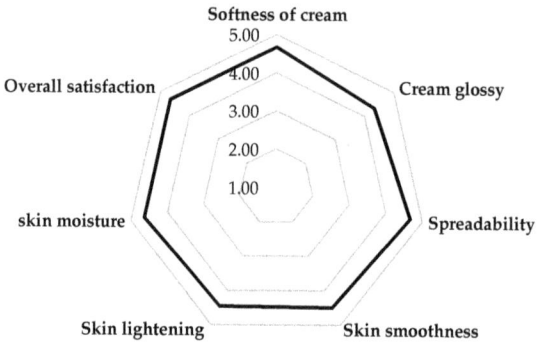

Figure 4. The satisfaction of the volunteers with the FL1 cream.

4. Conclusions

The present study demonstrated that both the flower and leaf extracts of *E. elatior* could potentially be a natural whitening ingredient for commercial cosmetics. In our previous study, aqueous extracts of the flowers and leaves revealed the presence of isoquercetin, catechin, and gallic acid [21], which are capable of inhibiting tyrosinase activity, leading to a skin lightening effect useful in cosmetic applications [37–39]. The results revealed that with the use of the cream, the melanin content decreased and the L^* value increased compared with initial values. The data showed an increased melanin reduction after application of FL1 to the skin when compared to an untreated area. The FL1 cream was found to be safe, with no reported irritation of the skin of the volunteers, and it was also found to be satisfactory by the volunteers. Therefore, FL1 cream containing *E. elatior* flower and leaf extracts might be an effective whitening cosmetic for improving skin appearance.

Author Contributions: Conceptualization, N.W., and D.A.; methodology, N.W., D.A., and, L.M.; formal analysis, N.W. and D.A.; investigation, N.W., D.A., and, L.M.; resources, D.A., and K.M.; supervision, D.A., L.M., and K.M.; writing—original draft, N.W., and D.A.

Funding: This research was funded by the Thailand Research Fund (TRF) under the program of Research and Researcher for Industry (RRi), grant number PHD59I0032.

Acknowledgments: The authors are grateful to the Center of Excellence in Agricultural Innovation for Graduate Entrepreneur, Graduate School of Maejo University for their material support.

Conflicts of Interest: The authors declare no conflict of interest.

References

1. D'Orazio, J.; Jarrett, S.; Amaro-Ortiz, A.; Scott, T. UV radiation and the skin. *Int. J. Mol. Sci.* **2013**, *14*, 12222–12248. [CrossRef] [PubMed]

2. Kim, C.S.; Noh, S.G.; Park, Y.; Kang, D.; Chun, P.; Chung, H.Y.; Jung, H.J.; Moon, H.R. A potent tyrosinase inhibitor, (E)-3-(2,4-Dihydroxyphenyl)-1-(thiophen-2-yl)prop2-en-1-one, with anti-melanogenesis properties in α-MSH and IBMX-induced B16F10 melanoma cells. *Molecules* **2018**, *23*, 2527. [CrossRef] [PubMed]
3. Diwaker, G.; Klump, V.; Lazova, R.; Pawelek, J. Evidence for glycosylation as a regulator of the pigmentary system: key roles of sialyl(α2-6)gal/GalNAc-terminated glycans in melanin synthesis and transfer. *Glycoconj J.* **2015**, *32*, 413–420. [CrossRef] [PubMed]
4. Ortonne, J.P.; Bissett, D.L. Latest insights into skin hyperpigmentation. *JIDSP* **2008**, *13*, 10–14. [CrossRef] [PubMed]
5. Zolghadri, S.; Bahrami, A.; Hassan Khan, M.T.; Munoz-Munoz, J.; Garcia-Molina, F.; Garcia-Canovas, F.; Saboury, A.A. A comprehensive review on tyrosinase inhibitor. *J. Enzyme Inhib. Med. Chem.* **2019**, *34*, 279–309. [CrossRef] [PubMed]
6. Baswan, S.M.; Leverett, J.; Pawelek, J. Clinical evaluation of the lightening effect of cytidine on hyperpigmented skin. *J. Cosmet. Dermatol.* **2019**, *18*, 278–285. [CrossRef] [PubMed]
7. Baswan, S.M.; Yim, S.; Leverett, J.; Pawelek, J. LB1591 In-vitro and in-vivo evaluation of skin lightening efficacy of cytidine. *J. Investig. Dermatol.* **2018**, *138*, B21. [CrossRef]
8. Baswan, S.M.; Yim, S.; Leverett, J.; Scholten, J.; Pawelek, J. Cytidine decreases melanin content in a reconstituted three-dimensional human epidermal model. *Arch. Dermatol. Res.* **2019**, *311*, 249–250. [CrossRef]
9. Lorz, L.R.; Yoo, B.C.; Kim, M.Y.; Cho, J.Y. Anti-wrinkling and anti-melanogenic effect of *Pradosia mutisii* methanol extract. *Int. J. Mol. Sci.* **2019**, *20*, 1043. [CrossRef]
10. Sahin, S.C. The potential of *Arthrospira platensis* extract as a tyrosinase inhibitor for pharmaceutical or cosmetic applications. *S. Afr. J. Bot.* **2018**, *119*, 236–243. [CrossRef]
11. Wang, G.H.; Chen, C.Y.; Lin, C.P.; Huang, C.L.; Liu, C.H.; Cheng, C.Y.; Chung, Y.C. Tyrosinase inhibitor and antioxidant activities of three *Bifidobacterium bifidum*-fermented herb extracts. *Ind. Crops Prod.* **2016**, *89*, 376–382. [CrossRef]
12. Ribeiro, A.S.; Estanqueiro, M.; Oliveira, M.B.; Lobo, J.M.S. Main benefits and applicability of plant extracts in skin care products. *Cosmetics* **2015**, *2*, 48–65. [CrossRef]
13. Mukherjee, P.K.; Maity, N.; Nema, N.K.; Sarkar, B.K. Bioactive compounds from natural resources against skin aging. *Phytomedicine* **2011**, *19*, 64–73. [CrossRef] [PubMed]
14. Li, F.X.; Li, F.H.; Yang, Y.X.; Yin, R.; Ming, J. Comparison of phenolic profiles and antioxidant activities in skins and pulps of eleven grape cultivars (*Vitis vinifera* L.). *J. Integr. Agric* **2019**, *18*, 1148–1158. [CrossRef]
15. Działo, M.; Mierziak, J.; Korzun, U.; Preisner, M.; Szopa, J.; Kulma, A. The potential of plant phenolics in prevention and therapy of skin disorders. *Int. J. Mol. Sci.* **2016**, *17*, 160. [CrossRef] [PubMed]
16. Soto, M.L.; Falqué, E.; Domínguez, H. Relevance of natural phenolics from grape and derivative products in the formulation of cosmetics. *Cosmetics* **2015**, *2*, 259–276. [CrossRef]
17. Ghasemzadeh, A.; Jaafar, H.Z.E.; Rahmat, A.; Ashkani, S. Secondary metabolites constituents and antioxidant, anticancer and antibacterial activities of *Etlingera elatior* (Jack) R.M.Sm grown in different locations of Malaysia. *BMC Complement. Altern. Med.* **2015**, *15*, 335. [CrossRef] [PubMed]
18. Chan, E.W.C.; Lim, Y.Y.; Wong, S.K. Phytochemistry and pharmacological properties of *Etlingera elatior*: A review. *Phcog. J.* **2011**, *3*, 6–10. [CrossRef]
19. Chan, E.W.C.; Lim, Y.Y.; Tan, S.P. Standardised herbal extract of chlorogenic acid from leaves of *Etlingera elatior* (Zingiberaceae). *Phcog. Res.* **2011**, *3*, 178–183. [CrossRef]
20. Lachumy, S.J.T.; Sasidharan, S.; Sumathy, V.; Zuraini, Z. Pharmacological activity, phytochemical analysis and toxicity of methanol extract of *Etlingera elatior* (torch ginger) flowers. *Asian Pac. J. Trop. Med.* **2010**, 769–774. [CrossRef]
21. Whangsomnuek, N.; Mungmai, L.; Mengamphan, K.; Amornlerdpison, D. Anti-aging and whitening properties of bioactive compounds from *Etlingera elatior* (Jack) R.M.Sm. flower and leaf extracts for cosmetic applications. *Maejo. Int. J. Sci. Tech.* In Press.
22. Masuda, T.; Yamashita, D.; Takeda, Y.; Yonemori, S. Screening for tyrosinase inhibitors among extracts of seashore plants and identification of potent inhibitors from *Garcinia. subelliptica*. *Biosci. Biotechnol. Biochem.* **2005**, *69*, 197–201. [CrossRef] [PubMed]
23. Censi, R.; Peregrina, D.V.; Lacava, G.; Agas, D.; Lupidi, G.; Sabbieti, M.G.; Martino, P.D. Cosmetic formulation based on an açai extract. *Cosmetics* **2018**, *5*, 48. [CrossRef]

24. Leelapornpisid, P.; Mungmai, L.; Sirithunyalug, B.; Jiranusornkul, S.; Peerapornpisal, Y. A novel moisturizer extracted from freshwater macroalga [*Rhizoclonium hieroglyphicum* (C.Agardh) Kützing] for skin care cosmetic. *Chiang Mai. J. Sci.* **2014**, *41*, 1195–1207.
25. Bashir, S.J.; Maibach, H.I. In vivo irritation. In *Handbook of Cosmetic Science and Technology*, 3rd ed.; Barel, A.O., Paye, M., Maibach, H.I., Eds.; Taylor and Francis Group: Vanderbilt Avenue, New York, NY, USA, 2009; pp. 471–479.
26. Jaros, A.; Zasada, M.; Budzisz, E.; Dębowska, R.; Gębczyńska-Rzepka, M.; Rotsztejn, H. Evaluation of selected skin parameters following the application of 5% vitamin C concentrate. *J. Cosmet. Dermatol.* **2019**, *18*, 236–241. [CrossRef] [PubMed]
27. Pillaiyar, T.; Manickam, M.; Namasivayam, V. Skin whitening agents: medicinal chemistry perspective of tyrosinase inhibitors. *J. Enzyme Inhib. Med. Chem.* **2017**, *32*, 403–425. [CrossRef] [PubMed]
28. Pintus, F.; Spanò, D.; Corona, A.; Medda, R. Antityrosinase activity of Euphorbia characias extracts. *PeerJ* **2015**, *3*, e1305. [CrossRef]
29. Brenner, M.; Hearing, V.J. The protective role of melanin against UV damage in human skin. *Photochem. Photobiol.* **2008**, *84*, 539–549. [CrossRef]
30. Smit, N.; Vicanova, J.; Pavel, S. The hunt for natural skin whitening agents. *Int. J. Mol. Sci.* **2009**, *10*, 5326–5349. [CrossRef]
31. Limtrakul, P.; Yodkeeree, S.; Thippraphan, P.; Punfa, W.; Srisomboon, J. Anti-aging and tyrosinase inhibition effects of Cassia fistula flower butanolic extract. *BMC Complement. Altern. Med.* **2016**, *16*, 497. [CrossRef]
32. Petrillo, A.D.; González-Paramás, A.M.; Era, B.; Medda, R.; Pintus, F.; Santos-Buelga, C.; Fais, A. Tyrosinase inhibition and antioxidant properties of *Asphodelus microcarpus* extracts. *BMC Complement. Altern. Med.* **2016**, *16*, 453. [CrossRef]
33. Wu, L.; Chen, C.; Cheng, C.; Dai, H.; Ai, Y.; Lin, C.; Chung, Y. Evaluation of tyrosinase inhibitory, antioxidant, antimicrobial, and antiaging activities of Magnolia officinalis extracts after Aspergillus niger fermentation. *BioMed Res. Int.* **2018**. Available online: https://www.hindawi.com/journals/bmri/2018/5201786/ (accessed on 5 July 2019). [CrossRef]
34. Chan, C.F.; Wu, C.T.; Huang, W.Y.; Lin, W.S.; Wu, H.W.; Huang, T.K.; Chang, M.Y.; Lin, Y.S. Antioxidation and melanogenesis inhibition of various Dendrobium tosaense extracts. *Molecules* **2018**, *23*, 1810. [CrossRef]
35. Lee, J.Y.; Cho, Y.R.; Park, J.H.; Ahn, E.K.; Jeong, W.; Shin, H.S.; Kim, M.S.; Yang, S.H.; Oh, J.S. Anti-melanogenic and anti-oxidant activities of ethanol extract of Kummerowia striata: Kummerowia striata regulate anti-melanogenic activity through down-regulation of TRP-1, TRP-2 and MITF expression. *Toxicol. Rep.* **2019**, *6*, 10–17. [CrossRef] [PubMed]
36. Weather Online. Available online: https://www.weatheronline.co.uk/weather/maps/city (accessed on 15 June 2019).
37. Su, T.R.; Lin, J.J.; Tsai, C.C.; Huang, T.K.; Yang, Z.Y.; Wu, M.O.; Zheng, Y.Q.; Su, C.C.; Wu, Y.J. Inhibition of melanogenesis by gallic acid: possible involvement of the PI3K/Akt, MEK/ERK and Wnt/β-catenin signaling pathways in B16F10 cells. *Int. J. Mol. Sci.* **2013**, *14*, 20443–20458. [CrossRef] [PubMed]
38. Hong, Y.H.; Jung, E.Y.; Noh, D.O.; Suh, H.J. Physiological effects of formulation containing tannase-converted green tea extract on skin care: physical stability, collagenase, elastase, and tyrosinase activities. *Integr. Med. Res.* **2014**, *3*, 25–33. [CrossRef] [PubMed]
39. De Freitas, M.M.; Fontes, P.R.; Souza, P.M.; Fagg, W.C.; Guerra, E.N.S.; de Medeiros Nóbrega, Y.K.; Silveira, D.; Fonseca-Bazzo, Y.; Simeoni, L.A.; Homem-de-Mello, M.; et al. Extracts of Morus nigra L. leaves standardized in chlorogenic acid, rutin and isoquercitrin: tyrosinase inhibition and cytotoxicity. *PLoS ONE* **2016**. Available online: https://www.ncbi.nlm.nih.gov/pubmed/27655047 (accessed on 5 July 2019). [CrossRef]

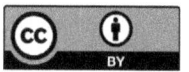

© 2019 by the authors. Licensee MDPI, Basel, Switzerland. This article is an open access article distributed under the terms and conditions of the Creative Commons Attribution (CC BY) license (http://creativecommons.org/licenses/by/4.0/).

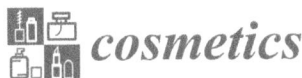

Article

Effects of a Phenol-Enriched Purified Extract from Olive Mill Wastewater on Skin Cells

Peggy Schlupp [1,*], Thomas M. Schmidts [1], Axel Pössl [1], Sören Wildenhain [1], Gianni Lo Franco [2], Antonio Lo Franco [2] and Bandino Lo Franco [2]

1. RSC Pharma LTD & Co. KG—Anwenderzentrum Technische Hochschule Mittelhessen—University of Applied Science, Gutfleischstr. 3-5, 35390 Giessen, Germany; schmidts@rscpharma.com (T.M.S.); axel.poessl@lse.thm.de (A.P.); wildenhain@rscpharma.com (S.W.)
2. Fattoria la Vialla, Via di Meliciano, 26, 52029 Castiglion Fibocchi AR, Arezzo, Italy; fattoria@lavialla.it
* Correspondence: schlupp@rscpharma.com; Tel.: +49-641-309-2554; Fax: +49-641-309-2957

Received: 4 March 2019; Accepted: 30 April 2019; Published: 7 May 2019

Abstract: Olive trees (Olea europaea) and their processed products, such as olive oil, play a major role in the Mediterranean way of life. Their positive impact on human health is being intensely investigated. One research topic is the identification of new application areas of olive mill wastewater (OMWW). OMWW is characterized by the high content of polyphenols possessing many positive health effects. Thus, the phenol-enriched OMWW extract offers the potential for the treatment of skin disorders and for cosmetic application. The aim of the present study was to evaluate cell viability and proliferation, the anti-inflammatory and anti-oxidative properties of a phenol-enriched OMWW extract on an immortal keratinocyte cell line (HaCaT cells). Moreover, the influence on the growth of various microorganisms was investigated; furthermore, the effects on normal human epidermal keratinocytes (NHEK) and human melanoma cells (A375) were studied in a commercially available tumor invasion skin model. The phenol-enriched OMWW extract showed excellent antimicrobial activity. Moreover, a noticeable reduction in reactive oxygen species formation as well as Interleukin-8 release in HaCaT cells were observed. Finally, the inhibited growth of A375 melanoma nodules in the melanoma skin model could be shown. Our results indicate that the OMWW extract is a promising ingredient for dermal applications to improve skin health and skin protection as well as having a positive impact on skin ageing.

Keywords: HaCaT cells; NHEK cells; ROS-assay; tumor invasion skin model; IL-8; antimicrobial effects

1. Introduction

Olive trees (Olea europaea) and their processed products, such as olive oil, play a major role in the Mediterranean way of life. In Mediterranean countries, a significant decline in cancer risk has been shown in several studies [1]. This is associated with the Mediterranean diet and its associated phenol-rich nutrition. Olive fruits, especially olive oil and the by-products of the manufacturing process, are the focus of many research groups [2–5]. In addition to the oil phase, a large quantity of aqueous phase (olive mill wastewater, OMWW) and small quantities of pomace (plant fibers) are formed during the olive grinding process [4,6]. The disposal of these by-products is cost-intensive. Thus, the search for alternative applications is of great interest. In particular, OMWW seems to be very promising due to a high amount of polyphenols [7] which can further be enriched by extraction [8]. The quantity and the compositions of the phenols largely depend on the cultivation conditions of the olive trees, the manufacturing process of the olive oil, and the extraction method for the purification of OMWW [8]. These are essential for the biological activity of the final product. Polyphenols are attributed to many health-promoting effects, such as anti-inflammatory [9], anti-microbiological [10], anti-oxidative [11], and potentially chemo-preventive properties [12]. Due to these properties, polyphenols are very promising for dermal applications. So far, though, only a few studies have been conducted with regard to OMWW application on the skin. Di Mauro et al. [13] investigated a sugar- and mineral-enriched fraction from OMWW for a cosmeceutical application and have shown its moisturizing properties in vivo. Therefore, the aim of the present study was to evaluate cell viability and proliferation, and the anti-inflammatory and anti-oxidative properties of a phenol-enriched OMWW extract on HaCaT cells. Furthermore, the influence on the growth of various microorganisms was investigated. Finally, the effects on normal human epidermal keratinocytes (NHEK) and human melanoma cells (A375) were studied in a tumor invasion skin model.

2. Materials and Methods

2.1. Preparation of the Olive Mill Wastewater (OMWW)

The olive mill wastewater (OMWW) used for the studies was provided by Agriturismo La Vialla (Castiglion Fibocchi (Arezzo), Italy). The phenol-enriched purified extract (OMWW extract) was obtained from Massimo and Daniele Pizzichini according to Patent formulation (Patent 8815815) [14]. The composition of the batch was provided by a certificate of analysis of Fattoria LaVialla (Table 1). The extract, originating from the aqueous part of olive oil production was filtered using a ceramic membrane, and concentrated by reverse osmosis [14]. Prior to use, the concentrate was centrifuged at $500\times g$ for 20 s and filtrated (0.2 µm). Final dilutions were completed in a cell culture growth medium.

Table 1. Quantification of the phenolic ingredients in the olive mill wastewater (OMWW) extract, n.d. = not detected.

Phenolic Ingredient	Concentration/g·L^{-1}
hydroxytyrosol glycoside	2.01
hydroxytyrosol	2.52
tyrosol and derivates of glycosids	0.80
chlorogenic acid	0.10
caffeic acid	n.d.
β-hydroxy-verbascoside isomer 1	0.29
β-hydroxy-verbascoside isomer 2	0.26
rutin	n.d.
Verbascoside	1.04
luteolin-7-glucoside	n.d.
nüzhenide	n.d.
Isoverbascoside	n.d.
3,4-DHPEA-EDA (oleacein)	n.d.
oleuropein aglycon	0.71
p-coumaroyl-secologanoside	0.38
Oleocanthal	not analyzed
total absorption (280 nm)	14.67

2.2. Cell Viability Assay

The cell viability was determined with a calorimetric WST-1 assay (Roche Diagnostics Mannheim, Germany); the conditions were adapted to the respective issue. The cell viability of an immortalized human keratinocyte cell line (HaCaT cells, AddexBio, San Diego, CA, USA) was determined after 72 h to exclude negative effects in the anti-inflammatory assay. HaCaT cells were inoculated with 20,000 cells per well (96-well plate) in growth medium (DMEM low glucose with 10% FCS, Capricorn Scientific GmbH, Germany) and incubated for 24 h at 37 °C with 8.5% CO_2. After a visual inspection of the intact monolayer, the cells were washed twice with phosphate buffer, and 200 µL of the OMWW extract dilutions in the growth medium as well as growth medium in case of the untreated control were applied for 72 h. At the end of incubation, the cells were washed twice with the phosphate buffer, and 100 µL of 5% WST-1 reagent in the growth medium was applied onto the cells and incubated for 4 h. Samples were measured at 450 and 630 nm (reference wavelength), using the Synergy HTX microplate reader (BioTek Instruments Inc., Germany). Cell viability was calculated in relation to the untreated control. The following changes in the protocol were done for the human malignant melanoma cell line A375 (Sigma-Aldrich, Taufkirchen, Germany) and the human epidermal keratinocytes neonatal NHEK (MatTek Corporation, Ashland, MA, USA) to estimate the application concentration for the tumor invasion model. The growth medium for A375 cells was DMEM with high glucose (4.5 g/L) (DMEM-HXA, 8.5% CO_2, Capricorn Scientific GmbH, Ebsdorfergrund, Germany) supplemented with 10% FCS, 2% glutamine (200 mM) and 1% sodium pyruvate (100 mM), respectively, and keratinocyte growth medium 2 (5% CO_2) delivered by PromoCell GmbH (Heidelberg, Germany) for NHEK cells. Both cell lines were inoculated with 40,000 cells per well (96-well plate), and sample incubation was done with 100 µL of the OMWW extract dilutions for 24 h. All experiments were carried out three times with at least six repetitions.

2.3. Anti-Inflammatory Assay In Vitro

HaCaT cells were cultured in a 24-well plate (20,000 cells per well) in 1 mL of growth medium overnight (24 h) at 37 °C and 8.5% CO_2. Prior to sample application (sample size: 1 mL in growth medium), the cells were washed twice with phosphate buffer. The inflammatory response was induced by the co-application of 10 ng/mL TNF-α (R&D Systems, Wiesbaden, Germany). The anti-inflammatory drug hydrocortisone (10^{-7} M) was used as a positive control. Cell-free supernatants were collected, and the Interleukin-8 (IL-8) concentration was determined by the commercially available ELISA kit (Life Technologies GmbH, Darmstadt, Germany). All experiments were carried out three times with at least three repetitions.

2.4. Assessment of the Antimicrobial Properties

For the testing of the antimicrobial properties of the OMWW concentrate, a time-modified assay was used, according to the European Pharmacopoeia (Ph. Eur.) method. Therefore, the inhibitory properties of the OMWW extract on the growth of various bacterial and mold organisms (Table 2) were determined by the suspension method, the punch hole method and the paper disk method. The cultivation and evaluation of the test organisms was based on the Pharmacopeia Europaea protocol [15]. Therefore, 10 mL of the OMWW extract was inoculated with the individual microorganism (MO), a bacterial concentration between 10^5 and 10^6 CFU/g and a mold concentration between 10^4 and 10^5 CFU/g. These samples were incubated at 25 ± 1 °C, and growth control was performed immediately after inoculation, i.e., after two days and one week of incubation with the dilution series determining the colony-forming units (CFU). Furthermore, the antimicrobial effectiveness was determined by the agar diffusion test. Two procedures were performed: the punch hole test and the paper disc method. With respect to the test organism, the medium was inoculated with 10^5 to 10^7 CFU per plate. Subsequently, a hole with a diameter of 11 mm was punched into the agar and filled with 0.5 mL of the OMWW extract (punch hole test), respectively, and an absorbent paper disc (⌀ 9 mm) soaked with 250 µL of the OMWW extract was placed onto the agar (paper disc method). The plates were incubated as described in the Ph. Eur.: bacteria for 18 to 24 h at 35 °C (depending on the bacterium: aerobic/anaerobic), *Candida albicans* for 48 h at 25 °C, and *Aspergillus brasiliensis* for 5 days at 25 °C. The results were obtained by measuring the inhibition zone.

Table 2. Overview of the test organism and the used broth.

Test Organism, Strain ID	Broth
Staphylococcus aureus, WDCM 00035	Casein soya peptone agar
Escherichia coli, DSMZ 301	Casein soya peptone agar
Pseudomonas aeruginosa, WDCM 00026	Casein soya peptone agar
Candida albicans, WDCM 00054	Sabouraud dextrose agar without antibiotic supplements
Aspergillus brasiliensis, WDCM 00053	Sabouraud dextrose agar without antibiotic supplements
Staphylococcus epidermidis, WDCM 00036	Casein soya peptone agar
Propionibacterium acnes, DSMZ 1897	Casein soya peptone agar

2.5. Reactive Oxygen Species (ROS) Assay In Vitro

42,000 HaCaT cells per well (100 µL of growth medium without phenol red) were grown in a black 96-well plate with a clear bottom overnight (37 °C and 8.5% CO_2). The next day, the cell monolayer was washed twice with phosphate buffer, and 100 µL of the OMWW extract dilution or ascorbic acid (100 µM) plus 50 µM 2,7-Dichlorodihydrofluorescein diacetate (DCFH-DA) sample per well were applied for 30 min. Then, the cells were washed with PBS buffer, and 100 µM H_2O_2 in phosphate buffer was added to the cells for 45 min (at 37 °C and 8.5% CO_2). A final washing step with phosphate buffer was done before measuring the fluorescence intensity (ex./em. 485/528 nm), using the microplate reader (100 µL of phosphate buffer, bottom read). To calculate the reduction of oxidative stress, the measurement signal of the control (cells treated with H_2O_2 only) is set to 100%. All experiments were done three times with at least five repetitions.

2.6. Tumor Invasion in a Full-Thickness Skin Model In Vitro

The influence of the OMWW extract on tumor invasion was examined using the commercially available Melanoma skin model "MLNM-FT-A375" (MatTek Corporation, Ashland, USA). Based on the "Testing of Anti-Melanoma Drugs" protocol, provided by MatTek Corporation, the skin models were prepared for a long-time treatment (12 days) after delivery. The treatment of the skin samples with 1:400 dilutions of the OMWW extract (with cell culture medium) started on day 1 and was renewed every other day. As a positive control, the same number of skin samples was treated with the cell culture medium only. On day 3, 7 and 12 (plus day 0 for positive control), two skin samples per time point and treatment were prepared for a histology characterization: formalin fixation and Hematoxylin and Eosin (H&E) staining. Hematoxylin stains the cell nuclei violet/dark blue, while eosin stains cell cytoplasm and most connective tissue fibers in varying shades and intensities of pink/red.

2.7. Data Analysis and Statistics

Data are given as arithmetic mean values ± standard deviation. In order to verify differences, data were subjected to the nonparametric Kruskal–Wallis test, followed by the Dunn's multiple comparison test, in case of significance (GraphPad Prism® version 8.1.0(325), GraphPad Software, San Diego, CA, USA). Thus $p \leq 0.05$ is regarded to indicate a difference.

3. Results

3.1. Phenol-Enriched OMWW Extract Reduces Interleukin-8 Release in Epidermal Skin Cells (In Vitro)

First, the influence of the OMWW extract on HaCaT cell viability was investigated over 72 h. The decrease in HaCaT viability depends on the OMWW extract concentration. The OMWW extract dilution of 1:100 showed a slight decrease in cell viability (70.9% ± 10.2%) after 72 h (Figure 1). An OMWW extract dilution of 1:200 to 1:1000 showed no negative effect on HaCaT cell viability (viability ≥ 100%) compared to the untreated sample (Figure 1). Therefore, the anti-inflammatory assay was carried out with the OMWW extract dilutions of 1:200, 1:400 and 1:600.

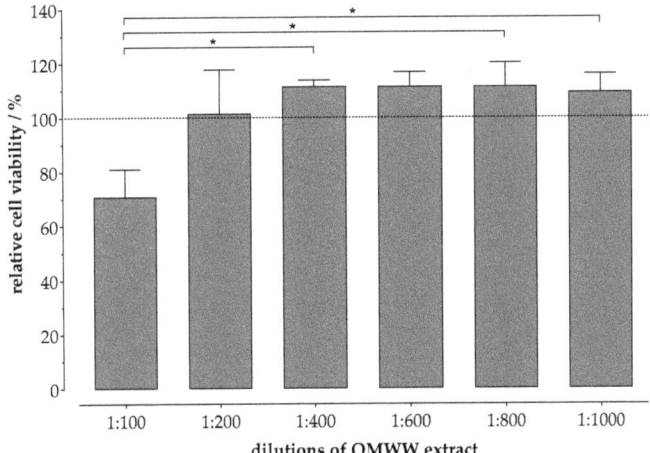

Figure 1. Viability of HaCaT cells (20,000 cells per well, 96-well plate) after treatment with the OMWW extract dilutions (1:100–1:1000) for 72 h, MW ± SD, $n = 3$, * $p \leq 0.05$ (each 6-fold). Indication of the viability is shown in relation to the untreated control (100% viability).

To study the possibility of an application of the OMWW extract in cases of inflammatory skin diseases, the modulation of Interleukin-8 (IL-8) release was studied in HaCaT cells. The stimulation of HaCaT cells with TNF-α (10 ng/mL) resulted in an increased release of IL-8 compared to the untreated control (Figure 2). Depending on the incubation period, the IL-8 concentration increased from 465.8 ± 31.0 pg/mL (24 h) to 2362.4 ± 35.9 pg/mL (72 h) after a TNF-α application. Furthermore, the sensitivity of the assay was controlled by the standard anti-inflammatory agent hydrocortisone (10^{-7} M), resulting in a reduction of 40% of IL-8 release compared to the TNF-α-treated sample after 72 h (Figure 2).

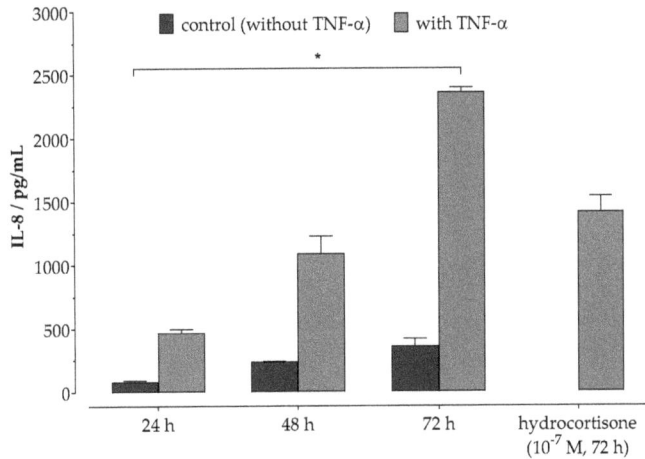

Figure 2. Pre-studies for Interleukin-8 (IL-8) release of HaCaT cells after treatment with 10 ng/mL TNF-α as a function of incubation time and treatment with hydrocortisone (10^{-7} M) for 72 h. MW ± SD, $n = 3$, * $p \leq 0.05$ (each in triplicates).

Stimulation of HaCaT cells with TNF-α resulted in a 4.8-fold higher release of IL-8 compared to the untreated control after 72 h (Figure 3). Co-administration of TNF-α and the OMWW extract led to a reduction in IL-8 release up to 73.4 ± 10.4% (1:200) compared to the control with TNF-α. The reduction in IL-8 release depended on the concentration, 45.2 ± 5.8% (1:400), and 37.2 ± 8.4% (1:600) respectively. Already, the unstimulated samples showed a positive effect on IL-8 release in HaCaT cells. IL-8 production was reduced up to 72.4% (1:200) (Figure 3).

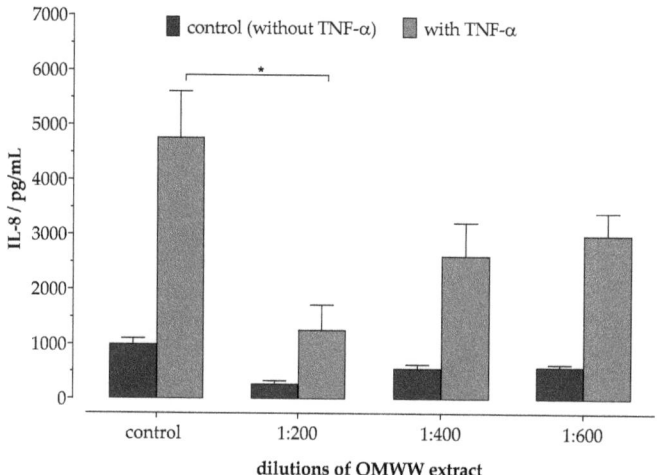

Figure 3. Determination of IL-8 release in HaCaT cells after treatment with 10 ng/mL TNF-α (controls without TNF-α) and incubation with the OMWW extract dilutions for 72 h. MW ± SD, $n = 3$, * $p \leq 0.05$ (each in triplicates).

The studies carried out on HaCaT cells showed that the OMWW extract positively influenced IL-8 release in vitro, thus demonstrating an anti-inflammatory effect on skin cells.

3.2. Phenol-Enriched OMWW Extract Inhibits the Growth of Selected Pathogenic Skin Organism

The influence of the OMWW extract on microbial growth was investigated by the suspension method (Table 3) and a determination of the inhibition zone (punch hole and paper disk) by the agar diffusion method (Tables 4 and 5). The OMWW extract showed excellent antimicrobial activity against *Staphylococcus aureus*, *Staphylococcus epidermidis* (both Gram-positive bacteria), *Escherichia coli*, *Pseudomonas aeruginosa* (both Gram-negative bacteria), *Candida albicans* (yeast), and *Propionibacterium acnes* (anaerobic Gram-positive bacteria). The antimicrobial activity against *Aspergillus brasiliensis* (mold) was less pronounced after 7 days of incubation, using the suspension method (Table 3).

Table 3. Studies on the antimicrobial effects of the OMWW extract on various microorganisms by the suspension method.

Test Organism	CFU/g (Start)	2 d		7 d	
		CFU/g Sample	Reduction in %	CFU/g Sample	Reduction in %
S. aureus	4.30×10^5	<10	>99.99	<10	>99.99
E. coli	1.06×10^6	<10	>99.99	<10	>99.99
P. aeruginosa	8.70×10^5	<10	>99.99	<10	>99.99
C. albicans	3.20×10^5	<10	>99.99	<10	>99.99
A. brasiliensis	8.00×10^4	3500	95.63	not determined	not determined
S. epidermidis	1.16×10^6	<10	>99.99	<10	>99.99
P. acnes	1.20×10^6	<10	>99.99	<10	>99.99

Table 4. Studies on the antimicrobial effects of the OMWW extract on various microorganisms by detection of the inhibition zone, by the punch hole and the paper disk method. The dashed line identifies the inhibition zone.

	Punch Hole Method	Paper Disk Method
S. aureus:		
E. coli:		
P. aeruginosa:		
C. albicans:		
A. brasiliensis:		
S. epidermidis:		
P. acnes:		

Table 5. Quantification of the inhibition zone formed, depending on the microorganism and its inoculation density for the punch hole method and paper disc method.

Organism	Inoculation CFU/g Sample	Inhibition Zone/mm (Punch Hole Method)	Inhibition Zone/mm (Paper Disc Method)
S. aureus	4.30×10^6	3.0	2.0
E. coli	1.06×10^7	4.0	2.5
P. aeruginosa	8.70×10^6	3.5	3.0
C. albicans	3.20×10^6	0	0
A. brasiliensis	8.00×10^5	0	0
S. epidermidis	1.16×10^7	7.0	3.1
P. acnes	1.20×10^6	9.0	7.0

In more detail, the variable potency in growth-inhibiting efficacy of the OMWW extract was observed by the detection of the inhibition zone (Tables 4 and 5). The OMWW extract showed an antibiotic effect against all the bacterial strains tested and was most effective against *S. epidermidis* and *P. acnes*. No growth-inhibiting properties could be detected against *C. albicans* and *A. brasiliensis*.

Considering these results, the OMWW extract revealed very good antimicrobial activity and a moderate effectiveness against the yeast and the mold.

3.3. Phenol-Enriched OMWW Extract Reduce the Formation of Free Radicals In Vitro

The anti-oxidative property was studied by the ability of the OMWW extract to reduce the formation of free radicals in HaCaTs cells. Reactive oxygen species (ROS) generation in HaCaT cells was induced by the application of H_2O_2 (100 µM). Based on Rossi et al. [14], the OMWW extract was applied in a concentration of 1:250 and 1:500. In the presence of the OMWW extract, ROS generation was clearly reduced and even more effective than the application of 100 µM ascorbic acid (Figure 4). Thus, the OMWW extract showed anti-oxidative properties in vitro.

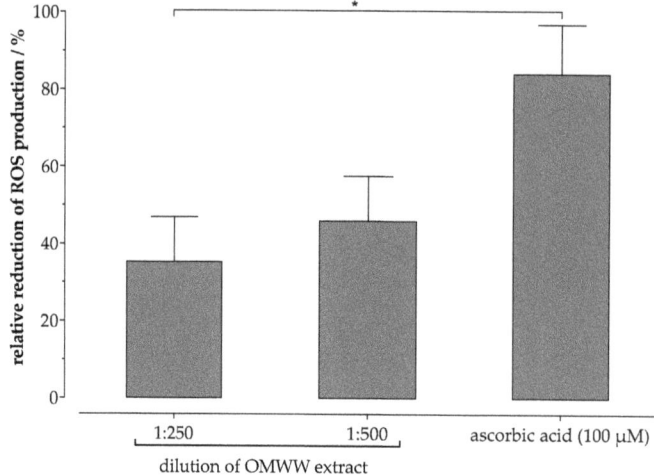

Figure 4. Treatment (30 min) of HaCaT cells with each OMWW extract dilution (1:250 and 1:500) and ascorbic acid (100 µM) after ROS induction by H_2O_2 (100 µM) for 15 min; MW ± SD, $n \geq 3$, * $p \leq 0.05$ (with five replications). HaCaT cells, only treated with H_2O_2, represent 100% of the generated reactive oxygen species (ROS).

3.4. The Phenol-Enriched OMWW Extract Modulates the Invasion of Tumor Cells in the Skin In Vitro

The melanoma skin model is a tool to study the influence of substances on the growth of A375 cells, human metastatic melanoma cells, within a full-thickness skin model consisting of normal human-derived epidermal keratinocytes (NHEK) and normal human-derived dermal fibroblasts. Skin models are more physiologically relevant and predictive than 2D cultures (monolayer) [16,17]. First, we investigated the influence of the OMWW extract on the viability of A375 and NHEK cells. The results showed a concentration-related effect of the OMWW extract on the cell viability of NHEK and A375 cells. NHEK cells treated with the OMWW extract showed clear increased cell proliferation, up to 189.1% with the 1:200 OMWW compared to the untreated control (Figure 5, dark grey bars). In comparison, the viability of A375 cells was approximately 90.1% (1:100) to 115.7% (1:400) after an OMWW extract treatment and, thus, comparable to the untreated control (Figure 5, light grey bars).

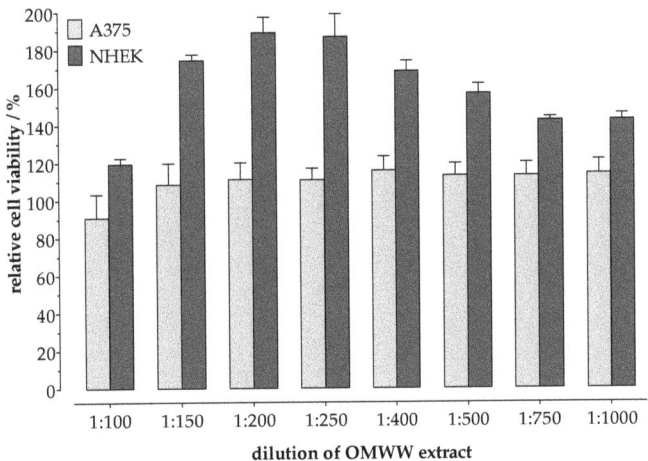

Figure 5. Viability of NHEK and A375 cells (40,000 cells per well, 96-well plate) depending on treatment with the OMWW extract dilutions (1:100–1:1000) after 24 h. MW ± SD, $n = 3$ (with six replications). An indication of the viability is shown in relation to the untreated control (=100% viability).

The melanoma skin model can be used to study the invasion of tumor cells (A375) into the dermis. In brief, the cultivation of an untreated skin sample results in the development of nodes by the incorporated metastatic melanoma cell line (A375) within 12 days (Figure 6). By applying potent substances, modulation in tumor invasion can be detected. The control of day 0 (Figure 6 left) shows the different layers of the skin (dermis with fibroblasts, epidermis with keratinocytes and the *stratum corneum*) and the membrane of the tissue culture inserts. Arrows indicate the melanoma cell clusters at the epidermal–dermal junction. On day 12 (Figure 6 right), the melanoma nodes are large and clearly visible in the control skin sample.

The following pictures (Figure 7) show the results of the treatment of the Melanoma skin model with an OMWW extract dilution (1:400) compared to the untreated control of 12 days. Each treatment was done in duplicate, and the representative section from each treatment is presented (10× magnification). The OMWW extract apparently affects the growth of melanoma cells and the formation of melanoma nodes within the three-dimensional skin models, respectively. The A375 cell clusters were smaller in size. These results suggest that the OMWW extracts reduce the growth of A375 melanoma nodules in vitro compared to the untreated samples as determined by a reduction in cell cluster size.

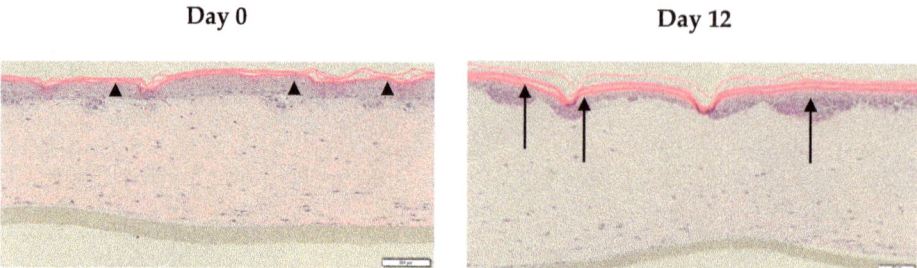

Figure 6. MatTek Melanoma skin model (MLNM-FT-A375) cultivation without treatment. Day 0 (**left**) and day 12 (**right**) of cultivation in our labs. Short arrows indicate the incorporated A375 cells; long arrows indicate some of the melanoma cell clusters at the epidermal–dermal junction, H&E staining, 10× magnification; scale bar 100 µm.

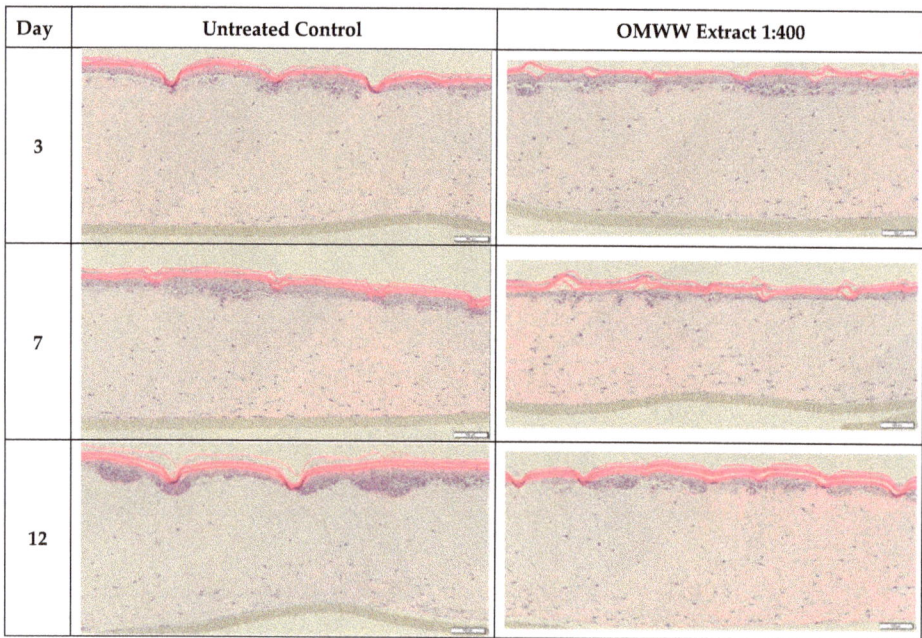

Figure 7. Results of the tumor invasion investigation of the MatTek Melanoma skin model. Skin section with H&E staining, 10× magnification; scale bar 100 µm. Two skin samples per time point and treatment were prepared for histology characterization; a representative cross section is shown.

4. Discussion

Olive mill wastewater is a by-product of olive oil production. Due to the high content of polyphenol in OMWW, the potential health properties are widely discussed and investigated [5,18]. The main polyphenols present in our purified and phenol-enriched OMWW extract are hydroxytyrosol, hydroxytyrosol glycoside, verbascosides, tyrosol, and oleuropein aglycon [Table 1]. The composition of the OMWW extract is essential for health-promoting effects, and strongly depends on the cultivation conditions of olive trees as well as on the applied preparation techniques [8]. Previous studies using this phenol-enriched OMWW extract revealed the anti-angiogenic and angiopreventive activity in endothelial cells [14] and the potential chemo-preventive properties in colon cancer [12]. Polyphenols are associated with several positive effects on cell viability and proliferation, inflammatory processes, microbiological growth and the formation of reactive oxygen species [18]. Therefore, the phenolic-enriched OMWW extract has great potential for dermal application. Based on the experimental conditions of the bacterial count reduction assay by the European Pharmacopoeia [15], a good antibacterial effect against Gram-negative (*E. coli*, *P. aeruginosa*) and Gram-positive bacteria (*S. aureus*, *S. epidermidis*, *P. acnes*) was detected. Regarding the inhibition zone determination, the Gram-negative bacteria were less susceptible to an application of the OMWW extract. This is well in accordance with other published data [19] and might be due to the outer membrane layer of Gram-negative bacteria, which serves as an additional barrier hindering the entrance of antibiotics [19]. The anti-fungal activity against *C. albicans* (yeast) and *A. brasiliensis* (mold) was less pronounced, and an inhibition of growth could be detected using the suspension method. Mahmoudi et al. [19] have already shown the less pronounced anti-microbiological effect of *C. albicans* and *A. brasiliensis* compared to Gram-positive and Gram-negative bacteria with the leaf extract of *Ficus carica*. The difference between the suspension and agar plate method is probably due to the dilution of the OMWW extract by diffusion into the agar medium. The excellent antibacterial activity and moderate anti-fungal activity is based on the high content of hydroxytyrosol and oleuropein in our OMWW extract [3,20]. Due to this antimicrobial effect, the OMWW extract can act as a booster for preservatives in dermal formulations to prevent contamination. Furthermore, this effect may have a positive impact on pathogenic germs on the skin, which are involved in various skin diseases, such as psoriasis or atopic dermatitis. Skin cells are constantly exposed to free radicals and other reactive oxygen species (ROS) caused by normal metabolic processes in the human body or from external sources like UV-radiation, cigarette smoke and air pollutants. An undesirable excess of ROS, called oxidative stress, is involved in inflammatory processes, skin aging and alteration of DNA resulting in skin cancer. Hydroxytyrosol, the major component of the phenol-enriched OMWW extract, is well known for anti-oxidant, anti-inflammatory and anti-tumor effects [18]. Thus, we verified these properties in vitro on human skin cells. The application of the OMWW extract clearly reduced H_2O_2-induced ROS formation in HaCaT cells in a dose-dependent manner; this is in accordance with the results in human umbilical vein endothelial cells by Rossi et al. [14]. Rossi et al. [14] have demonstrated that this phenol-enriched OMWW extract is even more effective in inhibiting ROS formation compared to the polyphenol hydroxytyrosol alone. Among others, inflammatory processes are involved in skin wounds; an excessive or permanent immune reaction can lead to chronic wounds [21]. The regulation of inflammatory mediators such as IL-8 may facilitate the healing process of these skin defects. The TNF-α-induced formation of IL-8 in HaCaT cells was down-regulated by the OMWW extract in a dose-dependent manner. This result is in accordance with the reported down-regulation of IL-8 in colon cancer cells by OMWW and hydroxytyrosol [12]. Several studies reported the anti-tumor activity of polyphenols [14,22,23] and discussed different chemo-preventive mechanisms [24]. Therefore, we investigated the influence of the OMWW extract in a commercially available melanoma skin model (Mattek MLNM FT A375) containing keratinocyte and fibroblast layers with melanoma nodules [25]. The growth and migration of A375, a metastatic melanoma cell line, were restricted during the 12 days. The OMWW extract seems to selectively eliminate the melanoma cells in the full-thickness skin model. Studies on the influence of the OMWW extract on cell viability (monolayer) revealed enhanced NHEK proliferation in contrast to A375 cells after 24 h. Comparable effects have been shown for polyphenols of black tea [26] as well as an induction of apoptosis in several cancer cells by the polyphenol epigallocatechin-3-gallate [27]. Among others, oleuropin and hydroxytyrosol are responsible for this antitumoral effect [28,29].

5. Conclusions

We presented a purified and phenol-enriched OMWW extract, a natural source of polyphenols, as a promising compound for dermal application. Due to its considerable anti-microbial, anti-inflammatory, anti-oxidative and anti-tumor activity, several fields of application are possible. This study evaluated the application of the OMWW extract in a melanoma 3D skin model for the first time. The superiority of the complex polyphenol mixture over the pure substances should be the subject of further investigations with skin cells.

Author Contributions: Conceptualization: P.S. and T.M.S.; Methodology: P.S. and A.P.; Investigation: A.P., S.W. and P.S.; writing—original draft preparation: P.S.; writing—review and editing: A.P., T.M.S., S.W. and P.S.; project administration: T.M.S.; sponsor and funding acquisition: G.L.F., A.L.F. and B.L.F.

Funding: This research received no external funding.

Acknowledgments: We thank Adriana Albini, Department of Medicine and Surgery, University Milano-Bicocca, Milan, Italy and Scientific and Technology Pole, IRCCS MultiMedica, Milan, Italy for her scientific support of the project. We are grateful to Massimo Pizzichini (Genelab srl, ENEA) for the phenol rich purified extract (OMWW extract, A009). We thank Michael Merzhäuser (Biodermic Health & Beauty GmbH & Co. KG, Giessen) for fruitful comments that greatly assisted the cosmetic research.

Conflicts of Interest: The authors declare no conflict of interest and that the sponsors have no role in design of the studies, data collection, analysis and interpretation; in the writing of the manuscript, or in the decision to publish the results.

References

1. Psaltopoulou, T.; Kosti, R.I.; Haidopoulos, D.; Dimopoulos, M.; Panagiotakos, D.B. Olive oil intake is inversely related to cancer prevalence: A systematic review and a meta-analysis of 13800 patients and 23340 controls in 19 observational studies. *Lipids Health Dis.* **2011**, *10*, 127. [CrossRef] [PubMed]
2. Barbaro, B.; Toietta, G.; Maggio, R.; Arciello, M.; Tarocchi, M.; Galli, A.; Balsano, C. Effects of the olive-derived polyphenol oleuropein on human health. *Int. J. Mol. Sci.* **2014**, *15*, 18508–18524. [CrossRef] [PubMed]
3. Bisignano, G.; Tomaino, A.; Cascio, R.L.; Crisafi, G.; Uccella, N.; Saija, A. On the in-vitro antimicrobial activity of oleuropein and hydroxytyrosol. *J. Pharm. Pharmacol.* **1999**, *51*, 971–974. [CrossRef]
4. Caporaso, N.; Formisano, D.; Genovese, A. Use of phenolic compounds from olive mill wastewater as valuable ingredients for functional foods. *Crit. Rev. Food Sci. Nutr.* **2018**, *58*, 2829–2841. [CrossRef] [PubMed]
5. Cicerale, S.; Lucas, L.; Keast, R. Biological activities of phenolic compounds present in virgin olive oil. *Int. J. Mol. Sci.* **2010**, *11*, 458–479. [CrossRef]
6. Souilem, S.; El-Abbassi, A.; Kiai, H.; Hafidi, A.; Sayadi, S.; Galanakis, C.M. Olive oil production sector: Environmental effects and sustainability challenges. *Olive Mill Waste* **2017**. [CrossRef]
7. Mulinacci, N.; Romani, A.; Galardi, C.; Pinelli, P.; Giaccherini, C.; Vincieri, F.F. Polyphenolic content in olive oil waste waters and related olive samples. *J. Agric. Food Chem.* **2001**, *49*, 3509–3514. [CrossRef]
8. Frankel, E.; Bakhouche, A.; Lozano-Sánchez, J.S.; Segura-Carretero, A.; Fernández-Gutiérrez, A. Literature review on production process to obtain extra virgin olive oil enriched in bioactive compounds. Potential use of byproducts as alternative sources of polyphenols. *J. Agric. Food Chem.* **2013**, *61*, 5179–5188. [CrossRef]
9. Ambriz-Pérez, D.L.; Leyva-López, N.; Gutierrez-Grijalva, E.P.; Heredia, J.B. Phenolic compounds: Natural alternative in inflammation treatment. A Review. *Cogent Food Agric.* **2016**, *2*, 1131412.
10. Daglia, M. Polyphenols as antimicrobial agents. *Curr. Opin. Biotechnol.* **2012**, *23*, 174–181. [CrossRef]
11. Raederstorff, D. Antioxidant activity of olive polyphenols in humans: A review. *Int. J. Vitam. Nutr. Res.* **2009**, *79*, 152–165. [CrossRef] [PubMed]
12. Bassani, B.; Rossi, T.; Stefano, D.D.; Pizzichini, D.; Corradino, P.; Macrì, N.; Noonan, D.M.; Albini, A.; Bruno, A. Potential chemopreventive activities of a polyphenol rich purified extract from olive mill wastewater on colon cancer cells. *J. Funct. Foods* **2016**, *27*, 236–248. [CrossRef]
13. Di Mauro, M.D.; Tomasello, B.; Giardina, R.C.; Dattilo, S.; Mazzei, V.; Sinatra, F.; Caruso, M.; D'Antona, N.; Renis, M. Sugar and mineral enriched fraction from olive mill wastewater for promising cosmeceutical application: Characterization, in vitro and in vivo studies. *Food Funct.* **2017**, *8*, 4713–4722. [CrossRef]
14. Rossi, T.; Bassani, B.; Gallo, C.; Maramotti, S.; Noonan, D.; Albini, A.; Bruno, A. Effect of a purified extract of olive mill waste water on endothelial cell proliferation, apoptosis, migration and capillary-like structure in vitro and in vivo. *J. Bioanal. Biomed.* **2015**, *12*, 006.
15. Europäisches Arzneibuch (Pharmacopeia Europaea). *5.1.3 Prüfung auf Ausreichende Antimikrobielle Konservierung*; Ausgabe, Grundwerk 2017; Deutscher Apotheker Verlag: Stuttgart, Germany, 2017; Volume 9.
16. Sun, T.; Jackson, S.; Haycock, J.W.; MacNeil, S. Culture of skin cells in 3D rather than 2D improves their ability to survive exposure to cytotoxic agents. *J. Biotechnol.* **2006**, *122*, 372–381. [CrossRef] [PubMed]

17. Ravi, M.; Paramesh, V.; Kaviya, S.R.; Anuradha, E.; Solomon, F.D. 3D cell culture systems: Advantages and applications. *J. Cell. Physiol.* **2015**, *230*, 16–26. [CrossRef]
18. Obied, H.K.; Prenzler, P.D.; Omar, S.H.; Ismael, R.; Servili, M.; Esposto, S.; Taticchi, A.; Selvaggini, R.; Urbani, S. Pharmacology of olive biophenols. In *Advances in Molecular Toxicology*; Elsevier: Amsterdam, The Netherlands, 2012; pp. 195–242.
19. Mahmoudi, S.; Khali, M.; Benkhaled, A.; Benamirouche, K.; Baiti, I. Phenolic and flavonoid contents, antioxidant and antimicrobial activities of leaf extracts from ten Algerian *Ficus carica* L. varieties. *Asian Pac. J. Trop. Biomed.* **2016**, *6*, 239–245. [CrossRef]
20. Visioli, F.; Bellomo, G.; Galli, C. Free radical-scavenging properties of olive oil polyphenols. *Biochem. Biophys. Res. Commun.* **1998**, *247*, 60–64. [CrossRef]
21. Mast, B.A.; Schultz, G.S. Interactions of cytokines, growth factors, and proteases in acute and chronic wounds. *Wound Repair Regen.* **1996**, *4*, 411–420. [CrossRef]
22. Fabiani, R.; de Bartolomeo, A.; Rosignoli, P.; Servili, M.; Selvaggini, R.; Montedoro, G.F.; di Saverio, C.; Morozzi, G. Virgin olive oil phenols inhibit proliferation of human promyelocytic leukemia cells (HL60) by inducing apoptosis and differentiation. *J. Nutr.* **2006**, *136*, 614–619. [CrossRef]
23. Sirianni, R.; Chimento, A.; Luca, A.d.; Casaburi, I.; Rizza, P.; Onofrio, A.; Iacopetta, D.; Puoci, F.; Andò, S.; Maggiolini, M. Oleuropein and hydroxytyrosol inhibit MCF-7 breast cancer cell proliferation interfering with ERK1/2 activation. *Mol. Nutr. Food Res.* **2010**, *54*, 833–840. [CrossRef]
24. Nichenametla, S.N.; Taruscio, T.G.; Barney, D.L.; Exon, J.H. A Review of the Effects and Mechanisms of Polyphenolics in Cancer. *Crit. Rev. Food Sci. Nutr.* **2006**, *46*, 161–183. [CrossRef]
25. Klausner, M.; Kaluzhny, Y.; Ayehunie, S. Reconstructed human skin model to study melanoma at different stages of progression. *J. Investig. Dermatol.* **2011**, *131*, 75.
26. Halder, B.; Bhattacharya, U.; Mukhopadhyay, S.; Giri, A. Molecular mechanism of black tea polyphenols induced apoptosis in human skin cancer cells: Involvement of Bax translocation and mitochondria mediated death cascade. *Carcinogenesis* **2008**, *29*, 129–138. [CrossRef] [PubMed]
27. Ahmad, N.; Feyes, D.K.; Nieminen, A.L.; Agarwal, R.; Mukhtar, H. Green tea constituent epigallocatechin-3-gallate and induction of apoptosis and cell cycle arrest in human carcinoma cells. *J. Natl. Cancer Inst.* **1997**, *89*, 1881–1886. [CrossRef]
28. Imran, M.; Nadeem, M.; Gilani, S.A.; Khan, S.; Sajid, M.W.; Amir, R.M. Antitumor Perspectives of Oleuropein and Its Metabolite Hydroxytyrosol: Recent Updates. *J. Food Sci.* **2018**, *83*, 1781–1791. [CrossRef] [PubMed]
29. Carrera-González, M.; Ramírez-Expósito, M.J.; Mayas, M.; Martínez-Martos, J.M. Protective role of oleuropein and its metabolite hydroxytyrosol on cancer. *Trends Food Sci. Technol.* **2013**, *31*, 92–99. [CrossRef]

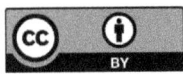

© 2019 by the authors. Licensee MDPI, Basel, Switzerland. This article is an open access article distributed under the terms and conditions of the Creative Commons Attribution (CC BY) license (http://creativecommons.org/licenses/by/4.0/).

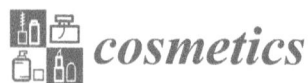

Review

Hop By-Products: Pharmacological Activities and Potential Application as Cosmetics

Olívia R. Pereira [1,2,*], Gleiciara Santos [3] and Maria João Sousa [1,2]

[1] Centro de Investigação de Montanha (CIMO), Instituto Politécnico de Bragança, Campus de Santa Apolónia, 5300-253 Bragança, Portugal
[2] Laboratório Associado para a Sustentabilidade e Tecnologia em Regiões de Montanha (SusTEC), Instituto Politécnico de Bragança, Campus de Santa Apolónia, 5300-253 Bragança, Portugal
[3] School of Health Science, Polytechnic Institute of Bragança, Av. D. Afonso V, 5300-121 Bragança, Portugal
* Correspondence: oliviapereira@ipb.pt; Tel.: +351-273-330-950

Abstract: Hops (*Humulus lupulus* L.) are known worldwide as a raw material in beer production due their flavor and preservative values. The beneficial properties of the plant have been mostly associated with the female hop inflorescences (cones), which is also the part used in the brewing industry. However, some studies indicate the presence of compounds associated with health benefits in the vegetative parts of hops or small-caliber cones, which discarded in hop collection. Moreover, large quantities of by-products remain in the forms of spent grains and spent hops/hot trub and are produced by breweries raising environmental and economic sustainability concerns. This review focuses on the phytochemicals and biological and pharmacological activities of hop and their potential use in skin care products and also intends to explore the potential of the hop' discarded parts and brewery industry by-products for production in the cosmetics industry.

Keywords: *Humulus lupulus* L.; hop; cosmetic; waste valorization; innovative functional ingredients; antioxidant activity; anti-inflammatory activity; antimicrobial activity

Citation: Pereira, O.R.; Santos, G.; Sousa, M.J. Hop By-Products: Pharmacological Activities and Potential Application as Cosmetics. *Cosmetics* **2022**, *9*, 139. https://doi.org/10.3390/cosmetics9060139

Academic Editor: Othmane Merah

Received: 6 November 2022
Accepted: 7 December 2022
Published: 10 December 2022

Publisher's Note: MDPI stays neutral with regard to jurisdictional claims in published maps and institutional affiliations.

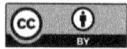

Copyright: © 2022 by the authors. Licensee MDPI, Basel, Switzerland. This article is an open access article distributed under the terms and conditions of the Creative Commons Attribution (CC BY) license (https://creativecommons.org/licenses/by/4.0/).

1. Introduction

The *Humulus lupulus* L. (hop) plant is dioecious (i.e., the male and female flowers usually develop on separate plants); occasional fertile monoecious individual plants have been reported. For brewing beer, viable seeds are undesirable; therefore, only female plants are grown in hops fields to prevent pollination. Female plants are propagated vegetatively, and male plants are culled if plants are grown from seeds. Under natural conditions, the flowers are wind pollinated and the female inflorescence develops to form a strobile (or cone). The strobiles of the female plants are able to develop the lupulin glands that secrete a fine yellow resinous powder. These glands secrete predominantly bitter acids and essential oils, the constituents of which include prenylflavonoids [1,2].

In Europe, there is evidence of the use of *H. lupulus* since prehistoric times. The ancient Romans employed its leaves and inflorescences in some food preparations as well as in textiles and cosmetic products [2]. Afterwards, the use of hop rapidly increased in the Middle Ages, presumably because of their developed utilization in the brewing process. Cultivation of hop began in the mid-ninth century AC in Germany, then spread throughout the Central Europe [3].

According to the latest Food and Agriculture Organization (FAO) estimates, the global area devoted to hop cultivation was around 65,500 ha in 2019, with a production that exceeded 130,000 tons. The European continent contributed decisively to this production, with a volume of almost 68,000 tons, representing 52% of the world hops production [4].

Hop plants are grown almost exclusively for the brewing industry, in which the resins and essential oils from female cones are used for aroma [5]. Female hop flowers, also known as cones or hops, are primarily used in brewing beer; most of the bitter flavor and characteristic zesty beer aromas arise from hop cones added at various points during wort boiling, secondary fermentation, and the aging process [6]. At harvest, one-third is valuable product (hop cones) and two-thirds is leftover biomass, consisting primarily of leaves, stems, and unremoved hop cones [7].

However, the plant has been well-known for its beneficial properties for human health since ancient times. This is due to the plethora of its bioactive compounds (bitter acids, prenyl chalcones, polyphenols, terpenoids, etc.), which are mainly associated with the female inflorescences [8]. On addition to the application in the brewing industry, hop have for a long time been used for various medicinal purposes [9,10]. The beneficial effects of hop polyphenols in various chronic diseases, such as insomnia, inflammation, diabetes, as well as in menopause and as antifungal, have been scientifically proven in many studies [11,12]. In recent years, the antioxidant and anti-inflammatory activities of hop extracts have attracted attention and have been widely studied [9,13].

In order to fill the void in knowledge, the present review provides insight into the valorization of high-volume brewery by-products as well as of leaves, stems, and small-caliber cones, which are commonly discarded in the hops harvest, and we also explore their potential use in cosmetics.

2. Materials and Methods

PubMed, Web of Science (WOS), and Scopus databases were used to perform this review. The keywords used were "*Humulus lupulus*", "hop", "hops", "hops AND waste", "hops by-products", "hops AND bioactivity", "hops AND antioxidant", "hops AND anti-inflammatory", "hops AND antimicrobial", "hops AND cosmetic". We obtained 638 documents with full text access that were published in the last 10 years: 235 in PubMed, 386 in WOS, and 17 in Scopus. Two documents from 2007 and 2009 were added due their relevance to the review. After elimination of duplicates, the documents were selected based on the title, the abstract, and whenever necessary, by reading the whole document, which resulted in 51 documents, including articles, review articles, book chapters and a monograph.

3. Results and Discussion

3.1. By-Products of H. lupulus

Millions of tons of residues are produced in the brewing process. On other hand, large amounts of vegetal material such as leaves, stems, and small-caliber cones are discarded in the harvest process. The recovery or extraction of high-value bioactive compounds from the by-products or non-used parts of *H. lupulus* in the brewing industry has been a strategy emphasized by the recent literature in order to solve this ecological and economical issue [14–16]. In fact, the by-products and parts of the plant discarded in the hops harvest are a source of potential nutritional and pharmacological compounds that could be used as functional and cosmetic ingredients [17]. The traditional methods using organic solvents have concerns related to the environment and also related to health. Still, new eco-friendly extraction methods should be developed to increase the yield and the selectivity of the compounds [14]. Natural, deep eutectic solvents and emerging extraction technologies such as ultrasound-assisted, microwave-assisted, pressurized liquid, and supercritical fluid extraction are emerging solutions to the sustainable extraction and isolation of natural compounds [2,18].

Many components of the hop by-products of interest are proteins, carbohydrates, fiber, phenolic compounds, vitamins, or minerals that have been explored for applications in the food industry [14,16] but less so for the development of skin care products.

3.1.1. Brewery By-Products

Generally, in beer production, chemical and biochemical reactions occur and the process involves the main stages of malting, mashing, lautering, boiling, fermenting, conditioning, filtering, and bottling [14]. During this process, spent grains, spent hops/hot trub, and spent yeast are produced (Figure 1), constituting the main marketable by-products with potential interest for the food, pharmaceutical, cosmetics, agriculture, and chemical industries.

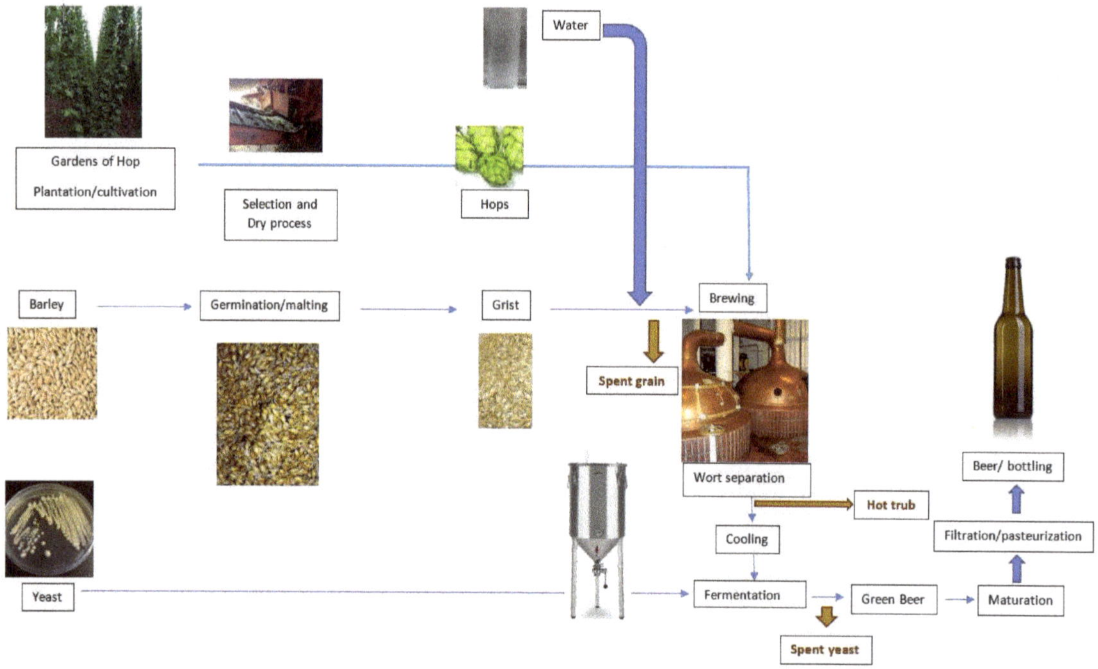

Figure 1. By-products generated in brewing process. Adapted from [14,16].

Spent brewer's grain is formed after the malt mashing process, and in some brewing regimens, some residues of hops are introduced during mashing. Spent brewer's grain is the main solid brewery by-product (accounting for approx. 85% of all residues) which can be used wet and dry as direct animal feed or for further preparation of silage, both used specially for cattle but also for poultry, pigs, goats, and as fish food [14], and less frequently, it is used in human food [19]. Even so, large amounts of spent brewer's grain are discarded despite it being rich in valuable compounds such as proteins (more than 20%), fiber, lipids and fatty acids, carbohydrates, polyphenols (mainly hidroxycinnamic acids), and minerals. In addition to that, it enhances aroma-binding properties and has gelling, emulsifying, and film-forming properties [19].

Approximately 85% of the hops constituents used by beer production become spent hop material. The hot trub are insoluble sediments formed during the wort boiling process [14].

These hops by-products (spent hops or hot trub) have been used as a fertilizer due to the high nitrogen content, as a low-grade fuel, and for animal feed when mixed with spent grain [20].

Although currently the possible markets for spent hops are restricted, hops constitute a by-product rich in interesting compounds such as proteins, lipids, polyphenols, minerals, flavors, carbohydrates, and organic acids [21].

Spent yeast is the second largest by-product from the brewing industry and is obtained after filtration or centrifuging. Originally applied as baker's yeast, currently it is used as fertilizer and as a feedstock for fuel and industrial ethanol production and mixed with spent brewers' grain as a feed material [22].

The chemical composition of spent yeast includes carbohydrates, free amino acids, ash, vitamins and minerals, and fatty acids; it also constitutes an excellent source of high-quality protein [22].

3.1.2. Non-Recovered Parts of *H. lupulus*

As only the hop cones have been used in the beer making industry, hop leaves are an agricultural by-product currently discarded as waste (like the stems and small-caliber cones that are discarded in the hop harvest process) [6].

Leaf sampling from wild-growing hop plants is a far simpler task than collecting cones, which are located up to 10 m off the ground in heavily wooded and overgrown areas and are only present late in the growing season. Additionally, male hop plants do not generate cones. Hop leaves are composed of flavanol glycosides (quercetin and kaempferol derivatives) ranging in total concentration from 0.28% to 2.77% dw (quercetin-3-O-rutinoside equivalents), although the total values are highly dependent on the phenological development stage, sampling date, and physical location [6]. The work of Macchioni et al. [4] showed the presence of significant quantities of soluble polyphenolic compounds and antioxidant pigments in the non-phenolic fraction of hop leaves.

3.2. Bioactivity of H. lupulus

3.2.1. Antioxidant Effects

Hop flavonoids xanthohumol, quercetin, and kaempferol are most responsible for the antioxidant properties of hop [9]. The total phenolic and antioxidant activities of hop extracts are generally determined by well-established methods.

The *H. lupulus* extracts have been explored for a range of biological effects, including antioxidant ability. Studies compiling such criteria are summarized in Table 1.

Acetone extract of cones cultivated in the Czech Republic showed good in vitro antioxidant and anti-adipocyte effects and are dependent on different polyphenols that vary with the time and year of harvest. Concerning individual compounds, the highest percentage of antioxidant capacity, determined with the DPPH radical method among compounds present in hop cones, was demonstrated for procyanidin B2, while xanthohumol showed the highest anti-NO production activity and isorhamnetin showed the best anti-adipocyte differentiation effects [11].

The Cascade variety of hop was also investigated by antioxidant activity using DPPH and ORAC methods. In detail, the study was performed to measure the impact of copper-based fungicides on the antioxidant quality of polar hops extracts (Cascade var.) observed no differences between hops treatments with copper (II) hydroxide [23].

Phenolic-enriched extracts obtained from pellets were also investigated for antioxidant effect by Wu at al. (2020). Ethanolic extracts have shown better antioxidant effects than hot water extracts in DPPH, TEAC, and reducing power assays, which were attributed to higher total phenolic and/or flavonoid compounds [13]. Similar conclusions have been drawn after antioxidant experiments with three Poland hop cultivars. The cones of Magnum demonstrated higher antioxidant activity, which is consistent with the higher phenolic acids and flavonol contents [24].

Table 1. Antioxidant activities of hop extracts.

Hop Variety/Part of Plant	Solvent Extraction (Compounds)	Methods/Studied Effects	Results of Assay	Ref.
Saaz hops/cones	Acetone/water (70:30, v/v) (polyphenols)	In vitro DPPH	DPPH (% of inhibition) = 45–60 (at 25 µg/mL)	[11]
Cascade var./cones	Aqueous ethanol (80:20 v/v)	In vitro DPPH ORAC	DPPH (µmol Trolox/g extract): 1.47 ± 0.11 (control), 1.50 ± 0.11 (low copper) 1.52 ± 0.14 (high copper) ORAC (µmol Trolox/g extract): 501.4 ± 45.69 (control), 490.7 ± 61.79 (low copper) and 491.3 ± 33.03 (high copper)	[23]
Pellets/cones	Hops hot water (HWE); Hops ethanol (HEE) (polyphenols, flavonoids)	In vitro DPPH TEAC RP	DPPH, IC_{50} (µg mL^{-1}): 93.12 (95% HEE) TEAC, IC_{50} (µg mL^{-1}): 948.55 (55% HEE); 956.43 (95% HEE); RP, %: 8.78 (55% HEE)	[13]
Magnum var. (M), Lubelski var. (L), and Marynka var. (Ma)/cones	Hot water and aqueous ethanol (60:40) (v/v) extracts (Phenolic acids, epicatechin and rutin)	In vitro Chelating activity DPPH ABTS	Chelating activity (%): ~90 for M ethanol extract at 2000 ppm DPPH (EC_{50}, µg/mL): 0.31, 0.38 and 0.44 for L, Ma, and L water extracts, respectively ABTS (EC_{50}, µg/mL): 0.92, 0.93, and 0.99 for M, L and Ma ethanol extracts, respectively	[24]
Aurora var. and Hallertauer Magnum var./leaves and cones	Ethanol extracts	In vitro DPPH FRAP	DPPH (IC_{50} mg/mL): ~0.01–0.043 (leaves); ~0.005–0.017 (cones) FRAP (mL µgferric ions): 0.055–0.2 (leaves); 0.05–0.33 (cones)	[25]
Young hop shoots	Methanol (flavonol glycosides)	In vitro DPPH Photochemiluminescence assay (PCL-ACL)	DPPH: 0.3–0.5 mg Trolox equivalents/g PC-L-ACL: 1.1–0.7 mg Trolox equivalents/g	[26]
Brewing spent grains (BSGs), Brewing spent hops (BSH)	Spent grains (phenolic acids), Spent hop (phenolic acids)	In vitro FRAP DPPH ABTS	FRAP, DPPH, ABTS (EC_{50}, g/L): BSG-IRA: 7.00, 23.09 and 8.52, respectively BSG-BSA: 5.18, 11.61 and 4.67, respectively BSH-IRA: 7.28, 12.35 and 5.40, respectively BSH-BSA: 6.11, 9.14 and 4.38, respectively	[21]

Table 1. Cont.

Hop Variety/Part of Plant	Solvent Extraction (Compounds)	Methods/Studied Effects	Results of Assay	Ref.
Cones	Aqueous ethanol (60:40) v/v (Proanthocyanidins, flavonoid glycosides, xanthohumol)	In vitro DPPH •OH– $O_2^{\bullet-}$ DNA oxidative damage In vivo TBARS, SOD and GSH-Px activity in mouse liver	DPPH, •OH–, $O_2^{\bullet-}$ (IC_{50} (μg mL^{-1}): 6.7, 34.0, and 690.0, respectively DNA oxidation damage: inhibited by extract TBARS (nmol mg^{-1} protein): 8.73 (HPE200), 6.20 (HPE400), 5.93 (HPE800) SOD (U mg^{-1} protein): 630.9 (HPE200), 658.9 (HPE400), 686.6 (HPE800) GSH-Px (U mg^{-1} protein): 657.1 (HPE200), 822.0 (HPE400), 838.3 (HPE800)	[27]
Cones	Supercritical hop CO_2-extract (Humulone, lupulone)	In vitro Irradiated human primary keratinocytes (HPKs)	↓ formation of ROS-induced dichlorofluorescein IC_{50} (μg/mL) = 29.43	[28]
Chinook var., Centennial var., Comet var., Columbus var., Cascade var./Leaves	Ethanol (oven drying (OD) at 45 °C and freeze-drying (FD))	In vitro DPPH ABTS	DPPH (EC_{50}, μg/mL) = 103–291 μg mL^{-1} (Chinook var. FD and Columbus var. OD, respectively) ABTS (EC_{50}, μg/mL): 1.15–15.6 μg mL^{-1} (Columbus var. FD and Comet var. OD, respectively)	[4]
Hop by-products	Water and aqueous ethanol (30:70) (v/v)	In vitro DPPH, FRAP, ABTS keratinocytes HaCaT cells	Spent malt: DPPH (μmol TE/g): 10.24 ± 1.35 (ethanol extract, Maior); ABTS (μmol TE/g): 21.72 ± 2.16 (ethanol extract, Alter); FRAP (μmol TE/g): 67.71 ± 1.44 (Water extract, Ego) Spent hops: DPPH (μmol TE/g): 7.579 ± 0.436 (ethanol extract, Ego); ABTS (μmol TE/g): 8.26 ± 1.32 (water extract, Ego); FRAP (μmol TE/g): 102.66 ± 3.99 (water extract, Ego) Spent yeast: DPPH (μmol TE/g): 58.68 ± 11.57 (ethanol extract, Ubi); ABTS (μmol TE/g): 51.31 ± 3.05 (water extract, Triplo malto); FRAP (μmol TE/g): 136.72 ± 2.91 (water extract, ubi) HaCaT cells: decrease mitochondrial activity; reduction of intracellular ROS formation	[29]

ABTS—2,2'-azino-bis-(3-ethylbenzothiazoline-6-sulphonic acid) radical scavenging assay; BSGs—brewing spent grains; BSH—brewing spent hop; BSA—Belgian strong ale beers; DPPH—2,2-diphenyl-1-picrylhydrazyl radical scavenging assay; EC_{50}—Half-maximal effective concentration; FRAP—ferric reducing antioxidant power; FD—freeze-drying; GSH-Px—gglutathione peroxidase; HPKs—human primary keratinocytes; HWE—hops water extract; HEE—hops ethanol extract; IC_{50}—Half-maximal inhibitory concentration; IRA—brewing of imperial red ale beer; PCL-ACL—photochemiluminescence assay; TBARS—thiobarbituric acid reactive substances assay; SOD—superoxide dismutase; •OH—hydroxyl radical scavenging assay; $O_2^{\bullet-}$—superoxide radical scavenging assay; ORAC—oxygen radical absorbance capacity; OD—oven-drying; RP—reducing power; ROS—reactive oxygen species; TE—Trolox equivalent; TEAC—Trolox equivalent absorbance capacity; TPA—12-O-Tetradecanoylphorbol-13-acetate; ↓—decrease.

Despite most studies being carried out on cones, there are some experiments performed with the non-recovered parts of *H. lupulus* and with brewery by-products. In more detail, hop young shoots from northern regions of Italy, composed of quercetin and kaempferol glycosides, have been studied in terms of antioxidant activity by means of PCL-ACL and DPPH assays. Vicchio hop shoot samples had the greatest number of antioxidants, followed by Santa Maria in Punta and Cologna. In addition, the data regarding antioxidant activity have a good correlation with the total flavonol content (r^2 of 0.9577) [26].

The antioxidant properties of hop leaf were investigated for ethanolic extracts, concluding that the antioxidant activity was lower for leaves than for hop cones [25]. An antioxidant study performed on the leaves of four varieties of hop showed the best antioxidant activities for freeze-dried extracts of Chinook var. and Columbus varieties and for oven-dried extracts of Columbus and Comet varieties [4].

On the other hand, the brewing by-products, spent grains, and spent hops have shown high antioxidant activity and the authors attributed the effect to the content of the phenolic compounds, mainly in Belgian strong ale samples [21].

Hop cones extracts rich in polyphenols, such as proanthocyanidins, flavonoid glycosides, and xanthohumol, have demonstrated important in vitro and in vivo protection from oxidation and from mutagenesis, with similar effects to green tea polyphenols [27].

3.2.2. Anti-Inflammatory Effects

Table 2 describes the anti-inflammatory effects of hop and spent hops extracts. When the inflammatory response occurs, excess NO production accelerates the formation of superoxide to damage tissues and DNA and further cause diseases. Therefore, scavenging NO is beneficial to decrease the damage. A cellular assay performed in murine macrophage J774.1 cells by Inui et al. showed anti-NO production activity of cones extract and also anti-adipocyte differentiation effects in murine pre-adipocyte 3T3-L1 cells (at 75 µg/mL for both assays). Moreover, xanthohumol and isorhamnetin were indicated as important compounds in those effects [11].

During the inflammatory response, pro-inflammatory cytokines such as tumor necrosis factor-α (TNF-α), IL-1β, and IL-6 are released and involved in the development of inflammatory and pathological diseases [2]. Therefore, the inhibition of pro-inflammatory cytokines is a method to improve inflammatory symptoms. Phenolic-enriched hot water extract and ethanol extract of hops pellets have been investigated for anti-inflammatory activities, and both have demonstrated the in vitro capacity to decrease NO production. Moreover, the hot water extract decreased the pro-inflammatory cytokines TNF-α and IL-6 secretion, while the ethanol extract decreased IL-1β and IL-6 secretion [13].

Table 2. Anti-inflammatory activities of hop extracts.

Hop Variety/Part of Plant	Solvent Extraction (Compounds)	Methods/Studied Effects	Results of Assay	Ref.
Cones	Acetone/water (70:30, v/v) (polyphenols)	In vitro Anti-NO murine macrophage J774.1 cells Anti-adipocyte differentiation (Murine pre-adipocyte 3T3-L1 cells)	Anti-NO production activity (%) = 20–60 (at 75 µg/mL), anti-adipocyte differentiation (%) = 15–70 (at 75 µg/mL)	[11]
Pellets/Cones	Hops hot water (HWE); Hops ethanol (HEE) (polyphenols)	In vitro NO production Pro-inflammatory cytokine secretion	↓ NO production: 20 and 40 µg mL^{-1} (HEE) Pro-inflammatory cytokine secretion ↓ TNF-α: up to 400 µg mL^{-1} (HWE) ↓ IL-1β: 5 to 40 µg mL^{-1} (HEE) ↓ IL-6: 50 to 400 µg mL^{-1} (HWE); 5 to 40 µg mL^{-1} HEE)	[13]
META060/Hops extract	Reduced iso-α acid	In vitro Endothelial and monocyte cell models	Inhibited cell adhesion (10 µg/mL) Inhibited expression of IL-6, IL-8, MCP-1, RANTES, IL-1β, IL-10, MIP-1α, and MMP-9 (1–20 µg/mL)	[30]
Hallertauer Magnum var./Cones	Hexane and methanol (phloroglucinol derivatives), xanthohumol, flavanones, flavonol glycosides, triterpenoids)	In vivo TPA-Induced Inflammation in mice	Anti-inflammatory activity similar to indomethacin: ID$_{50}$ = 0.13–1.06 µmol/ear (All studied compounds except astragallin and quercitrin) ID$_{50}$ = 0.91 µmol/ear (indomethacin)	[31]
Cascade var./Cones	Methanol/water (80:20) (v/v) and acetone (prenylated compounds)	In vitro Pro-inflammatory enzymes, microsomal mPGES-1 5-LO	5-LO cell-free (IC$_{50}$, µM) = 2.1 (xanthohumol); 5.9 (4-hydroxycolupulone) 5-LO cell-based (IC$_{50}$, µM) = 2.9 (xanthohumol); >10 (4-hydroxycolupulone) mPGES-1 (residual activity at 10 µM) = 32.3 (xanthohumol); 32.8 (4-hydroxycolupulone)	[32]
Cones	Supercritical hops CO$_2$-extract (humulone, lupulone)	In vitro Irradiated human primary keratinocytes (HPKs)	↓ IL-6 expression: IC$_{50}$: 0.8 µg/mL	[28]
Spent hops	Basal diet supplemented with 1% spent hops	Randomized, controlled trial in pigs	↓ Expression of pro-inflammatory genes: IL1β, IL8, and TNF	[33]

HPKs—human primary keratinocytes; HWE—hops water extract; HEE—hops ethanol extract; IC$_{50}$—half-maximal inhibitory concentration; ID$_{50}$—inhibitory dose; IL—interleukin; 5-LO—5-lipoxygenase; mPGES-1—microsomal prostaglandin E2 synthase; MCP-1—monocyte chemoattractant protein-1; MIP-1α—macrophage inflammatory protein 1α; MMP-9—matrix metallopeptidase 9; NO—nitric oxide; RANTES—regulated on activation, normal T cell expressed and secreted; TPA—12-O-Tetradecanoylphorbol-13-acetate; TNF-α—tumor necrosis factor α; ↓—decrease.

META060, a reduced iso-α acid derived from an extract of *H. lupulus*, showed anti-inflammatory effects in endothelial and monocyte cell models. In detail, it was effective for inhibiting TNF-α-induced expression of many inflammatory factors such as IL-1β, MCP-1, RANTES in HAECs, and THP-1 cells. In addition to that, META060 inhibited expression and activity of MMP-9 [30]. A randomized, controlled trial aimed to determine the effect of spent hops on the expression of pro-inflammatory genes in the intestine of pigs showed the reduction of the mRNA concentrations of IL1β and IL8 in the duodenum, of IL1β and IL8 in the ileum, and of IL1β and TNF in the colon in pigs fed with spent hops [33].

The potential anti-inflammatory activity of a hop cone CO_2 extract composed of 50% humulone and lupulone was determined. After solar irradiation of human primary keratinocytes, the extract showed a reduction in IL-6 expression with an IC_{50} of 0.8 µg/mL [28].

Compounds obtained from cones of the Cascade var. of hop exerted marked effects on key enzymes of eicosanoid biosynthesis. In detail, xanthohumol and 4-hydroxycolupulone showed a capacity to inhibit in vitro the pro-inflammatory target enzymes prostaglandin E2 synthase (mPGES)-1 and 5-lipoxygenase (5-LO) [32]. Xanthohumol showed an effective inhibition of 5-LO with an IC_{50} of 2.9 µM, and together with 4-hydroxycolupulone, were the two most active compounds in inhibiting mPGES-1. The phenolic compounds isolated from an extract of the Magnum var. of hops, i.e., phloroglucinol derivatives, xanthohumol, flavanones, flavonol glycosides, and triterpenoids, have shown important anti-inflammatory activity in TPA-induced inflammation in a mouse model. In fact, almost all of the isolated compounds showed anti-inflammatory activities (ID_{50} = 0.13–1.06 µmol/ear) similar to or higher than indomethacin (ID_{50} = 0.91 µmol/ear), which was used as positive control [31].

3.2.3. Antimicrobial Effects

Antimicrobial effects have been described for the hop plants and its components (Table 3). In detail, a hops CO_2 extract was proved to be effective against bacteria responsible for acne, such as *Propionibacterium acnes* (*P. acnes*) and *Staphylococcus aureus* (*S. aureus*), including MRSA (methicillin-resistant strains), and also *Bacillus anthracis*, *Bacillus subtilis*, *Corynebacterium diphteriae*, *Sarcina lutea* and *Lactobacillus brevis*. In addition to that, a gel formulation with 0.3% hops extract (w/w) showed antibacterial activity superior to that of the placebo gel [28].

S. aureus and *Staphylococcus epidermidis* were sensitive mainly to aqueous extracts of the cones of Magnum, Lubelski, and Marynka varieties [24]. Low values of minimal inhibitory concentrations (MICs) against *S. aureus* of ethanol extracts from different countries of hop cones of cv. 'Aurora' and cv. 'H. Magnum' showed high antimicrobial activities [25].

A hydroalcoholic extract obtained from female inflorescences (hops) of *H. lupulus* has shown the inhibition bacterial capacity by diffusion methods. In detail, from the Gram-positive bacterial strains tested, the larger inhibition area was observed against *B. subtilis* (~8mm), similar to the positive control vancomycin (30 µg) and for *S. aureus* (~4.5mm for the extract; ~6mm for the same positive control). A similar effect was observed for *E. coli* (gram negative bacteria) with ~4.5mm of the inhibition zone against ~14mm rifampicin used as positive control [34].

Table 3. Antimicrobial activities of hop extracts.

Hop Variety/Part of Plant	Solvent Extraction (Compounds)	Methods/Studied Effects	Results of Assay	Ref.
Magnum var., Lubelski var., Marynka var./Cones	Ethanol/water (40%), Water, 85 °C (chlorogenic acid, o-coumaric, p-coumaric, cinnamic, and syringic acid, epicatechin, rutin, quercetin and kaempferol)	In vitro Well-diffusion method	*Staphylococcus aureus* ATCC 25923 Inhibition growth area [mm] = 18, 27, 39 (water extracts of Lubelski, Marynka, and Magnum varieties, respectively) *Staphylococcus aureus* clinical isolates Inhibition growth area [mm] = 11, 22, 28 (water extracts of Lubelski, Marynka, and Magnum varieties, respectively) *Staphylococcus epidermidis* ATCC 12228 Inhibition growth area [mm] = 12, 31, 34 (water extracts of Lubelski, Marynka, and Magnum varieties, respectively) *Staphylococcus epidermidis* clinical isolates Inhibition growth area [mm] = 8, 26, 25 (water extracts of Lubelski, Marynka, and Magnum varieties, respectively)	[24]
Cones	Supercritical hops CO_2-extract (humulone, lupulone)	In vitro Broth microdilution method	*P. acnes* MIC = 3.1 µg/mL Inhibition growth area gel = 5.5 mm *S. aureus* MIC = 9.4 µg/mL Inhibition growth area gel = 3 mm	[28]
Cones	Ethanol/water (70:20) (v/v)	In vitro Disc diffusion method	*B. subtilis* Inhibition growth = ~8mm *S. aureus* and *E. coli* Inhibition growth = ~4.5mm (for both)	[34]
Cones/prenylated phenolic compound	Hydro-ethanolic	In vitro Antibacterial; Antiparasitic	*Corynebacterium*, *Enterococcus*, *Mycobacterium*, *Staphylococcus* and *Streptococcus* strains MICs = 39–156 µg/mL *T. brucei* IC_{50} = <1 to 11 µg/mL	[35]
Aurora var. and Hallertauer Magnum var./Leaves and cones	Ethanol	In vitro Broth microdilution method	*S. aureus* MIC = 0.0013–0.0029 mg/mL (cones); 0.22–0.44 mg/mL (leaves) *E. coli* MIC = 0.19–0.43 mg/mL (cones); 0.16–0.44 mg/mL (leaves)	[25]

Table 3. Cont.

Hop Variety/Part of Plant	Solvent Extraction (Compounds)	Methods/Studied Effects	Results of Assay	Ref.
Hop/Isoxanthohumol	Ethanol	In vitro Mycelium growth inhibition method	Antifungal activity: 37.01~51.52% (*H. lupulus* at 500 µg/mL) EC_{50} = 4.32, 14.52 and 16.50 µg/mL (Isoxanthohumol agains *B. cinerea*, *S. sclerotiorum* and *F. graminearum*, respectively)	[12]
Cones	Hydro-ethanolic (rutin, syringic acid)	In vitro Anti-influenza activity	Antiviral effect during the 1 h infection PR8, NWS, and ULSTER strains (46%, 50%, and 29% of inhibition, respectively). Antiviral effect after the infection pH1N1, PR8, and ULSTER titer (75%, 44% and 29% reduction, respectively).	[36]
Purified hop fractions	(α-bitter acids, β-bitter acids and xanthohumol)	In vitro Standard testing protocols EUCAST	Antibacterial effect: xanthohumol MICs = 4–7.5 mg/L β-bitter acids MICs = 0.5–15 mg/L α-bitter acids MICs = 30–60 mg/L	[37]
Aerial parts	Supercritical carbon dioxide ($scCO_2$) extracts and 75% ethanol extracts (cohumulinic acid, dehydrocohumulinic acid, hulupone, lupulone)	In vitro CellTiter-Glo® LuminescencenAssay	*E. coli* $scCO_2$ extracts are more active than the ethanol extracts	[38]
Hallertauer Magnum var./Cones	Supercritical hops extract	In vitro Agar-dilution assay	MICs = 6.25 and 25 µg/mL (*Corynebacterium xerosis* and *S. epidermidis*, respectively)	[39]
Hop bract polyphenols (HBP)	Mouthrinse containing 0.1% HBP	Randomized, controlled trial Patient hygiene Performance score	Reduction amount of plaque score ($p < 0.001$) Reduction the number of *Mutans streptococci* in the plaque samples ($p < 0.05$)	[40]
Hallertauer Magnum var./Cones	Hops and zinc ricinoleate	Clinical study ASTM method E 1207-87 in 42 human volunteers	Malodor score: 6.28 (±0.70) (control) to: 1.80 (±0.71) (8 h of extract application), 1.82 (±0.74) (12 h of extract application), 2.24 (±0.77) (24 h of extract application)	[39]

EC_{50}—Half-maximal effective concentration; EUCAST—European Committee on Antimicrobial Susceptibility Testing; HBP—hops bract polyphenols; MIC—minimum inhibitory concentration; NWS—A/NWS/33 H1N1; pH1N1—pandemic A/California/04/09 H1N1; PR8—human A/Puerto Rico/8/34 H1N1; ULSTER—avian Parrot/Ulster/73 H7N1.

In another study, the antibacterial properties of the *H. lupulus* were tested against *Escherichia coli* (*E. coli*), a standard model for bacteria studies. The extracts were tested on bacterial cells starting from a concentration of 40 mg/mL with a serial two-fold dilution. In detail, hops leaf supercritical carbon dioxide (scCO$_2$) extracts inhibited the growth of bacterial cells more than 75% while ethanol extracts never exceeded 60% of growth inhibition. In addition to that, the scCO$_2$ extraction of hop leaves could be used to obtain innovative functional ingredients by valorizing low-value agro-waste [38]. In these extracts, cohumulinic acid, dehydrocohumulinic acid, hulupone, and lupulone are the more representative compounds that may play an important role in the antibacterial effect. In fact, Weber et al. identified hops bitter acids α- and β-acids and their derivatives as important antimicrobial agents, probably due to their highly hydrophobic character that induces leakage of the bacterial membrane [28].

Essential oils have been described as potent antimicrobial agents. In fact, Jeliazkova et al. [41] reported that *E. coli* and *S. aureus* were strongly inhibited by essential oil fractions of hops after 0 to 30 min.

Mizobuchi reported that xanthohumol and 6-isopentenylnaringenin can inhibit the growth of *S. aureus* with an MIC value of 6.25 μg/mL, while that of isoxanthohumol is 50.0 μg/mL. According to Bocquet et al., it was possible to demonstrate that desmethylxanthohumol in *H. lupulus* has antifungal activity against *Zymoseptoria tritici* (MIC value of 0.63 g/L) [42]. Additionally, it was found that xanthohumol can inhibit the growth of three *Fusarium* species, with MIC values from 0.015 to 0.100 mg/mL [43]. Additionally, Yin-Fang Yan showed in his work that ethanolic extracts of *H. lupulus* showed moderate antifungal activity against pathogenic fungi, while isoxanthohumol, an isoprene flavonoid from *H. lupulus*, showed high antifungal activity, in particular against *B. cinerea*. The study suggests isoxanthohumol as a potential botanical fungicide for the management of phytopathogenic fungi [12].

The results of Bocquet and co-workers also showed an inhibition close to 100% at the MIC for the selected MRSA clinical isolate. In addition, it was also demonstrated that a previous formation of the biofilm does not prevent hops compounds from acting on bacteria. In both cases, desmethylxanthohumol and lupulone seem to be more effective than xanthohumol, with an inhibition of the biofilm formation and a biofilm destruction at sub-inhibitory concentrations [35].

According to Sotto et al. the hydroalcoholic extract from *H. lupulus* (female inflorescences) have the ability to directly counteract viral replication and viral protein synthesis and indirectly increase host cell defense due to its phenolic content [36].

In 2018, Bogdanova and co-workers showed that a purified fractions of hop composed by α-bitter acids (humulones), β-bitter acids (lupulones), and xanthohumol were effective against reference strains of Gram-positive bacteria and also against their methicillin- and vancomycin-resistant variants, although no effect was detected against Gram-negative bacterial strains. Xanthohumol was the hop fraction with more antimicrobial activity. Hop compounds have antimicrobial effects at concentrations lower than the determined MICs, with the biggest effect from α-bitter acids on enterococci [37].

3.3. H. lupulus and By-Products as Cosmetics

Herbal products and/or it active compounds have been used as ingredients for cosmetics formulations [44]. Recent scientific studies confirm the use of hop extracts for treating acne, loose skin, stretch marks and sagging, preventing skin aging, and as hair cosmetics [2,45,46].

As previous described, hop cones and also other parts of the plant or brewery by-products have been described as enriched in antioxidant, anti-inflammatory and antimicrobial compounds, with these properties being crucial for skincare formulations [44]. Other properties such as antioxidant protective effects in keratinocytes models, in vitro and cellular tyrosinase inhibition, intracellular melanin inhibition, and anti-odor and anti-acne effects, have been reported.

In detail, trehalose, a polysaccharide that could be used as bio-protectant in cosmetic formulations, has been recovered from spent hops [18]. Moreover, the improvement in the mitochondrial activity and the prevention of oxidative stress of spent hops extracts and yeast extracts was proved in an in vitro assay in keratinocytes HaCaT [29].

The antimicrobial effects of hop and their constituents against oral pathogens such as *Streptococcus mutans*, *S. salivarius*, *S. sanguinis*, *Porphyromonas gingivalis*, *Lactobacilli* and also *Candida albicans* have also been described [47].

A randomized controlled trial performed with 29 healthy male volunteers showed the inhibitory effects of a mouthrinse containing 0.1% hops bract polyphenols. In fact, a significant reduction in the mean amount of plaque was verified after volunteers used the mouthrinse [40].

The deodorant effect of hops extracts has been demonstrated in in vitro and in vivo studies. In detail, antibacterial activity of a *H. lupulus* extract against *Corynebacterium xerosis* and *Staphylococcus epidermidis* showed minimum inhibitory concentration values of 6.25 and 25 µg/mL in an agar-dilution assay. The in vivo axillary deodorant effect was evaluated with the ASTM method E 1207-87 Standard Practice for the Sensory Evaluation of Axillary Deodorancy of a hops/zinc ricinoleate-containing formulation. The mean malodor score dropped from 6.28 (±0.70) to 1.80 (±0.71), 1.82 (±0.74), and 2.24 after 8 h, 12 h, and 24 of the application, respectively [39].

In a recent study, a gel formulation with 0.3% hops extract (w/w) showed antibacterial activity in the agar-diffusion test against *P. acnes* and *S. aureus* (inhibition zone values: 5.5 mm and 3 mm, respectively). Therefore, hops extract might be an alternative treatment option for acne-prone skin [28]. A formulation of shower gels based on CO_2 extracts of hop cones was created, and its skin-conditioning properties were attributed to their bioactive compounds [48].

Weber et al. performed an in vitro assay on a human primary keratinocytes (HPKs) model with a supercritical hops CO_2 extract rich in hops bitter acids α- and β-acids. The extract was shown to be able to reduce the formation ROS induced in a concentration-dependent manner, and with similar effect to the flavonoid luteolin. In adition to that, the extract showed strong inhibitory effects in reducing pro-inflammatory cytokine IL-6 production, with an effect comparable to the positive control luteolin [28].

Another described effect of hops is their tyrosinase inhibition ability, which makes them promising whitening agents for the cosmetics industry. A study performed by Liu et al., showed a tyrosinase inhibition of hops-enriched tannins extract with a comparable effect to kojic acid, recognized as stronger tyrosinase inhibitor (IC_{50} = 76.52 ± 6.56 µM and 49.54 ± 2.08 µM, respecytively) [49]. In cellular assays, the tannin extract showed intracellular tyrosinase inhibition and intracellular melanin inhibition in a dose-dependent manner (70% and 35% for 10 µM, respectively). Another study showed the in vitro depigmenting effect of xanthohumol, a prenylated flavonoid of hops. In fact, low micromolar concentrations of xanthohumol were able to inhibit melanogenesis in human melanocytes by targeting melanin export and also by melanin degradation [50].

Although the limited scientific data related to the application of hop ingredients in skin products, the properties described for hop plant extracts or brewery by-products and also for their active compounds makes hop a promising ingredient for skincare cosmetics. However, some studies suggest occupational dermatitis related to hop harvesting, and there are some questions about oral animal ingestion. This point must also be better explored before proposing any extract or component as a cosmetics ingredient [47,51].

In this context, the extracts or isolated compounds must fulfil the Cosmetics Regulation related to the safety of cosmetics ingredients (EC 1223/2009) and also the Directive 2004/24/EC if the natural ingredients are used as herbal medicinal products. The regulations cover the choice of the ingredients, manufacturing (according to Good Manufacturing Practices), and product commercialization. The Cosmetics Regulation ensures the equality and immediate access to the market and the free circulation throughout the European Union. Additionally, define the 'responsible person' comprising a person or company who places the cosmetic product on the market and is responsible for that product ensures the safety of the product and compliance with the Cosmetics Regulation requirements.

4. Conclusions

In hop cultivation as a brewery industry raw material, just the hop cones are the valuable product, leaving about two-thirds of the crop as almost unexploited biomass. On the other hand, applying the high-volume brewery by-products to develop new innovative products would be useful for waste management and the environment. Hop plant and brewery by-products are sources of bioactive compounds with proved antioxidant, anti-inflammatory, and antimicrobial activities. In addition, extracts of hop have been proposed as whitening, anti-odor, and anti-acne agents. Polar extracts obtained by hop or their by-products are rich in polyphenols (e.g., phenolic acids, phloroglucinol derivatives, flavanones, flavonol glycosides and terpenes), while supercritical carbon dioxide extracts contain mainly hop bitter acids (α- and β-acids). These compounds, along with those present in essential oils, have been the most associated with the described effects. However, this review showed that the beneficial effects of hop plants and their by-products have been mainly assessed in in vitro experiments, emphasizing the need to be tested in animal models and further with randomized, double-blind and placebo-controlled studies.

Author Contributions: G.S. contributed to the literature review and the initial draft; O.R.P. and M.J.S. contributed to supervision and writing—reviewing and editing. All authors have read and agreed to the published version of the manuscript.

Funding: The authors are grateful to the Foundation for Science and Technology (FCT, Portugal) for financial support through national funds FCT/MCTES (PIDDAC) to CIMO (UIDB/00690/2020, UIDP/00690/2020 and EXPL2021CIMO_06) and SusTEC (LA/P/0007/2020).

Institutional Review Board Statement: Not applicable.

Informed Consent Statement: Not applicable.

Data Availability Statement: Not applicable.

Conflicts of Interest: The authors declare no conflict of interest.

References

1. Committee on Herbal Medicinal Products Assessment report on *Humulus lupulus* L., flos. *Eur. Med. Agency* **2014**, *44*, 1–38.
2. Astray, G.; Gullón, P.; Gullón, B.; Munekata, P.E.S.; Lorenzo, J.M. *Humulus lupulus* L. as a natural source of functional biomolecules. *Appl. Sci.* **2020**, *10*, 5074. [CrossRef]
3. Santagostini, L.; Caporali, E.; Giuliani, C.; Bottoni, M.; Ascrizzi, R.; Araneo, S.R.; Papini, A.; Flamini, G.; Fico, G. *Humulus lupulus* L. cv. Cascade grown in Northern Italy: Morphological and phytochemical characterization. *Plant Biosyst.* **2020**, *154*, 316–325. [CrossRef]
4. Macchioni, V.; Picchi, V. Hop Leaves as an Alternative Source of Health-Active Compounds: Effect of Genotype and Drying Conditions. *Plants* **2022**, *11*, 99. [CrossRef] [PubMed]
5. Almaguer, C.; Schönberger, C.; Gastl, M.; Arendt, E.K.; Becker, T. *Humulus lupulus*—A story that begs to be told. A review. *J. Inst. Brew.* **2014**, *120*, 289–314. [CrossRef]
6. Mccallum, J.L.; Nabuurs, M.H.; Gallant, S.T.; Kirby, C.W.; Mills, A.A.S. Phytochemical Characterization of Wild Hops (*Humulus lupulus* ssp. lupuloides) Germplasm Resources from the Maritimes Region of Canada. *Front. Plant Sci.* **2019**, *10*, 1438. [CrossRef]
7. Hrnčič, M.K.; Španinger, E.; Košir, I.J.; Knez, Ž.; Bren, U. Hop compounds: Extraction techniques, chemical analyses, antioxidative, antimicrobial, and anticarcinogenic effects. *Nutrients* **2019**, *11*, 257. [CrossRef]
8. Muzykiewicz, A.; Nowak, A.; Zielonka-brzezicka, J.; Duchnik, W.; Klimowicz, A. Comparison of antioxidant activity of extracts of hop leaves harvested in different years. *Herba Pol.* **2019**, *65*, 1–9. [CrossRef]
9. Zugravu, C.; Bohiltea, R.; Salmen, T.; Pogurschi, E. Antioxidants in Hops: Bioavailability, Health Effects and Perspectives for New Products. *Antioxidants* **2022**, *11*, 241. [CrossRef]
10. Liu, M.; Hansen, P.E.; Wang, G.; Qiu, L.; Dong, J.; Yin, H.; Qian, Z.; Yang, M.; Miao, J. Pharmacological profile of xanthohumol, a prenylated flavonoid from hops (*Humulus lupulus*). *Molecules* **2015**, *20*, 754–779. [CrossRef]
11. Inui, T.; Okumura, K.; Matsui, H.; Hosoya, T.; Kumazawa, S. Effect of harvest time on some In Vitro functional properties of hop polyphenols. *Food Chem.* **2017**, *225*, 69–76. [CrossRef]
12. Yan, Y.-F.; Wu, T.-L.; Du, S.-S. The Antifungal Mechanism of Isoxanthohumol from *H. lupulus* Linn. *Int. J. Mol. Sci.* **2021**, *22*, 10853. [CrossRef]

13. Wu, C.N.; Sun, L.C.; Chu, Y.L.; Yu, R.C.; Hsieh, C.W.; Hsu, H.Y.; Hsu, F.C.; Cheng, K.C. Bioactive compounds with anti-oxidative and anti-inflammatory activities of hop extracts. *Food Chem.* **2020**, *330*, 127244. [CrossRef]
14. Fărcaş, A.C.; Socaci, S.A.; Mudura, E.; Dulf, F.V.; Vodnar, D.C.; Tofană, M.; Salanță, L.C. Exploitation of Brewing Industry Wastes to Produce Functional Ingredients. *Brew. Technol.* **2017**, *13*, 137–156.
15. Kerby, C.; Vriesekoop, F. An Overview of the Utilisation of Brewery By-Products as Generated by British Craft Breweries. *Beverages* **2017**, *3*, 24. [CrossRef]
16. Rachwał, K.; Waśko, A.; Gustaw, K.; Polak-berecka, M. Utilization of brewery wastes in food industry. *PeerJ* **2020**, *8*, e9427. [CrossRef]
17. del Río, J.C.; Prinsen, P.; Gutiérrez, A. Chemical composition of lipids in brewer's spent grain: A promising source of valuable phytochemicals. *J. Cereal Sci.* **2013**, *58*, 248–254. [CrossRef]
18. Olivares-Galván, S.; Marina, M.L.; García, M.C. Extraction of valuable compounds from brewing residues: Malt rootlets, spent hops, and spent yeast. *Trends Food Sci. Technol.* **2022**, *127*, 181–197. [CrossRef]
19. Jackowski, M.; Niedźwiecki, Ł.; Jagiełło, K.; Uchańska, O.; Trusek, A. Brewer's spent grains—valuable beer industry by-product. *Biomolecules* **2020**, *10*, 1669. [CrossRef]
20. Habschied, K.; Krstanovi, V.; Karlovi, A.; Juri, A. By-Products in the Malting and Brewing Industries—Re-Usage Possibilities. *Fermentation* **2020**, *6*, 82.
21. Bravi, E.; De Francesco, G.; Sileoni, V.; Perretti, G.; Galgano, F.; Marconi, O. Brewing by-product upcycling potential: Nutritionally valuable compounds and antioxidant activity evaluation. *Antioxidants* **2021**, *10*, 165. [CrossRef] [PubMed]
22. Mussatto, S.I. Brewer's spent grain: A valuable feedstock for industrial applications. *J. Sci. Food Agric.* **2014**, *94*, 1264–1275. [CrossRef] [PubMed]
23. Chrisfield, B.J.; Hopfer, H.; Elias, R.J. Impact of copper-based fungicides on the antioxidant quality of ethanolic hop extracts. *Food Chem.* **2021**, *355*, 129551. [CrossRef] [PubMed]
24. Kobus-cisowska, J.; Szymanowska-powałowska, D.; Szczepaniak, O.; Cielecka-piontek, J.; Smuga-kogut, M.; Szulc, P. Composition and In Vitro Effects of Cultivars of *Humulus lupulus* L. Hops on Cholinesterase Activity and Microbial Growth. *Nutrients* **2019**, *11*, 1377. [CrossRef] [PubMed]
25. Abram, V.; Čeh, B.; Vidmar, M.; Hercezi, M.; Lazić, N.; Bucik, V.; Možina, S.S.; Košir, I.J.; Kač, M.; Demšar, L.; et al. A comparison of antioxidant and antimicrobial activity between hop leaves and hop cones. *Ind. Crops Prod.* **2015**, *64*, 124–134. [CrossRef]
26. Maietti, A.; Brighenti, V.; Bonetti, G.; Tedeschi, P.; Prencipe, F.P.; Benvenuti, S.; Brandolini, V.; Pellati, F. Metabolite profiling of flavonols and in vitro antioxidant activity of young shoots of wild *Humulus lupulus* L. (hop). *J. Pharm. Biomed. Anal.* **2017**, *142*, 28–34. [CrossRef]
27. Wang, X.; Yang, L.; Yang, X.; Tian, Y. In Vitro and In Vivo antioxidant and antimutagenic activities of polyphenols extracted from hops (*Humulus lupulus* L.). *J. Sci. Food Agric.* **2014**, *94*, 1693–1700. [CrossRef]
28. Weber, N.; Biehler, K.; Schwabe, K.; Haarhaus, B.; Quirin, K.W.; Frank, U.; Schempp, C.M.; Wölfle, U. Hop extract acts as an antioxidant with antimicrobial effects against Propionibacterium acnes and Staphylococcus aureus. *Molecules* **2019**, *24*, 223. [CrossRef]
29. Censi, R.; Peregrina, D.V.; Gigliobianco, M.R.; Lupidi, G.; Angeloni, C.; Pruccoli, L.; Tarozzi, A.; Di Martino, P. New Antioxidant Ingredients from Brewery By-Products for Cosmetic Formulations. *Cosmetics* **2021**, *8*, 96. [CrossRef]
30. Desai, A.; Darland, G.; Bland, J.S.; Tripp, M.L.; Konda, V.R. META060 attenuates TNF-α-activated inflammation, endothelial-monocyte interactions, and matrix metalloproteinase-9 expression, and inhibits NF-κB and AP-1 in THP-1 monocytes. *Atherosclerosis* **2012**, *223*, 130–136. [CrossRef]
31. Akazawa, H.; Kohno, H.; Tokuda, H.; Suzuki, N.; Yasukawa, K.; Kimura, Y.; Manosroi, A.; Manosroi, J.; Akihisa, T. Anti-inflammatory and anti-tumor-promoting effects of 5-deprenyllupulonol C and other compounds from hop (*Humulus lupulus* L.). *Chem. Biodivers.* **2012**, *9*, 1045–1054. [CrossRef]
32. Forino, M.; Pace, S.; Chianese, G.; Santagostini, L.; Werner, M.; Weinigel, C.; Rummler, S.; Fico, G.; Werz, O.; Taglialatela-Scafati, O. Humudifucol and Bioactive Prenylated Polyphenols from Hops (*Humulus lupulus* cv. "cascade"). *J. Nat. Prod.* **2016**, *79*, 590–597. [CrossRef]
33. Fiesel, A.; Gessner, D.K.; Most, E.; Eder, K. Effects of dietary polyphenol-rich plant products from grape or hop on pro-inflammatory gene expression in the intestine, nutrient digestibility and faecal microbiota of weaned pigs. *BMC Vet. Res.* **2014**, *10*, 196. [CrossRef]
34. Arsene, A.L.; Rodino, S.; Butu, A.; Petrache, P.; Iordache, O.; Butu, M. Study on antimicrobial and antioxidant activity and phenolic content of ethanolic extract of *Humulus lupulus*. *Farmacia* **2015**, *63*, 851–857.
35. Bocquet, L.; Sahpaz, S.; Bonneau, N.; Beaufay, C.; Mahieux, S.; Samaillie, J.; Roumy, V.; Jacquin, J.; Bordage, S.; Hennebelle, T.; et al. Phenolic Compounds from *Humulus lupulus* as Natural Antimicrobial Products: New Weapons in the Fight against Methicillin Resistant Staphylococcus aureus, Leishmania mexicana and Trypanosoma brucei Strains. *Molecules* **2019**, *24*, 1024. [CrossRef]
36. Di Sotto, A.; Checconi, P.; Celestino, I.; Locatelli, M.; Carissimi, S.; De Angelis, M.; Rossi, V.; Limongi, D.; Toniolo, C.; Martinoli, L.; et al. Antiviral and Antioxidant Activity of a Hydroalcoholic Extract from *Humulus lupulus* L. *Oxidative Med. Cell. Longev.* **2018**, *2018*, 5919237. [CrossRef]

37. Bogdanova, K.; Kolar, M.; Langova, K.; Dusek, M.; Mikyska, A.; Bostikova, V.; Bostik, P. Inhibitory effect of hop fractions against Gram-positive multi-resistant bacteria. A pilot study. *Biomed. Pap. Med. Fac. Univ. Palacky Olomouc. Czech Repub.* **2018**, *162*, 276–283. [CrossRef]
38. Campalani, C.; Chioggia, F.; Amadio, E.; Gallo, M.; Rizzolio, F.; Selva, M.; Perosa, A. Supercritical CO_2 extraction of natural antibacterials from low value weeds and agro-waste. *J. CO2 Util.* **2020**, *40*, 101198. [CrossRef]
39. Dumas, E.R.; Michaud, A.E.; Bergeron, C.; Lafrance, J.L.; Mortillo, S.; Gafner, S. Deodorant effects of a supercritical hops extract: Antibacterial activity against *Corynebacterium xerosis* and *Staphylococcus epidermidis* and efficacy testing of a hops/zinc ricinoleate stick in humans through the sensory evaluation of axillary deodorancy. *J. Cosmet. Dermatol.* **2009**, *8*, 197–204. [CrossRef]
40. Shinada, K.; Tagashira, M.; Watanabe, H.; Sopapornamorn, P.; Kanayama, A.; Watanabe, H.; Sopapornamorn, P.; Ikeda, M.; Kawaguchi, Y. Hop Bract Polyphenols Reduced Three-day Dental Plaque Regrowth. *J. Dent. Res.* **2007**, *86*, 848–851. [CrossRef]
41. Jeliazkova, E.; Zheljazkov, V.D.; Kačániova, M.; Astatkie, T.; Tekwani, B.L. Sequential elution of essential oil constituents during steam distillation of hops (*Humulus lupulus* L.) and influence on oil yield and antimicrobial activity. *J. Oleo Sci.* **2018**, *67*, 871–883. [CrossRef] [PubMed]
42. Bocquet, L.; Sahpaz, S.; Hilbert, J.L.; Rambaud, C.; Rivie, C. *Humulus lupulus* L., a very popular beer ingredient and medicinal plant: Overview of its phytochemistry, its bioactivity, and its biotechnology. *Phytochem. Rev.* **2018**, *17*, 1047–1090. [CrossRef]
43. Stompor, M.; Świtalska, M.; Podgórski, R.; Uram, Ł.; Aebisher, D.; Wietrzyk, J. Synthesis and biological evaluation of 4′-O-acetylisoxanthohumol and its analogues as antioxidant and antiproliferative agents. *Acta Biochim. Pol.* **2017**, *64*, 577–583. [CrossRef] [PubMed]
44. Hoang, H.T.; Moon, J.; Lee, Y. Natural Antioxidants from Plant Extracts in Skincare Cosmetics: Recent Applications, Challenges and Perspectives. *Cosmetics* **2021**, *8*, 106. [CrossRef]
45. Ivana, B.; Viktor, L.; Milanka, L.; Jelena, M.; Dusan, S. Skin Ageing: Natural Weapons and Strategies. *Evid.-Based Complement. Altern. Med.* **2013**, *2013*, 1–10.
46. Hoffmann, J.; Gendrisch, F.; Schempp, C.M.; Wölfle, U. New herbal biomedicines for the topical treatment of dermatological disorders. *Biomedicines* **2020**, *8*, 27. [CrossRef]
47. Abiko, Y.; Paudel, D.; Uehara, O. Hops components and oral health. *J. Funct. Foods* **2022**, *92*, 105035. [CrossRef]
48. Vogt, O.; Sikora, E.; Ogonowski, J. The effect of selected supercritical CO_2 plant extract addition on user properties of shower gels. *Polish J. Chem. Technol.* **2014**, *16*, 51–54. [CrossRef]
49. Liu, J.; Chen, Y.; Zhang, X.; Zheng, J.; Hu, W.; Teng, B. Hop Tannins as Multifunctional Tyrosinase Inhibitor: Structure Characterization, Inhibition Activity, and Mechanism. *Antioxidants* **2022**, *11*, 772. [CrossRef]
50. Goenka, S.; Simon, S.R. Depigmenting effect of Xanthohumol from hop extract in MNT-1 human melanoma cells and normal human melanocytes. *Biochem. Biophys. Rep.* **2021**, *26*, 100955. [CrossRef]
51. Spiewak, R.; Dutkiewicz, J. Occupational airborne and hand dermatitis to hop (*Humulus lupulus*) with non-occupational relapses. *Ann. Agric. Environ. Med.* **2002**, *9*, 249–252.

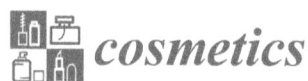

Review

From Traditional Knowledge to Modern Formulation: Potential and Prospects of *Pistacia atlantica* Desf. Essential and Fixed Oils Uses in Cosmetics

Asma El Zerey-Belaskri [1,2,*], Nabila Belyagoubi-Benhammou [3] and Hachemi Benhassaini [2]

[1] Laboratoire de Recherche: Biotechnologie des Rhizobiums et Amélioration des Plantes, Faculté des Sciences de la Nature et de la Vie, Université Ahmed Ben Bella Oran 1, Oran 31000, Algeria

[2] Laboratoire de Recherche: Biodiversité Végétale: Conservation et Valorisation, Université Djillali Liabes, Sidi Bel Abbes 22000, Algeria

[3] Laboratory of Natural Products, Department of Biology, Faculty of Natural and Life Sciences, Earth and Universe, University Abou-Bekr Belkaïd, Tlemcen 13000, Algeria

* Correspondence: asma.elzerey.belaskri@gmail.com

Abstract: *Pistacia atlantica* Desf. (Atlas pistachio) is one of the most widely distributed wild species of the genus. It is an Irano–Touranian species with a large geographic area that extends from the Canary Islands to Pamir Mountains. Since ancient times, atlas pistachio gum-like resin and fruits, very rich in essential oils (EOs) and fixed oils (FOs), respectively, were used in traditional medicine and included in different traditional cosmetics and health and beauty products. Since then, Atlas pistachio fixed oil is incorporated into several soaps, creams and shampoos to benefit from its medicinal properties. Atlas pistachio fixed oils, resin and leaf essential oils are constituted by several bioactive compounds such as monoterpenes with α-pinene and β-pinene in the resin, terpinen-4-ol, elemol, sesquiterpenes with *D*-germacrene and *E*-caryophyllene in the leaves and oxygenated monoterpenes (bornyl acetate) in the fruits. The unsaturated fatty acids (oleic, linoleic, palmitic and stearic acid), sterols (β-sitostero) and tocopherols represented the principal compounds in fatty oil fruits. All these compounds exhibit great therapeutic and cosmetic virtues. Unlike lentisk oil uses in cosmetology, the cosmetic potentials of Atlas pistachio oils remain less valued. In the current review, we seek to highlight the characteristics and properties of Atlas pistachio oils in the prospects of the development of new and different cosmetic formulations as well as an innovative valuation of active ingredients and products inspired by indigenous knowledge and practices.

Keywords: *Pistacia atlantica* Desf.; essential oils; fixed oils; cosmetic formulation; indigenous knowledge

Citation: El Zerey-Belaskri, A.; Belyagoubi-Benhammou, N.; Benhassaini, H. From Traditional Knowledge to Modern Formulation: Potential and Prospects of *Pistacia atlantica* Desf. Essential and Fixed Oils Uses in Cosmetics. *Cosmetics* **2022**, *9*, 109. https://doi.org/10.3390/cosmetics9060109

Academic Editor: Othmane Merah

Received: 30 December 2021
Accepted: 19 October 2022
Published: 25 October 2022

Publisher's Note: MDPI stays neutral with regard to jurisdictional claims in published maps and institutional affiliations.

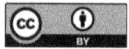

Copyright: © 2022 by the authors. Licensee MDPI, Basel, Switzerland. This article is an open access article distributed under the terms and conditions of the Creative Commons Attribution (CC BY) license (https://creativecommons.org/licenses/by/4.0/).

1. Introduction

When Aristotle gave the living creature's classification using 'the soul' as a 'principal', he put human beings in a unique class based on their 'rational soul'. Aristotle (De Anima, III,7431b, 14–17) considers that this soul enables the human to have a manner of perception of 'images'. He continues and cites that " ... whenever it affirms or denies that something is good or bad, it pursues or avoids. Consequently, the soul never thinks without an image ... ". So, man is that creature who thinks, describes, distinguishes, and gives values. Among these values, we cite 'beauty'. The 'beauty' is the one which has from ancient times interested and fascinated man leading him to continuously look for products and rituals to take care of external body appearance but also for his wellbeing and welfare. Five thousands years earlier, the Egyptians, Sumerians, Assyrians and Babylonians used mud, plasters, ointments and plants in their spiritual rituals and personal grooming. Many Artifacts from these civilisations attest to this such as mirrors, cosmetic jars, combs, hairbrushes, and toothbrushes [1].

In 7000 BC, beauty and health-care products such as pomades and oils based on animal and vegetable fats were already in use in Kish and Mesopotamia, although seed pressing and nut oils extraction had not yet begun [2]. Scented products and fragrances would have been elaborated using oil and fat bases. The fragrance industry was well developed in Egypt, Mesopotamia, Crete and mainland Greece [3]. Since then, this know-how has spread throughout the world, giving a great interest to the content and the container. In fact, the art of fragrance has always kept a great place. The containers were in glass, bronze, lead, or precious metals such as silver and gold. The flakes could be, therefore, decorated with precious gemstones (Figure 1).

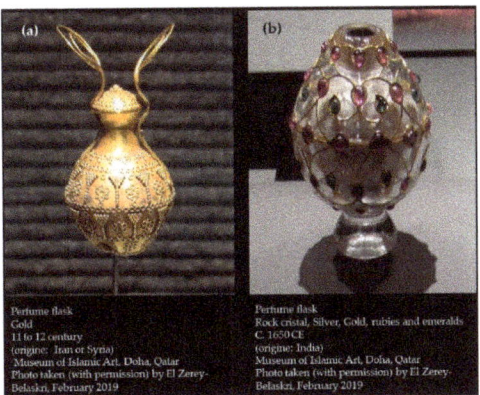

Figure 1. Ancient perfume flasks witnessing the luxury of fragrance bottles: (**a**) perfume flask in gold, decorated with a bold geometric pattern; (**b**) perfume flask in rock crystal, decorated with gold, silver, and precious gemstones, rubies and emeralds. Conservation: Museum of Islamic Art, Doha, Qatar. Personal photos taken by the first author with permission. February 2019.

The fragrance was obtained by the maceration of flowers, spices, barks, woods, and resins in oils. One of the oldest species used in healthcare products belongs to the genus *Pistacia*. It is assumed that resin obtained from several *Pistacia* species primarily from *P. atlantica* and *P. lentiscus* (Anacardiaceae) was the first natural chewing gum of the ancient world. Pistachio resin was known for its distinguishing flavour and therapeutic properties and was used subsequently to clean the teeth and freshen the breath [4]. Since the ancient Egyptian dynasties, Pistachio resin was a key ingredient in body-care practices and the mummification process and rituals. Several scientific analyses of pigments from ancient Egyptian tomb walls and funerary items showed a predominant presence of pistachio resin [5–7]. Brettell et al. [8] showed that resinous substances obtained from pistachio species were highly prized in the ancient world for use in Roman mortuary practices in acting to disguise the odour of decomposition. Wherever pistachio species occur, their fruits are appreciated mainly by the rural population for human consumption because of their oleaginous exocarp while the fatty oils are used either for consumption or traditional cosmetic recipes. The leaves are used principally for their medicinal virtues while young and fresh ones could be added to some traditional culinary preparations such as salads and bread [9]. In Palestine and some regions in Algeria, the fruits are crushed and added to the bread dough to give it an exceptional flavour [9].

Pistacia is not the only Anacardiaceae member known for exhibiting substances with cosmetic potentials; *Anacardium* species, mainly *A. humile* (monkey nut), *A. occidentale* (cashew tree) and *A. nanum*, *Rhus* species, the Burmese lacquer tree (*Gluta usitata*), *Mangifera indica* and several other members present advanced active ingredients for the pharmaceutical and cosmetic industries [10]. Bennett [11] placed the *Anacardiaceae* within the top 25 plant families of high economic importance.

In the current review, we attempt to expose *Pistacia atlantica* essential and fixed oil potentials in modern cosmetics but also to highlight craft use and traditional practices of this species with high patrimonial values.

2. Botanical Description and Variability of *P. atlantica*

One of the most widely distributed wild species of the genus, *Pistacia atlantica* Desf. is an Irano–Touranian species which occurs from the Canary Islands to Pamir Mountains [12]. In this large area, *P. atlantica* is known under several local names. It is called in the Arabic area (El bottom, btom, bettam, battach or botma for an individual tree) [13–15]. It is called by the Amazighs of the Maghreb (iggt, iqq, idj, tismelelt and tesemhalt [13,14], while it is named (Baneh) in persian, (Wana, Gwan, and Kasore) in different local dialects in Pakistan, (melengiç or atlantik sakizi) in Turkish, (Treminthos) in Italian [16], (Almácigo de Canarias) or (Lengua de oveja) in Spanish [17]. Atlas pistachio trees are strong and vigorous (Figure 2), characterized mainly by their dense foliage although the leaves are deciduous. The leaves are used by rural populations for dyeing textiles and to give a durable colouration, principally in traditional medicine [9,15,18]. In fact, the leaves are a rich source of bioactive compounds which interested researchers in several studies in the field of pharmacology.

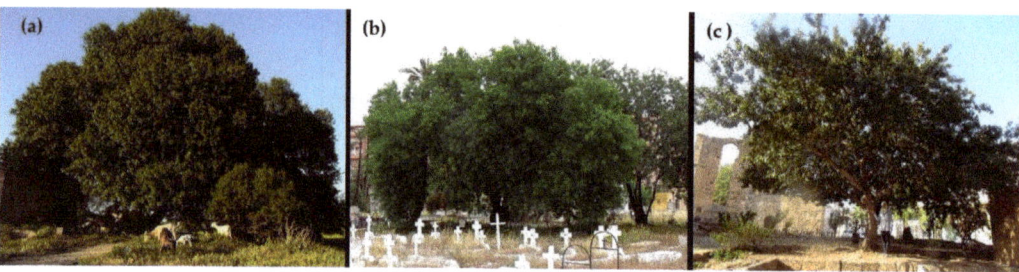

Figure 2. *Pistacia atlantica* trees in different countries: (**a**), a great *P. atlantica* tree (female) in the region of Sidi Bel abbes (Algeria), June 2016; (**b**) a vigorous *P. atlantica* within a dense wild population (here, in an ancient Christian graveyard) in the region of Marrakech, Morocco, March 2018; (**c**) a beautiful *P. atlantica* (male) in the town centre of Famagusta (Northern Cyprus), October 2017. Personal photos taken by the first author.

Pistacia atlantica is very variable, with three subspecies (*P. atlantica* subsp. *cabulica*, *P. atlantica* subsp. *mutica*, and *P. atlantica* subsp. *atlantica*) qualified as eco-geographical ecotypes [19,20]. We don't cite here (*P. atlantica* subsp. *kurdica*) since this subspecies was elevated to the species level and is considered a distinct species [21]. Additionally, the variability is not observed only at the subspecies level but also between the different populations of the same subspecies. Moreover, the variability doesn't concern only the morphological features [22] but also the chemical profile of leaf essential oils, oleoresin, fatty oils and their potential biological activities [23–31].

The morphological variability concerns the habitus, the leaves, the trunk and the fruits [12,22,32–36]. Furthermore, several studies on micro-morphological variability have been also undertaken [37–40] revealing an interesting micro-feature variability.

The leaves are spectacularly variable (Figure 3) [22,34,36] causing difficulties, principally to sometimes distinguish the three subspecies. In North Africa, this variability induced for a long time hypotheses [12,35,41] that more than one subspecies may occur in the region until the study undertaken by El Zerey-Belaskri [15] on the diversity of *P. atlantica* subsp. *atlantica* in Algeria, stating that the great morphological variability is mainly due to ecological, chemical and genetic factors and that *P.atlantica* is represented in Algeria by the only subspecies *P. atlantica* subsp. *atlantica*. The following botanical description can be found in the literature: the leaves are pinnate, oval glabrous almost sessile and dark green with seven to nine lance-shaped leaflets waxy impair-pinnate with petioles a little winged. While El Zerey-Belaskri and Benhassaini [36] updated the *P. atlantica* subsp. *atlantica* key describing more morphometric and morphological traits and new features; new leaf and leaflet shapes and new features have been observed (up to 18 leaflets, up to 24.5 cm leaf length, up to 21.9 cm leaf width). The terminal leaflet may be petiolulated [36]. According to this updated key, the leaves, reaching 24.5 cm long and 21.9 cm wide, are composed of one to nine leaflet pairs, imparipinnate, deciduous, leaf rachis winged. being sometimes paripinnate by losing the terminal or the pre-terminal leaflet. Leaflets (1–) 2–8 (−9) pairs; lanceolate, oval, elliptic, oblong, rhomboid, obovate, (falciform); obtuse, acute, acuminate, mucronated, emarginate, rounded, retuse, and attenuate apex leaflet. The terminal leaflet is sessile or petiolulated (0.1–3.4 cm long) [36].

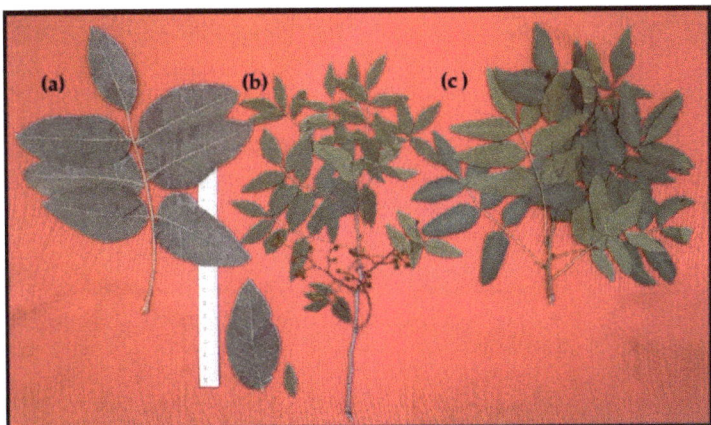

Figure 3. *Pistacia atlantica* leaves from different countries: (**a**) one of the largest *Pistacia atlantica* subsp. *atlantica* leaf, from Northwest Algeria, September 2014; (**b**) *Pistacia atlantica* subsp. *atlantica* branch with leaves and unripe fruits, from Marrakech, Morocco, March 2018; (**c**) branch with *Pistacia atlantica* leaves, in the town centre of Famagusta (Northern Cyprus), October 2017. Personal photo taken by the first author.

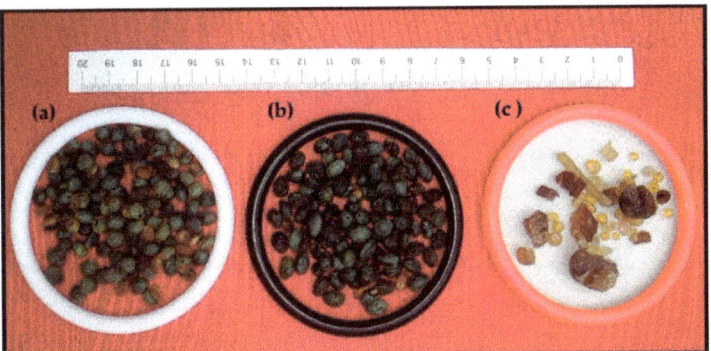

Figure 4. Atlas pistachio fruits from two countries and two different subspecies (**a** ≠ **b**) and resin: (**a**) *Pistacia atlantica* fruits from Iran. (**b**) *Pistacia atlantica* subsp. *atlantica* fruits from the region of El bayadh, Algeria; (**c**) *Pistacia atlantica* subsp. *atlantica* resin from the region of El bayadh, Algeria. Personal photo taken by the first author.

Likewise, the fruits are slightly variable. They (Figure 4a,b) are small (≤0.8/0.7 cm) with thin and oleaginous exocarp, and with a syncarp drupe, ovoid or ovoid-globose with an osseous endocarp of a green to dark green–blue or black colour when ripe [22,35,42,43]. The fruits are called by several vernacular names. In Algeria, they are called "Goddim" because of the hardness of their endocarp requiring strength to break them with teeth [15] and also "el khodiri" [35] because of their colour (from akhdar, green in Arabic). In other regions in Algeria, when the fruits are present in two colours (green and black), the rural people call the green ones "el khoddir" (from akhdar, in Arabic) and the black ones "el ko'hhil" (from ak'hal), black in Arabic [15]. Yaaqobi et al. [44] reported that the Atlas pistachio fruit is called 'Tikouaoueche' (an Amazigh noun) in Morocco. The fruit is edible and used traditionally in many recipes bringing power mainly because of its energetic fatty oil [45–47]. Belyagoubi-Benhammou et al. [48], evaluated the antioxidant activity of the flavonoid fractions of *Pistacia atlantica* fruit, stating that the fruits could be used as a source of natural antioxidants in food and pharmaceutical industries.

3. Potential Use of *Pistacia atlantica* Essential Oils (EOs) in Cosmetics

Essential oil, also defined as essence, volatile oil, etheric oil or aetheroleum, is a complex mixture of volatile constituents biosynthesised by living organisms [49]. If higher plants are the best-known and most important source of essential oils, some mosses, liverworts, seaweeds and some terrestrial and marine animals (sponges), insects, fungi, and microorganisms are also known to biosynthesise volatile compounds [50–52]. Interestingly, essential oils are added to cosmetics formulations for their pleasant aroma but principally for their valuable biological activities including anti-pathophysiological activity.

3.1. Chemical Composition and Variability

The volatile compounds of *P. atlantica* were investigated in the large area where the Atlas pistachio occurs, showing great variability in the chemical composition. Although the essential oil yield (Figure 5a) is quantitatively less important, regarding other aromatic plants, several chemical analyses were interested in this secondary compound present in mostly all the plant organs. In fact, *P. atlantica* EOs were found in ripe and unripe fruits [23], leaf-buds [24], twigs, flower galls [53,54] and in the resin, called consequently oleresin [23,55,56] (Figure 4c), nevertheless, the leaf essential oils remain the most targeted. Moreover, the leaf EO composition is characterized by high variability.

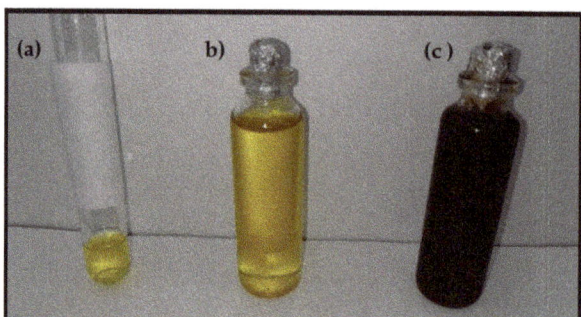

Figure 5. *Pistacia atlantica* subsp. *atlantica* oils: (**a**) essential oil obtained by hydrodistillation; (**b**) solvent fixed oil obtained by using a Soxhlet; (**c**) fixed oil obtained by using the traditional method; kindly provided by a friend from the region of El bayadh (Algeria). Personal photo taken by the first author.

Pistacia atlantica subsp. *atlantica*, is the only representative subspecies in the Maghreb, however, it occurs from the Canary Islands to Palestine, Syria, Jordan, Lebanon and Turkey in the Asian area [57]. It is "a characteristic tree" of the Saharan desert landscape in Algeria [58], and possesses a special consideration for people of all its distribution area [9]. This subspecies is the most studied regarding the essential oil compositions and biological activities, followed by *Pistacia atlantica* subsp. *mutica* (from Crimea, Turkey, Iran and the Caucus). *Pistacia atlantica* subsp. *cabulica* (from Afghanistan, Pakistan, and Iran) is not clearly mentioned in the chemical studies, nevertheless, it may be studied but cited as *Pistacia atlantica* without any precision of the subspecies. *Pistacia atlantica* subsp. *Kurdica* is not considered in the current review since, as noted below, it is elevated at the species level for *P. eurycarpa* as a specific name [21].

Pistacia atlantica subsp. *atlantica* leaf EOs from Algeria and Morocco have been deeply analysed, recording differently in α-pinene, terpinen-4-ol, germacrene D, E-caryophyllene, δ-3-carene, α-terpineol, γ-gurjunene/spathulenol/α-phellandrene as major compounds in several studies investigating seasonal, tree-sex and ecological variability factors [23,25,26,28–30,54,59]. Benhassaini et al. [56] analysed the chemical composition of the oleoresin, which was found to be dominated by α-pinene, β-pinene and carvacrol. Bornyl acetate was recorded as the major compound in fruit EO of *Pistacia atlantica* subsp. *atlantica*, in Morocco by Barrero et al. [23], while α-pinene, β-pinene and camphene dominated the chemical composition in Algerian *P. atlantica* [25].

From *Pistacia atlantica* subsp. *mutica* (in the Greek East Aegean islands, Kalimnos and Lesvos), leaf, bud-leaf and fruit essential oils were analysed. It was, therefore, reported that myrcene and terpinen-4-ol were found to be the predominant compounds in leaf EOs from female trees and terpinen-4-ol and *p*-mentha-1(7),8-diene in leaf EOs from male trees; terpinen-4-ol, myrcene and sabinene in unripe fruit EOs and *p*-mentha-1(7),8-diene, sabinene and α-pinene in leaf-buds EOs, while, sabinene, *p*-mentha-1(7),8-diene, germacrene D, terpinen-4-ol were found to be the major compounds in bud-leaf EOs [24]. In the same subspecies, widely distributed in Iran, the oleoresin was dominated by α-pinene [60] and by α-pinene followed by limonene oxide [61], while the fruit EOs showed α-pinene and camphene/β-myrcene/limonene as major compounds [53]. Eghbali-Feriz et al. [62] revealed that β-E-ocimene, myrcene, β-Z-ocimene, α-pinene, and E-caryophyllene composed principally the unripe fruit essential oil collected from *Pistacia atlantica* subsp. *mutica* from the Northeast of Iran.

On the other hand, Didehvar et al. [63] analysed oleoresin from Iranian *P. atlantica* (without any precision of the subspecies) and reported α-pinene, trans-pinocarveol, cis-limonene oxide, sabinene, and β-pinene as major compounds.

3.2. Potential of Pistacia atlantica EO Compounds in Cosmetics

Several conventional methods are used for essential oil extraction such as hydrodistillation, steam distillation, Soxhlet extraction, and solvent extraction while other advanced methods (microwave or SPME-based methods) are currently used to enhance oil yield with less sample amount. For *P. atlantica* EOs, hydrodistillation is still the most commonly used method although the efficiency of microwave techniques has been shown by using magnetic nanoparticle-assisted microwave (MW) distillation for *Pistacia vera* [64].

Essential oils are one of the most important natural products valorized for their organoleptic properties in the fragrance industry but principally for their various biological properties in cosmetics. They are composed of monoterpene and sesquiterpene hydrocarbons and their oxygenated derivatives, aldehydes, ketones, esters, ethers, oxides, lactones and coumarins, phenols [65]. The bioactivity of EOs is the sum of their constituents which act either in a synergistic or in an antagonistic way [66]. In addition to the smell and fragrance, essential oils are added to cosmetics products as preservatives particularly to prevent their oxidation. Their antioxidant potential acts as a protective agent in various products like moisturizers, lotions and cleaners, skin care cosmetics, conditioners, masks for anti-dandruff products, hair care products lipsticks, or fragrances in perfumery [67]. Preservatives are additionally, added to cosmetics to prevent microbial spoilage, as well as for the protection of consumers from potential infections.

3.2.1. Monoterpene Potentials

Monoterpenes are important fragrant molecules and suitable starting materials in the perfumery industry and cosmetic industries [65]. The monoterpenes in *P. atlantica* EOs are essentially represented by (α-pinene β-pinene α-thujene, camphene, terpinen-4-ol, δ-3-carene, *p*-cymene, limonene).

α and β-pinene are typically the most representative compounds of *P. atlantica* EOs although there is great chemical variability. These compounds are the most abundant bicyclic monoterpenes and are used as a fragrance substance to improve the odour of industrial products but also as precursors of important flavour and aroma compounds [68]. Additionally, monoterpenes are used in cosmetic products for their biological activities, α-Pinene is widely used as a fragrance in the cosmetics and household industry. *P. atlantica* leaf and resin EOs, being mostly an important source of α–pinene, were always evaluated for their microbial activities. Oleoresins, obtained from *P. atlantica* (from Iran) and *P. atlantica* subsp. *atlantica* (from Algeria), both dominated by α–pinene were tested, respectively, for their activity against *Helicobacter pylori* by Memariani et al. [60] and against *Candida albicans* by Benabdallah et al. [59]. According to Memariani et al. [60], all the tested *H. pylori* strains were susceptible to the essential oil. Furthermore, in a microscopic examination, *P. atlantica* oleoresin attenuated the destruction and necrosis of gastric tissue. On the other hand, Benabdallah et al. [59] revealed that the tested oleoresin showed bactericidal activity against *C. albicans*.

Helicobacter pylori is a common bacterium described first in the digestive tract as being the responsible agent for most ulcers in the stomach and small intestine. However, it is established that it also actually occurs in the oral cavity independently of stomach colonization [69]. Besides, *C. albicans* is considered to be the most common fungal pathogen of humans, manifesting itself in the oral cavity, causing oral candidiasis or thrush, female reproductive tract (commonly referred to as a yeast infection), and less commonly in the digestive tract. The bactericidal effect of pistachio EOs against buccal and stomachic flora remains the traditional use of pistachio resin and other organ plants.

Interestingly, it is known that the rural populations in the distribution area of Atlas pistachio used to chew the leaves and the resin of Atlas pistachio. This health and care practice is inherited from the ancient world where pistachio resin was used to clean the teeth and freshen the breath. Most compelling evidence shows that the indigenous knowledge regarding the medical use of Atlas pistachio corroborates the scientific findings.

Additionally, anti-Leishmania effects of *Syzygium cumini* leaf EOs and its major compound (α-pinene) were assessed by Rodrigues et al. [70] using MTT methods and macrophage cytotoxicity measurements. It has been shown that α-pinene exerts cytotoxic effects directly correlated with the different doses used against promastigotes of *Leishmania amazonensis* [70].

α-pinene and β-pinene showed cytotoxicity on tumour lymphocytes [71] while α–pinene revealed a positive antitumor activity in cell lines and in animal models of hepatocellular carcinoma [72], and a noticeable ability to induce, in vivo, apoptosis and antimetastatic properties [73]. In contrast, Buriani et al. [74] assessed human adenocarcinoma cell line sensitivity to EOs extracted from five *Pistacia* taxa (*P. lentiscus*, *P. lentiscus* var. *chia*, *P. terebinthus*, *P. vera*, and *P. integerrima*). According to the obtained results, they assumed that anti-tumoral activity was principally the effect exerted by the phytocomplex as a whole, which cannot be attributed to a single component but, rather, is likely the result of a complex network of simultaneous biological signals which contribute to the global cytotoxic effect.

Moreover, α-pinene and 1,8-cineole have been shown to present a beneficial effect on the equilibration of oxidant/antioxidant to protect against H_2O_2-induced oxidative stress in rat PC12 (rat pheochromocytoma) cells [75]. Pre-treatment with these monoterpenes inhibited the intracellular reactive oxygen species production and markedly enhanced the expression of antioxidant enzymes including catalase (CAT), superoxide dismutase (SOD), glutathione peroxidase (GPx), glutathione reductase (GR) and heme-oxygenase 1 (HO-1) [75].

β-pinene is known for its antimicrobial properties either purified or as part of essential oils [76–78]. β-pinene was one of the two main active principles of essential oil showing antidepressant-like and sedative-like activity and a clear potential in the treatment of sadness [79,80]. In fact, several essential oils are currently researched and in use as aromatherapy agents and cosmetics to relieve anxiety, stress, and depression.

Resources rich in terpinen-4-ol are used as antiseptics and antifungals to treat cuts, burns, abrasions and acne in a range of cosmetic products such as antiseptics, deodorants, shampoo and soaps. Thus, Huynh et al. [81] evaluated the antibacterial effect of two terpinen-4-ol-based cosmetic formulations against *Escherichia coli* and *Staphylococcus aureus*. They revealed, in fact, a higher antibacterial activity against *E. coli* than *S. aureus*. In addition, the formulated cosmetic products have been appreciated by 28 female customers and showed satisfactory microbial standards for the cosmetics field according to Ho Chi Minh City Pasteur Institute (Vietnam) [81].

Indeed, Benabdallah et al. [59] attempted to determine the antimicrobial activity of *Pistacia atlantica* subsp. *atlantica* leaf EO dominated by terpinen-4-ol against *S. aureus*, *E. coli*, *Klebsiella pneumoniae*, *Pseudomonas aeruginosa* and *E. albicans* and revealed a bactericidal effect against *S. aureus*, *C. albicans* and, *E. coli*.

Furthermore, Yang et al. [82] demonstrated that a solid-state terpinen-4-ol/β-CD inclusion complex, they prepared, clearly enhanced the antibacterial activity against *S. aureus*, *P. aeruginosa* and, *E. coli*. Although terpinen-4-ol is known for its antimicrobial activities, this improvement could be attributed to that terpinen-4-ol being easily volatile and, especially, its low solubility in water limits its inhibitory effect. The enhancement also could be explained by the interactions of β-CD with terpinen-4-ol to form intermolecular hydrogen bonds, which improved its controlled release and water solubility [82].

Demodex mites (*Demodex folliculorum*) is the most common ectoparasite found in the human skin extending to the eye. Looking for a cosmetic formulation against these mites, Tighe et al. [83] assessed the killing effect of terpinen-4-ol on *D. folliculorum*. They stated that even though terpinen-4-ol exhibited a significant synergistic effect with terpinolene, deployment of terpinen-4-ol alone should enhance its potency in killing *Demodex* mites by reducing the adverse and antagonistic effects from other EO ingredients. They conclude that terpinen-4-ol could be adopted in future formulations of acaricides to treat a number of ocular and cutaneous diseases caused by demodicosis.

δ-3-carene was recorded as major constituent in *P. atlantica* in the Saharan region of Algeria by Gourine et al. [26]. This compound occurs principally in Cupressaceae exhibiting a high antifungal activity; proving to be a fundamental compound for this activity and an emergent alternative as an antifungal agent against dermatophyte strains [84]. Essential oils from other conifers with a high content of δ-3-carene and α-pinene possess important antibacterial and anti-inflammatory activities mostly against acne-causing pathogens and have therapeutic potential for diseases involving skin infections.

Plants and EOs with an important content of δ-3-carene could be targeted for cosmetic formulations for therapeutic potential, mainly in fungal diseases involving mucosal and cutaneous infections. However, the autoxidation of δ-3-carene to the hydroperoxide leading to eczematogenic and allergenic effects should be taken into consideration [85]. On the other hand, these oils, rich in δ-3-carene exhibit variable levels of antioxidant activities, evaluated in vitro in several studies. This variability was highly correlated with the quality and quantity of oil which is influenced by the harvest season, tree sex and the plant organs [26,27,53,54,86,87].

In *P. atlantica* EO chemical compositions, other monoterpenes with appreciable amounts were identified, such as *p*-cymene and camphene:

p-cymene is widely involved in the preparation and synthesis of dyes, medicines, fragrances and perfumes. *p*-cymene is known for its safety. This compound doesn't show genotoxicity, repeated dose toxicity, reproductive toxicity, local respiratory toxicity, phototoxicity/photoallergenicity, or skin sensitization [88,89]. Furthermore, this compound was shown to possess anti-tumoral activity [90].

Camphene is used as a fragrance and flavouring substance as well as in the production of cleaning agents produced that aim to eliminate or mask unpleasant smells (mainly as toilet fragrances, air fresheners and deodorizers). Camphene is converted to alkyl isobornyl ether, which is used in the formulation of cosmetics and perfumes [91]. In fact, acid-catalysed alkoxylation of terpenes is an important synthesis route to valuable terpenic ethers with many applications in the perfumery and pharmaceutical industry. Interestingly, for medical uses, camphene known for its antioxidant and anti-inflammatory activities was found to be able to significantly increase cell viability as indicated by MTT assay and LDH release assay [92]. Furthermore, it is used for renal and hepatobiliary disorders.

In addition, it is important to highlight that the antioxidant properties of essential oils are due to the synergetic effect of large amounts of monoterpenes and oxygenated sesquiterpenes which exhibited a significant ability to scavenge free radicals using 2,2'- diphenyl-1-picrylhydrazyl (DPPH) free radical-scavenging, ferric reducing antioxidant power (FRAP), β-carotene bleaching test, thiobarbituric acid reactive species (TBARS) and Rancimat assays [26,27,53,86]. The highest antioxidant effect was also demonstrated for seven predominant terpenoids (i.e., α-pinene, limonene, myrcene, geraniol, linalool, nerol, and terpineol) [93].

Essential oil also acts as an anti-inflammatory agent. This activity is assumed to be correlated to their antioxidant activities and their interactions with several key enzymes, signalling cascades involving cytokines, and regulatory transcription factors [86,94]. For *P. atlantica*, its essential oil possesses potent sedative and anti-inflammatory properties in different mice and rat based models using the carrageenan-induced hind paw edema test [95]. Another study revealed the therapeutic effects of applied doses of oral gum as well as volatile oil to reduce all indices of colitis and myeloperoxidase activity in an animal model of ulcerative colitis [96]. In addition, the essential oil of resin showed angiogenesis and skin burn wound healing in rats. The results of this study demonstrated a concentration-dependent effect on the healing of burn wounds by increasing the concentration of basic fibroblast growth factor (bFGF) and platelet-derived growth factor (PDGF) and by enhancing angiogenesis after 14 days of treatment by the plant [97]. The anti-inflammatory activity of *P. atlantica* has been proven by a cream formulated that contains oleoresin, alone and in combination with other systemic drugs [98]. In this work, the cream reduced pain, inflammation and restrictions of joint movement in patients with mild to moderate (grades 2 and 3) knee osteoarthritis. This effect is attributed to the high percentage of α-pinene which revealed the best analgesic effect by inhibiting some enzymes involved in inflammation caused by osteoarthritis.

3.2.2. Sesquiterpenes Potentials

El Zerey-Belaskri et al. [29] described for the first time two sesquiterpenes (Germacrene D and E-caryophyllene) as major compounds in *P. atlantica* leaf EOs, in particular natural populations. These populations were found to be in a distinctive group based on a molecular analysis [99]. Bicyclogermacrene was observed with a remarkable percentage in some *P. atlantica* EOs from Algeria by [26,29] while spathulenol was recorded as one of the main sesquiterpenes in *P. atlantica* EOs in the south region of Algeria [26].

Germacrene is known to be a bitter sesquiterpene olefin produced by several plants with antifeedant, antimicrobial and insecticidal properties [100]. Mosquitoes are the deadliest vectors of parasites that cause diseases mainly in Africa. In our opinion, this compound could be valorized for the cream formulation of cosmetic products with repellent activity.

Aloysia virgata EOs from Cuba and Brasil, dominated by germacrene-D, bicyclogermacrene, and E-caryophyllene were found to possess antifungal activity against *Candida albicans*, and antibacterial activity against *Escherichia coli*, *Bacillus cereus* and *Staphylococcus aureus* [101,102].

E-caryophyllene is a bicyclic-sesquiterpene, with a strong woody and spicy odour, widely used in cosmetology and perfumery as a fragrance chemical for its aroma quality since the 1930s [103,104]. Furthermore, it is incorporated into the ingredients of several non-cosmetic products such as household cleaners and detergents [105].

E-Caryophyllene is known for its anti-inflammatory effect [106–109], antibacterial [102] antiallergic effect [108] and local anaesthetic properties [106]. It is very used in medical and pharmacological fields, also for its analgesic activity and cytoprotective gastric effect [106]. EOs containing E-caryophyllene as one of the main constituents, evidently, showed antinociceptive and analgesic effects without inducing gastric damage [109]. E-caryophyllene in *P. atlantica* EOs is potentially an important element for dermo-cosmetic products.

In concordance with the traditional use of Atlas pistachio leaves, this organ is often used by the local population as an efficient treatment for stomach and gastric diseases. Moreover, Atlas pistachio leaf-boiled-water is used as a finishing bath lotion to treat skin problems [9].

Regarding its safety (GRAS-FDA 21 CFR 121.11.64) and distinctive smell and aroma, this compound is approved by the U.S. Food and Drug Administration as a food additive and a harmless element for the cosmetic compositions of face creams, hair care products, body lotions and shampoos.

Moreover, EOs rich in β-pinene, germacrene D, *trans*-β-caryophyllene, and α-pinene showed a clear antioxidant activity promising an interesting potential for the utilization of the oil in the prevention of oxidative damage in cosmetic creams [110]. Oxidation of unsaturated substances in cosmetic cream can affect its odour and colour and denature its quality, eventually leading to the formation of harmful compounds to health as well as to the product [110].

4. Potential Use of *P. atlantica* Fixed Oils (FOs) in Cosmetics

Pistacia atlantica, like the other members of the genus *Pistacia* has oleaginous fruits considered by several researchers. Fruit oil was considered a new source for the production of vegetable oils (Figure 5b,c) concerning the high amount of mono-unsaturated and omega-3 fatty acids. The oil content varied between 29.45% to 40% [46,111,112]. Several methods are used in oil extraction. Both traditional methods and modern extraction techniques (such as microwave assisted extraction (MAE), ultrasonic-assisted extraction (UAE) and supercritical fluid extraction (SFE) methods) are utilized.

4.1. Physical and Chemical Characteristics

The oil content variation has been shown to vary largely according to the genotype and climatic conditions [113]. It is noted that NO plays a highly complex role in the regulation of plant development. It plays a key function in seed oil accumulation and fatty acid composition [114]. Moreover, the oil extraction methods influence greatly the oil content [111]. Likewise, the chemical modifications which affect the quality of the vegetable oils are mainly due to several forms such as the esterification/transesterification by rearranging the acyl moieties to synthesize trimesters; estolide formation by modifying the acyl group after the hydrolysis of triglyceride and elimination of glycerol and formation of new ester bonds between the fatty acid chains and the epoxidation by modifying double bonds and subsequent ring opening to synthesize different diesters [112]. Compared to that extracted by pressure and by hexane, the supercritical carbon dioxide (CO_2) produced better oil quality with interesting physicochemical and a higher antioxidant activity with the existence of unsaturated fatty acids, sterols, tocopherols and polyphenols [115]. The physico-chemical proprieties of oil *P. atlantica* seeds obtained by Soxhlet extractor are shown in Table 1 [116].

Table 1. Physico-chemical proprieties of oil *P. atlantica* seeds: according to Achheb et al. [116].

Properties	Oil Extracted by Hexane
Density (20 °C)	0.917 ± 0.002
Refractive index (20 °C)	1.472 ± 0.001
Viscosity 20 °C (Cp)	85.000 ± 0.750
Acidic index (mg KOH/g)	8.350 ± 0.120
Peroxide index (meq O_2/Kg)	9.950 ± 0.950
Iodine index (g I_2 100 g)	88.000 ± 0.010
Saponification value (mg KOH/g)	204.490 ± 0.040
Unsaponifiable matter (%)	1.740 ± 0.010

Oils with lower values of viscosity and density are highly appreciated by consumers. These parameters increase with high saturation and polymerization [117]. For the refractive index of oils, its value depends on the molecular weight, fatty acid chain length, degree of unsaturation, and degree of conjugation [118]. The refractive index of *P. atlantica* seed oil was 1.472, which was slightly higher than the value observed for *P. lentiscus* (1.468), however, it is closely similar to the standard range reported by Firestone [119] for *Pistacia vera* (1.467–1.470). The iodine value is highly correlated with the refractive index. Its value measures the degree of unsaturation in fats, oils and waxes. In *P. atlantica* fruit oil, the high iodine value (88 of I_2/100 g) indicated a high nutritional value. The acid index with low value is very appreciated in the cosmetics industry and is associated with the amount of free acid formed from enzymatic hydrolysis reactions of triglycerides. It is considered to be more representative of oil quality during harvesting, handling or processing [120]. The acid value of the *P. atlantica* oil was high (8.350 ± 0.120 mg KOH/g oil). This value is close to that reported for *P. lentiscus* (7 ± 0.3 mg KOH/g oil) [121]. The peroxide index (9.950 ± 0.950 meq O_2/kg) of *P. atlantica* oil reported in this study is slightly lower than the one noted for *P. lentiscus*, (10 ± 0.04 meq O_2/kg) [121]. For saponification (204.490 ± 0.040 mg KOH/g) and unsaponifiable matter (1.740 ± 0.010%), their values were higher than that reported for the same plant [119].

4.2. Chemical Composition and Variability

4.2.1. Fatty Acid Composition

Fatty acids composition of Atlas pistachio fruits was reported in several studies, showing a quantitative variability due to the extraction methods, maturity stage of fruits, Atlas pistachio subspecies and geographical origins (Table 2).

Table 2. Fatty acids composition of *P. atlantica* samples obtained by CG (%).

	Geographical Origins		Palmitic Acid	Palmitoleic Acid	Heptadecanoic Acid	Cis-10-Heptadecenoic Acid	Stearic Acid	Oleic Acid	Linoleic Acid	A-Linolenic Acid	Arachidic Acid	Cis-11-Eicosenoic Acid	Saturated Fatty Acids	Monounsaturated Fatty Acids	Poly-Unsaturated Fatty Acids
			C16:0	C16:1	C17:0	C17:1	C18:0	C18:1	C18:2	C18:3	C20:0	C20:1	SFA	MUFA	PUFA
Ziyad et al. [122]	Laghouat	Immature Fruits	18.8	0.35			0.84	55.4	21.9	0.74	ND		19.6	55.7	22.6
		Mature Fruits	14.7	0.39			2.6	53.5	24.9	0.71	0.26		17.5	53.8	25.6
	Ain oussera	Immature fruits	19.4	0.22			0.32	52.3	25.9	0.74	ND		19.7	52.5	26.6
		Mature fruits	12.7	1.1			1.6	51.6	29.4	0.61	0.22		14.7	52.7	30.0
Salhi et al. [115]	Elkharrouba (Tunisia)	Pressure extraction	11.32	0.12	0.07		2.36	56.80	28.83	0.32	0.18				
		Hexane extraction	11.30	0.23	0.07		2.41	56.67	28.82	0.35	0.15				
		Supercritical CO₂ extraction	11.42	0.15	0.05		2.33	56.12	29.45	0.33	0.15				
Hazrati et al. [123]	Kazerun (Iran)	kernel	20.20	2.97	0.06		2.02	53.15	20.41	0.71	0.15	0.32	22.59	56.44	21.12
Bentireche et al. [124]	Laghouat (Algeria)	Unripe	14.46	Tr			1.65	49.96	31.63	0.75	Tr	0.26	16.42	51.09	32.38
		Middle maturity	18.64	Tr			1.63	51.32	25.35	0.75	0.08	0.27	20.37	53.46	26.11
		Ripe	19.95	Tr			1.49	52.77	22.41	Tr	Tr	0.22	21.68	54.33	23.56
Labdelli et al. [111]	Djelfa	Seeds	26.7	1			2.1	40.9	26.8	1.1	0.1	0.2			27.9
Mohammadi et al. [125]	Shirez (Iran)	Hull	29.84	1.7			1.49	42.84	5.85	2.75			31.33	59.84	8.6
		Kernel	11.24	1.02			2.76	57.77	26.64	0.56			14	58.79	27.2
Gsallaoui et al. [126]	Tunisia	Seeds	11.16	0.23	0.04	0.03	2.42	56.35	28.74	0.35	0.14	0.46			
Guenane et al. [127]	Laghouat (Algeria)	Fruits mature	25.1	0.5			1.9	49.6	22.0	0.8	Tr	Tr	27.1	50.1	22.8
		Intermediate maturity	17.5	0.7			2.2	53.1	25.6	0.7	Tr	Tr	19.7	53.8	26.3
		Immature	13.9	0.3			2.2	51.7	30.8	0.8	Tr	Tr	16.2	52.0	31.7
Saber-Tehrani et al. [128]		Seeds	13.12	2.04	0.07	0.09	2.78	50.65	29.76		0.17		16.51	53.10	30.39
Yousfi et al. [45]	Algeria	Fruits	24	1.2			1.8	46	27.4	-					
Ghalem et al. [129]	Sidi Bel Abbes (Algeria)		12.2	1.8			2.4	54.2	28.8	0.4	0.1				29.3
Benhassaini et al. [46]	Tlemcen (Algeria)	Fruits	12.2	1.8			2.4	54.2	28.8	0.4	0.1				29.3

Tr: Trace.

Numerous studies reported that the fatty acid composition of *P. atlantica* oils shows a high content of unsaturated fatty acid, notably oleic acid from 40.9% to 81% [111,130–134] and linoleic acid from 20.41% to 29.4% [46,122,123].

Linolenic (C18:3), stearic (C18:0), and palmitoleic (C16:1) acid were less present in the fruit oil, while myristic (C14:0) and arachidic (C20:0) acid were only present in trace amounts [122]. These values varied according to the harvest month, which is in turn correlated to the maturation stage [122,124,133]. The ratio of unsaturated/saturated fatty acids was significantly higher in immature fruit oil (3.43–5.19) compared with the mature ones [123,124,128].

4.2.2. Phytosterol Composition

Phytosterols are naturally occurring in plants and cannot be synthesized in humans. They play major functions in several fields like pharmaceuticals (production of therapeutic steroids), nutrition (anti-cholesterol additives in functional foods, anti-cancer properties), and cosmetics (creams, lipstick) [135,136].

In comparison to other seed oils, pistachio oil had a typical distribution of sterols, characterized by a high content of β-sitosterol, and by a low content of campesterol and stigmasterol. Δ^5-Avenasterol had an intermediate distribution [130].

The major sterol of the *P. atlantica* seed oil is β-sitosterol (85 to 87%) [45,46,128,137]. The next major components are campesterol (4 to 4.35%) and Δ^5-avenasterol (2 to 4.35%). Each of the $\Delta^{5,24}$-stigmastadienol, Δ^7-avenasterol and stigmasterol amounted to about 1% of the total amount of sterols. The level of stigmasterol was absent in fruits harvested from *P. atlantica* from the southern region of Algeria but was twofold higher in the north (11%) [46]. Cholesterol is present at low levels (0.4%). The total sterol content in wild pistachio was 2164.5 mg kg^{-1} oil [128,137].

4.2.3. Tocopherol Composition

It was noticed that the tocols (tocopherols and tocotrienols) had potential health benefits, they contribute to the prevention of certain types of cancer, heart disease, and other chronic ailments [138]. In edible oil, the high concentration of these phenolic antioxidants plays a major role in preserving mono- and polyunsaturated fatty acids [139]. For that, research of vegetable oil as a source of natural antioxidants is very encouraged in cosmetic and pharmaceutical applications as therapeutics and skincare active moieties against collagenase and elastase activities [140,141].

Tocopherols and tocotrienols are monophenols, and exist in four different isoforms (α, β, γ and δ), that differ from each other by the number and location of methyl groups in their chemical structures [142]. In *P. atlantica*, the fruit oil appears to be richer in tocopherols which vary depending on the developmental stage and the maturation degree of the fruits [124,143]. Their contents had a high value in immature fruit oil (50.7 ± 7.9 mg/100 g oil) compared to intermediate (44.3 ± 8.1 mg/100 g) and mature fruits (34.1 ± 10.9 mg/100 g) [143]. The predominant tocopherol in wild pistachio cold-press oil was α- tocopherol with 379.68 mg/kg. The amounts of (γ + β)-tocopherol and δ-tocopherol were 20.70 and 9.59 mg/kg of oil [128]. On the other hand, the tocopherols analysis performed for eleven samples of *P. atlantica* fruit oils extracted by n-hexane showed a dominance of α- and γ-tocopherols [143]. These compounds contribute the highest antioxidant propriety of oil with the participation of phenolic compounds [124]. It may be noted that the extraction method did not affect the content of tocophenols in fruit oil of *P. atlantica* obtained by three techniques i.e., supercritical CO_2, organic solvent (hexane) and cold pressing [126].

4.2.4. Pigment Composition

Besides, their use as antioxidants in dietary supplements and pharmacological agents, the carotenoids can be employed in cosmetics against photoaging effects on the skin, irritation, acne and cancer. They play the role of a filter to absorb ultraviolet radiation [144]. The chlorophylls represent not only the most abundant natural pigment molecules intervening in photosynthesis, but they have numerous therapeutic properties on inflammation, oxidation, wound healing and cancer prevention [145]. Moreover, these molecules have also been used as colouring agents and anti-ageing components in cosmetic products where they are added to creams and soaps [146].

In *Pistacia atlantica* fixed oils, it is shown that tocopherols and carotenoids were the major constituents of the unsaponifiable matter [133]. Pheophytin a (12.02 mg/kg), and luteoxanthin (10.41 mg/kg) represent the major carotenoid components, followed by lutein (5.2 mg/kg). The compounds neoxanthin, violaxanthin, lutein isomers and pheophytin a were also present with low contents, ranging between 0.15 to 1.46 mg/kg. For chlorophylls, their amounts were 0.92 and 1.19 mg/kg for chlorophyll a' and chlorophyll a, respectively [128]. As tocopherols, the carotenoids showed the highest level in ripe fruit oil compared to other stages of development [133].

4.2.5. Total Phenol and Flavonoid Contents

Total phenolic and flavonoid contents of *P. atlantica* fatty oil were 130.77 ± 3.11 mg gallic acid equivalent/100 g oil and 126.91 ± 4.41 mg quercetin/100 g oil, respectively [123]. These contents decrease with fruit maturation from 2.51 to 0.13 mg GAE/100 g oil and 1.64 to 0.09 mg quercetin/100 g for phenolic and flavonoid contents, respectively.

According to Farhoosh et al. [147], the greatest total phenolic concentrations have been recorded in fruit oils of *P. atlantica* subsp. *mutica* (81.12 mg gallic acid equivalent/kg) and *kurdica* (56.51 mg gallic acid equivalent/kg).

Additionally, Saber-Tehrani et al. [128] stated that caffeic acid (1.96 ± 0.04 mg/kg oil), cinnamic acid (0.67 ± 0.02 mg/kg oil) and pinoresinol (0.64 ± 0.01 mg/kg) were the predominant phenolic compounds in *P. atlantica* oil obtained by cold-press. Other compounds such as ferulic acid, o-coumaric acid, vanillin and *p*-coumaric acid were present at low levels.

4.3. Biological Activities

Some reports cited above studied the biochemical composition of fruit oil which contains interesting nutritional properties such as a high oleic acid content, phytosterols, carotenoids, phenolics and tocopherols. These essential compounds contribute to human health benefits for their antimicrobial, antioxidant, anti-inflammatory, immunity correction, hypocholeserolaemic, antiatherogenic, anticancer, digestive etc. Given these elements, Atlas pistachio fruit oil could be a promising component for cosmetics.

4.3.1. Antimicrobial Activity

The previous studies reported the highest contents of oleic and linoleic acids in *P. atlantica* fatty oil. These compounds have potential antibacterial properties which are partly attributed to their unsaturated long-chain lengths with 12–18 carbons [148]. This observation is consistent with previous work carried out with *P. lentiscus* fatty oil and its phenolic extract [149]. Additionally, it is noted that linoleic and oleic acids showed their growth inhibition against the Gram-positive bacteria but were inactive against the Gram-negative ones [150].

4.3.2. Antioxidant Activity

The antioxidant activity of *P. atlantica* crude oils might be attributed to the presence of tocopherols, carotenoids, and unsaturated fatty acids in particular omega-three fatty acids [133]. Another study, carried out on the stage of development of *P. atlantica* fruits showed positive correlations between flavonoid contents and total antioxidant capacity for unripe and red fruits [151].

4.3.3. Anti-Inflammatory Activity

Pistachio oil had been reported to possess anti-inflammatory activity. The fruit oil constituted of linoleic acid, oleic acid and stearic acid, as the major components, exhibited significant wound healing and anti-inflammatory effects of oil-absorbed bacterial cellulose in an in vivo burn wound model [152]. This oil can be used as a potential bio-safe dressing for wound management. In addition, *P. atlantica* fruit oil may be efficient for ulcerative colitis [153]. Tanideh et al. [153] stated that a high dose of oil reduces colonic injury by suppressing oxidative damage in rats when administered orally and rectally.

The oil of wild pistachio may modulate hypothyroidism and its effects on serum lipid profile and leptin concentration, modulate hypothyroidism and its effects on serum lipid profile and leptin concentration [154].

In 2017, Hamidi et al. [155] revealed the effects of topical application of a gel formulation prepared with 5%, and 10% of *P. atlantica* oil on cutaneous wound healing in an experimentally induced cutaneous wound model in rats. This study showed a re-epithelialization with continuous stratum basalis and mature granulation tissue and adnexa (hair follicles and sweat gland) with Atlas pistachio oil gels (especially Bene 10%) at 21 days post-injury.

Interestingly, the fixed oils traditionally extracted by the rural populations from Atlas pistachio fruits are widely used and recommended for rheumatoid arthritis and joint pain. The oil is directly applied over the painful area with a light massage to heat it and for greater adherence.

4.3.4. Antihyperlipidemic Effects

Unsaturated fatty acids in *P. atlantica* fruit oil modulated serum leptin, thyroid hormones, and lipid profile in female rats with experimentally induced hypothyroidism caused by propyl thiouracil (PTU) [154]. Jamshidi et al. [156] revealed the preventive effects of *P. atlantica* subsp. *mutica* oil, *P. atlantica* subsp. *mutica* resin and mixture oils in reducing metabolic syndrome risk. By measuring the lipid profiles, glycaemic indices, oxidative stress and inflammatory parameters, the results showed that consuming *P. atlantica* subsp. *mutica* oil was more effective than other oils (wild pistachio resin and mixture oils) in preventing hyperglycaemia, hypertriglyceridemia, hypercholesterolaemia, inflammation and pancreatic secretory disorders.

Phytosterols are important micronutrients in human diets, they form the unsaponifiable part of *P. atlantica* oil. They play an essential role in the reduction of cholesterol in the blood and therefore decrease cardiovascular morbidity [157]. β β-sitosterol ester with linoleic acids and β-sitosterol self-microemulsions have positive hypolipidaemic effects on hyperlipidaemic mice [157].

4.3.5. Antidiabetic Activity

It was shown that the resin oil of *P. atlantica* represents the best wound healing agent in STZ-induced diabetic experimental rats [158]. This oil improves blood flow and vascularization by elevation of vascular endothelial growth factor (VEGF) levels and reduces harmful effects of diabetic oxidative status, as well as burn damage in the wound area.

4.3.6. Cytotoxic Activity

Thanks to its chemical composition, *P. atlantica* fruit oil may be used for its anticancer potential. It is well noted that the fatty acids [159], unsaponifiable fraction [160], α-terpineol [161] and β-sitosterol [162] have the potential to reduce the proliferation of and induce apoptosis. It has been investigated whether the vitamin E and its tocopherol members (α-, β-, γ-, δ-) and tocotrienols (α-, β-, γ-, δ-) showed a strong association with the prevention of cancer and inhibition of tumour, both in vitro and in vivo [163].

The traditional extraction of oils (Figure 5c) had limited its utilization to domestic consumption and use. Whereas, with the availability of electric grinder–extractors, many artisans currently extract the fatty oils and sell them in herbalist shops or using electronic trade (e-Commerce). Therefore, Atlas pistachio fatty oil is increasingly experienced and appreciated. It is used to treat hair and skin damage as it is recommended since ancient times. Furthermore, it is incorporated into several handicraft cosmetics products such as soaps, shampoos, and protective repair and moisturizing creams.

5. Innovation and Modern Formulations for the Cosmetics Industry

Nanotechnology is a burgeoning scientific approach in research and presents potential applications in diverse fields, including biomedical, pharmaceutical and cosmetics industries [164]. Among the various nanoparticles used since the development of nanotechnology applications, silver nanoparticles (AgNPs) have attracted the attention of researchers in the last two decades [165] due to their useful characteristics in several fields, principally in cosmetics and care products. *Pistacia atlantica* leaf extract from Iran was used to synthesize pure crystalline and spherical green AgNPs with a high surface area of about 27 nm average size [165]. The results suggest that the synthesized AgNPs act as an effective antibacterial agent (e.g., against *Staphylococcus aureus*) and are capable of rendering high antibacterial efficacy and so possess a great potential in the preparation of drugs used against bacterial diseases, but mostly in cosmetic products [165]. The authors state that *Pistacia atlantica* is a very good eco-friendly and nontoxic source for the synthesis of Ag-NPs as compared to conventional chemical/physical methods [165].

P. atlantica fruit oil is one of the most nutritious vegetable oils which can be used as a carrier in lipid formulations. The use of vegetable oils in lipid nanoparticle preparation constitutes a promising field to treat diverse pathologies. These therapeutic activities are a result of synergistic effects by interactions of vegetable oil lipid carriers and active compounds [166].

The nanoformulations based on unsaturated fatty acids, carotenoids, retinoids, and tocopherols are employed as excipients in cosmetics and personal care products to alleviate skin disorders like irritation and inflammation [167]. Among the major fatty acids with potential applications, linoleic acid (omega-6) and α-linolenic acid (omega-3) were used in the prevention and treatment of inflammatory skin diseases such as atopic dermatitis, psoriasis and acne [168].

6. Challenges of the Use of EOs and FOs of *Pistacia atlantica* in the Cosmetics Industry

Although essential oils are used for their biological activities (antibacterial, antifungal, anti-inflammatory, antioxidant) and preservative properties against contamination, the safety issues regarding the use of EOs should not be neglected. EOs may induce allergenic and chronic toxicity risks if they are not added based on an accurate assessment. Nevertheless, the essential oil of *Pistacia atlantica* is known for its low toxicity [169]. Indeed, EOs with α-pinene as a major constituent have very low toxicity and would be a good candidate for use in health products [170]. The chemical variability also constitutes a great challenge for the use of *P. atlantica* EOs in the cosmetics industry, mainly when the plant material is brought from natural populations or populations under different environmental conditions. In addition, regarding the use of *P. atlantica* VOs in the cosmetics industry, the principal challenge is how to provide sufficient plant material (the fruit) without over-exploitation. In this sense, one of the main challenges is that fruit over-exploitation may induce a conflict between socio–economic and industrial needs. However, the valuation of Atlas pistachio EOs and VOs remains a major opportunity for dynamic rural development.

At the end of this paper, we believe that natural resource utilization should receive all our consideration. Atlas pistachio regarding its spiritual, social and economic value, but also its alarming situation as a threatened species, needs to be given particular consideration. The species should be intensively and broadly included in reforestation schemes and programs in the whole of its wide area to ensure sustainable valorization and to provide sufficient production.

7. Conclusions

Because of their health problems, toxicity and carcinogenicity, the use of synthetic compounds in several fields such as the food industry, drug industry, and cosmetics is currently being limited. Consequently, the search for new natural sources and novel natural bioactive compounds has been very accentuated in recent years.

Pistacia atlantica essential and fixed oils have been valorized and used in traditional medicine for the treatment of various diseases. Fruits and fatty oils are widely consumed as a nutrient by the local populations. They constitute a major source of beneficial compounds such as fatty acids with a predominance of oleic and linoleic acids, phenolic compounds, and unsaponifiable matter with their active molecules (tocopherols, phytosterols and carotenoids) which exhibited a large panel of health benefits. Both *Pistacia atlantica* essential and fruit oils have not been widely used for industrial applications. Nevertheless, the traditional uses and the indigenous knowledge have recently inspired modern cosmetic formulations but also cosmetic handicraft products which currently represent an emergent market in natural-based beauty and care products.

To the best of our knowledge, the current paper is the first review focusing principally on the potential of the use of EOs and FOs of *P. atlantica* in cosmetics. The chemical compositions of Atlas pistachio essential and fixed oils present a promising source for potential applications in pharmaceuticals and cosmetics as a single product or nanoformulation in the form of moisturizers, anti-ageing serums, makeup removers and massage oil. Thus, further field investigations and ethnobotanical surveys will provide useful information about the valorization of Atlas Pistachio EOs and VOs. This data may help to draw several perspectives in using *Pistacia atlantica* EO and VO components in modern cosmetic products principally for their biological activities and therapeutic potential.

Author Contributions: Conceptualization, A.E.Z.-B.; validation, A.E.Z.-B., N.B.-B. and H.B.; writing—original draft preparation, A.E.Z.-B., N.B.-B. and H.B.; writing—review and editing, A.E.Z.-B., N.B.-B. and H.B.; supervision, A.E.Z.-B.; All authors have read and agreed to the published version of the manuscript.

Funding: This research received no external funding.

Institutional Review Board Statement: Not applicable.

Informed Consent Statement: Not applicable.

Conflicts of Interest: The authors declare no conflict of interest.

References

1. Dalley, S.S. Ancient mesopotamian gardens and the identification of the hanging gardens of babylon resolved. *Garden Hist* **1993**, *21*, 1–13. [CrossRef]
2. DeNavarre, M.G. Oils and fats, the historical cosmetics. *J. Am. Oil Chem. Soc* **1978**, *55*, 435–437. [CrossRef]
3. Nicholson, P.T.; Shaw, I. *Ancient Egyptian Materials and Technology*; Cambridge University Press: Cambridge, UK, 2000; p. 461.
4. EMA (European Medicines Agency). Assessment report on *Pistacia lentiscus* L., resin (mastix). EMA/HMPC/46756/2015. 2015. Available online: https://www.ema.europa.eu/en/documents/herbal-report/draft-assessment-report-pistacia-lentiscus-l-resin-mastic_en.pdf (accessed on 25 November 2021).
5. Serpico, M.; White, R. The use and identification of varnish on New Kingdom funerary equipment. In *Colour and painting in ancient Egypt*; The British Museum Press: London, UK, 2001; pp. 33–42.
6. Stern, B.; Heron, C.; Corr, L.; Serpico, M.; Bourriau, J. Compositional variations in aged and heated pistacia resin found in late bronze age canaanite amphorae and bowls from Amarna Egypt. *Archaeo* **2003**, *45*, 457–469. [CrossRef]
7. Fulcher, K.; Budka, J. Pigments, incense, and bitumen from the New Kingdom town and cemetery on Sai Island in Nubia. *J. Archaeol. Sci. Rep.* **2020**, *33*, 102550. [CrossRef]
8. Brettell, R.C.; Stern, B.; Reifarth, N.; Heron, C. The 'semblance of immortality'? Resinous materials and mortuary rites in Roman Britain. *Archaeo* **2014**, *56*, 444–459. [CrossRef]
9. El Zerey-Belaskri, A.; Benhassaini, H. 'El bottom' à travers l'existence des Homo: Récit entre altruisme et ingratitude. In Proceedings of the 1ere Journée d'Etude sur la Conservation et la Valorisation de la Biodiversité Végétale en Algérie, Sidi Bel Abbes, Algeria, 21 February 2017.
10. Lima, S.N.R.; Lima, R.J.; de Salis, C.; de Azevedo Moreira, R. Cashew-tree (*Anacardium occidentale* L.) exudate gum: A novel bioligand tool. *Biotech. Appl. Biochem.* **2002**, *35*, 45–53.
11. Bennett, B.C. Twenty-five Important Plant Families. In *UNESCO Encyclopedia of Life Support Systems*; Bennett, B.C., Ed.; Florida International University: Miami, FL, USA, 2007. Available online: https://www.eolss.net/Sample-Chapters/C09/E6-118-03.pdf (accessed on 20 December 2021).
12. Zohary, M. A monographical study of the genus *Pistacia*. Palestine. *J. Bot.* **1952**, *5*, 187–228.

13. Benhassaini, H. Contribution à L'étude de L'autoécologie de *Pistacia atlantica* Desf. ssp. *atlantica* et Valorisation. Ph.D. Thesis, University of Sidi Bel Abbes, Sidi Bel Abbes, Algeria, 2004.
14. Quezel, P.; Santa, S. *Nouvelle Flore de l'Algérie et Des Régions Désertiques Méridionales*; Centre National de la Recherche Scientifique: Paris, France, 1963; pp. 611–612.
15. El Zerey-Belaskri, A. A Multidisciplinary Approach for the Characterization of *Pistacia atlantica* Desf. subsp. *atlantica* Diversity in Northwest Algeria. Ph.D. Thesis, University of Sidi Bel Abbes, Sidi Bel Abbes, Algeria, 2016; 143p.
16. Gregoriou, C. Collection, conservation and utilization of Pistacia genetic resources in Cyprus. In *Project on Underutilized Mediterranean Species. Pistacia: Towards a Comprehensive Documentation of Distribution and Use of Its Genetic Diversity in Central & West Asia, North Africa and Mediterranean Europe*; Padulosi, S., Hadj-Hassan, A., Eds.; Report of the IPGRI Workshop: Irbid, Jordan, 2001.
17. Mansf Ency. *Mansfeld's Encyclopedia of Agricultural and Horticultural Crops*; Hanelt, P., Ed.; 2001; Volume 1–6. Available online: http://mansfeld.ipk-gatersleben.de/pls/htmldb (accessed on 19 November 2021).
18. Daoudi, A.; Boutou, H.; Ibijbijen, J.; Zair, T.; Nassiri, L. Etude éthnobotanique du pistachier de L'Atlas, *Pistacia atlantica*, dans la ville de Meknes—Maroc. *Sci. Lib* **2013**, *5*, 131113.
19. Rechinger, K.H. *Flora Des Iranischen Hochlandes und der Umrahmenden Gebirge*; Akademische Druck-u.: Graz, Austria, 1969.
20. Browicz, K. *Chorology of Trees and Shrubs in South-West Asia and Adjacent Regions*; Polish Scientific Publications: Poznan, Poland, 1988; Volume 6.
21. Yaltirik, F. Anacardiaceae. In *Flora of Turkey*; Davis, P.H., Ed.; Edinburgh University Press: Edinburgh, UK, 1967; Volume 2, pp. 544–548.
22. El Zerey-Belaskri, A. Taxonomic and botanical retrospective review of *Pistacia atlantica* Desf. (Anacardiaceae). *Arab. J. Arom. Med. Plants* **2019**, *5*, 47–77.
23. Barrero, A.F.; Herrador, M.M.; Arteaga, J.F.; Akssira, M.; Mellouki, F.; Belgarrabe, A.; Blàzquez, M. Chemical composition of the essential oils of *Pistacia atlantica* Desf. *J. Essent. Oil Res.* **2005**, *17*, 52–54. [CrossRef]
24. Tzakou, O.; Bazos, I.; Yannitsaros, A. Volatile metabolites of *Pistacia atlantica* Desf. from Greece. *Flavour Fragr. J.* **2007**, *22*, 358–362. [CrossRef]
25. Mecherara-Idjeri, S.; Hassani, A.; Casanova, J. Composition of leaf, fruit and gall essential oils of Algerian *Pistacia atlantica* Desf. *J. Essent. Oil Res.* **2008**, *20*, 215–219. [CrossRef]
26. Gourine, N.; Bombarda, I.; Nadjemi, B.; Yousfi, M.; Gaydou, E.M. Chemotypes of *Pistacia atlantica* leaf essential oils from Algeria. *Nat. Prod. Commun.* **2010**, *5*, 115–120. [CrossRef]
27. Gourine, N.; Yousfi, M.; Bombarda, I.; Nadjemi, B.; Stocker, P.; Gaydou, E.M. Antioxidant activities and chemical composition of essential oil of *Pistacia atlantica* from Algeria. *Ind. Crops Prod.* **2010**, *31*, 203–208. [CrossRef]
28. Ait Said, S.; Fernandez, C.; Greff, S.; Torre, F.; Derridj, A.; Gauquelin, T.; Mevy, J.P. Inter-population variability of terpenoid composition in leaves of *Pistacia lentiscus* L. from Algeria: A chemoecological approach. *Molecules* **2011**, *16*, 2646–2657. [CrossRef]
29. El Zerey-Belaskri, A.; Cavaleiro, C.; Romane, A.; Benhassaini, H.; Salgueiro, L. Intraspecific chemical variability of *Pistacia atlantica* Desf. subsp. *atlantica* essential oil from Northwest Algeria. *J. Essent. Oil Res.* **2017**, *29*, 32–41. [CrossRef]
30. Khiya, Z.; Oualcadi, Y.; Zerkani, H.; Gamar, A.; Amine, S.; Hamzaoui, N.E.; Berrekhis, F.; Zair, T.; Hilali, F.E. Chemical Composition and Biological Activities of *Pistacia atlantica* Desf. Essential Oil From Morocco. *J. Essent. Oil-Bear. Plants* **2021**, *24*, 254–265. [CrossRef]
31. Benguechoua, M.I.; Benguechoua, M.; Gourine, N.; Silva, A.M.S.; Saidi, M.; Yousfi, M. Harvest date and variability in lipid bioactive compounds in *Pistacia atlantica* Mediterranean. *J. Nutr. Metab.* **2021**, *14*, 173–190.
32. Al Yafi, J. New characters differentiating *Pistacia atlantica* subspecies. *Candollea* **1978**, *33*, 201–208.
33. Al Yafi, J. Approches Systématique et Ecologique du Genre *Pistacia* L. dans la région méditerranéenne. Ph.D. Thesis, Univ. D'Aix-Marseille St Jérome France, Marseille, France, 1979.
34. Behboodi, B.S. Ecological distribution study of wild pistachios for selection of roostock. In *XIII GREMPA Meeting on Almonds and Pistachios*; Oliveira, M.M., Cordeiro, V., Eds.; CIHEAM: Zaragoza, Spain, 2005; Volume 63, pp. 61–67.
35. Belhadj, S.; Derridj, A.; Auda, Y.; Gers, C.; Gauquelin, T. Analyse de la variabilité morphologique chez huit populations spontanées de *Pistacia atlantica* en Algérie. *Botany* **2008**, *86*, 520–532. [CrossRef]
36. El Zerey-Belaskri, A.; Benhassaini, H. Morphological leaf variability in natural populations of *Pistacia atlantica* Desf. subsp. *atlantica* along climatic gradient: New features to update *Pistacia atlantica* subsp. *atlantica* key. *Int. J. Biometeorol.* **2016**, *60*, 577–589. [CrossRef]
37. Behboodi, B.S.; Ghaffari, M. Pollen morphology and analysis of Iranian wild pistachio. In *XIII GREMPA Meeting on Almonds and Pistachios*; Oliveira, M.M., Cordeiro, V., Eds.; Série A. Séminaires Méditerranéens; CIHEAM: Zaragoza, Spain, 2005; Volume 63, pp. 123–127.
38. Belhadj, S.; Derridj, A.; Aigouy, T.; Gers, C.; Gauquelin, T.; Mevy, J.-P. Comparative morphology of leaf epidermis in eight populations of Atlas Pistachio (*Pistacia atlantica* Desf., Anacardiaceae). *Microsc. Res. Tech.* **2007**, *70*, 837–846. [CrossRef]
39. Belhadj, S.; Derridj, A.; Civeyrel, L.; Gers, C.; Aigouy, T.; Otto, T.; Gauquelin, T. Pollen morphology and fertility of wild Atlas pistachio (*Pistacia atlantica* Desf., Anacardiaceae). *Grana* **2007**, *46*, 148–156. [CrossRef]
40. Tirse, M.; Benhassaini, H.; Sail, K.; Bassou, G. Leaflets Epidermal Micro-Characters of *Pistacia atlantica* Desf. subsp. *atlantica* (Anacardiaceae) under Semi-Arid Environmental Factors. *Environ. Res. J.* **2014**, *7*, 433–447.
41. Monjauze, A. Le pays des dayas et *Pistacia atlantica* Desf. dans le Sahara algérien. *Rev. Forest. Franç.* **1982**, *34*, 277–289. [CrossRef]

42. Ozenda, P. *Flore du Sahara*; CNRS: Paris, France, 1983; 622.
43. Zohary, M. *Pistacia* L. Flora Palestine. Academy of Science and Humanities. *Jerusalem* **1972**, *2*, 297–300.
44. Yaaqobi, A.; El Hafid, L.; Haloui, B. Etude biologique de *Pistacia atlantica* Desf. de la région orientale du Maroc. *Biomatec. Echo.* **2009**, *6*, 39–49.
45. Yousfi, M.; Nedjmi, B.; Bellal, R.; Ben Bertal, D.; Palla, G. Fatty acids and sterols of *Pistacia atlantica* fruit oil. *J. Am. Oil Chem. Soc.* **2002**, *79*, 1049–1050. [CrossRef]
46. Benhassaini, H.; Bendahmane, M.; Benchalgo, N. The chemical composition of fruits of *Pistacia atlantica* desf. subsp. *atlantica* from Algeria. *Chem. Nat. Compd.* **2007**, *43*, 121–124. [CrossRef]
47. El Zerey-Belaskri, A.; Belyaagoubi-Benhammou, N.; Kendouli, I.; Gambaza, N.; Bennaoum, Z.; Lalout, J.; Oughilas, A.; Atik-Bekkara, F.; Benhassaini, H.; Rosa, A.; et al. Phenolic profile, physic-chemical properties, fatty acid composition and anti-oxydant activity of *Pistacia atlantica* Desf. subsp. *atlantica* fruit oil from Algeria. In Proceedings of the 6th International Congress of Aromatic and Medicinal Plants (CIPAM), Coimbra, Portugal, 29 May–1 June 2016.
48. Benhammou-Belyagoubi, N.; Belyagoubi, L.; El Zerey-Belaskri, A.; Atik-Bekkara, F. In vitro antioxidant properties of flavonoid fractions from *Pistacia atlantica* Desf. subsp. *atlantica* fruit using five techniques. *J. Mat. Environ. Sci.* **2014**, *6*, 1118–1125.
49. Hüsnü, K.; Başer, C.; Demirci, F. Chemistry of Essential Oils. In *Flavours and Fragrances*; Berger, R., Ed.; Springer: Hannover, Germany, 2007; pp. 43–86.
50. Katayama, T. Volatile constituents. In *Physiology and Biochemistry of Algae*; Lewln, R.A., Ed.; Academic: Cambridge, MA, USA, 1962; pp. 467–473.
51. Katayama, T. Chemical studies on volatile constituents of seaweeds VI. On volatile constituents of *Sargasswn* sp. *Bul. Jap. Soc. Sci. Fish.* **1955**, *21*, 425–428. [CrossRef]
52. Joshi, G.V.; Gowda, C.A. Seasonal variations in chemical composition of *Sargasswn ilicifolium* Grun, sea water. *Indian J. Mar. Sci.* **1975**, *4*, 165–168.
53. Rezaei, P.F.; Fouladdel, S.; Hassani, S.; Yousefbeyk, F.; Ghaffari, S.M.; Amin, G.; Azizi, E. Induction of apoptosis and cell cycle arrest by pericarp polyphenol-rich extract of Baneh in human colon carcinoma HT29 cells. *Food Chem. Toxicol.* **2012**, *50*, 1054–1059. [CrossRef]
54. Labed-Zouad, I.; Ferhat, M.; Öztürk, M.; Abaza, I.; Nadeem, S.; Kabouche, A.; Kabouche, Z. Essential Oils Composition, Anticholinesterase and Antioxidant Activities of *Pistacia atlantica* Desf. *Rec. Nat. Prod.* **2017**, *11*, 411–415.
55. Benha Ssaini, H.; Benabderrahmane, M.; Chikhi, K. Contribution à l'évaluation de l'activité antiseptique de l'oléorésine et des huiles essentielles du pistachier de l'Atlas sur certains souches microbiennes: *Candida albicans* (ATCC 20027), *Candida albican* (ATCC 20032) et *Saccharomyces cerevisiae*. *Ethnopharamcologia* **2003**, *30*, 38–46.
56. Benhassaini, H.; Bendeddouche, F.Z.; Mehdadi, Z.; Romane, A. GC/MS analysis of the essential oil from the oleoresin of *Pistacia atlantica* Desf. subsp. *atlantica* from Algeria. *Nat. Prod. Com.* **2008**, *3*, 929–932. [CrossRef]
57. Karimi, H.R.; Kafkas, S. Genetic relationships among *Pistacia* species studied by SAMPL markers. *Plant Syst. Evol.* **2011**, *297*, 207–212. [CrossRef]
58. Benhassaini, H.; Mehdadi, Z.; Hamel, L.; Belkhodja, M. Phytoécologie de *Pistacia atlantica* Desf. subsp. *atlantica* dans le Nord-ouest algérien. *Sécheresse* **2007**, *18*, 199–205.
59. Benabdallah, F.Z.; Kouamé, R.O.; El Bentchikou, M.; Zellagui, A.; Gherraf, N. Études ethnobotanique, phytochimique et valorisation de l'activité antimicrobienne des feuilles et de l'oléorésine du pistachier de l'atlas (*Pistacia atlantica* Desf.). *Phytothérapie* **2015**, *15*, 222–229. [CrossRef]
60. Memariani, Z.; Sharifzadeh, M.; Bozorgi, M.; Hajimahmoodi, M.; Farzaei, M.H.; Gholami, M.; Siavoshi, F.; Saniee, P. Protective effect of essential oil of *Pistacia atlantica* Desf. on peptic ulcer: Role of α-pinene. *J. Trad. Chin. Med.* **2017**, *37*, 57–63. [CrossRef]
61. Delazar, A.; Reid, R.G.; Sarker, S.D. GC-MS analysis of the essential oil from the oleoresin of *Pistacia atlantica* var. *mutica*. *Chem. Nat. Comp.* **2004**, *40*, 24–27. [CrossRef]
62. Eghbali-Feriz, S.; Taleghani, A.; Al-Najjar, H.; Emami, S.A.; Rahimi, H.; Asili, J.; Hasanzadeh, S.; Tayarani-Najaran, Z. Anti-melanogenesis and anti-tyrosinase properties of *Pistacia atlantica* subsp. *mutica* extracts on B16F10 murine melanoma cells. *Res. Pharm. Sci.* **2018**, *13*, 533–545. [CrossRef] [PubMed]
63. Didehvar, M.; Ebadi, M.T.; Ayyari, M. Qualitative and Quantitative Evaluation of *Pistacia atlantica* Desf. Essential Oil from Thirteen Natural Habitats. *Iran. J. Horti. Sci.* **2021**, *52*, 419–428.
64. Hashemi-Moghaddam, H.; Mohammdhosseini, M.; Salar, M. Chemical composition of the essential oils from the hulls of *Pistacia vera* L. by using magnetic nanoparticle-assisted microwave (MW) distillation: Comparison with routine MW and conventional hydrodistillation. *Anal. Methods* **2014**, *6*, 2572–2579. [CrossRef]
65. Scott, R.P.W. Essential oils. *Encycl. Anal. Sci.* **2005**, 554–561. [CrossRef]
66. Elshafie, H.S.; Mancini, E.; Sakr, S.; De Martino, L.; Mattia, C.A.; De Feo, V.; Camele, I. Antifungal Activity of Some Constituents of *Origanum vulgare* L. Essential Oil Against Postharvest Disease of Peach Fruit. *J. Med. Food* **2015**, *18*, 929–934. [CrossRef] [PubMed]
67. Guzmán, E.; Lucia, A. Essential Oils and Their Individual Components in Cosmetic Products. *Cosmetics* **2021**, *8*, 114. [CrossRef]
68. Bicas, J.L.; Dionisio, A.P.; Pastore, G.M. Bio-oxidation of Terpenes: An Approach for the Flavor Industry. *Chem. Rev.* **2009**, *109*, 4518–4531. [CrossRef]
69. Bürgers, R.; Schneider-Brachert, W.; Reischl, U.; Behr, A.; Hiller, K.A.; Lehn, N.; Schmalz, G.; Ruhl, S. *Helicobacter pylori* in human oral cavity and stomach. *Eur. J. Oral. Sci.* **2008**, *116*, 297–304. [CrossRef]

70. Rodrigues, K.A.; Amorim, L.V.; Dias, C.N.; Moraes, D.F.; Carneiro, S.M.; Carvalho, F.A. *Syzygium cumini* (L.) Skeels essential oil and its major constituent alpha-pinene exhibit anti-Leishmania activity through immunomodulation in vitro. *J. Ethnopharmacol.* **2015**, *160*, 32–40. [CrossRef]
71. Sonboli, A.M.A.; Esmaeili, A.; Gholipour, A.; Kanani, M.R. Composition, cytotoxicity and antioxidant activity of the essential oil of *Dracocephalum surmandinum* from Iran. *Nat. Prod. Commun.* **2010**, *5*, 341–344. [CrossRef] [PubMed]
72. Chen, W.; Liu, Y.; Li, M.; Mao, J.; Zhang, L.; Huang, R.; Jin, X.; Ye, L. Anti-tumor effect of α-pinene on human hepatoma cell lines through inducing G2/M cell cycle arrest. *J. Pharmacol. Sci.* **2015**, *127*, 332–338. [CrossRef] [PubMed]
73. Matsuo, A.L.; Figueiredo, C.R.; Arruda, D.C.; Pereira, F.V.; Scutti, J.A.B.; Massaoka, M.H.; Travassos, L.R.; Sartorelli, P.; Lago, J.H.G. α-Pinene isolated from *Schinus terebinthifolius* Raddi (Anacardiaceae) induces apoptosis and confers antimetastatic protection in a melanoma model. *Biochem. Biophys. Res. Commun.* **2011**, *411*, 449–454. [CrossRef]
74. Buriani, A.; Fortinguerra, S.; Sorrenti, V.; Dall'Acqua, S.; Innocenti, G.; Montopoli, M.; Gabbia, D.; Carrara, M. Human adenocarcinoma cell line sensitivity to essential oil phytocomplexes from *Pistacia* species: A multivariate approach. *Molecules* **2017**, *22*, 1336. [CrossRef] [PubMed]
75. Porres-Martínez, M.; González-Burgos, E.; Carretero, M.E.; Gómez-Serranillos, M.P. *In vitro* neuroprotective potential of the monoterpenes α-pinene and 1,8-cineole against H2O2-induced oxidative stress in PC12 cells. *Z. Nat. C* **2016**, *71*, 191–199. [CrossRef] [PubMed]
76. Leite, A.M.; de Oliveira Lima, E.; de Souza, E.L.; Diniz, M.F.F.M.; Trajano, V.N.; de Medeiros, I.A. Inhibitory effect of β-pinene, α–pinene and eugenol on the growth of potential infectious endocarditis causin gram-positive bacteria. *Rev. Bras. Ciências Farm.* **2007**, *43*, 121–126. [CrossRef]
77. Gavrilov, V.V.; Startseva, V.A.; Nikitina, L.E.; Lodochnikova, O.A.; Gnezdilov, O.I.; Lisovskaya, S.A.; Clushko, N.I.; Klimovitskii, E.N. Synthesis and antifungal activity of sulfides, sulfoxides, and sulfones based on (1 s)-(−)-β-pinene. *Pharm. Chem. J.* **2010**, *44*, 126–129. [CrossRef]
78. Silva, A.C.R.; Lopes, P.M.; Azevedo, M.M.B.; Costa, D.C.M.; Alviano, C.S.; Alviano, D.S. Biological activities of α–pinene and β-pinene enantiomers. *Molecules* **2012**, *17*, 6305–6316. [CrossRef]
79. Guzman-Gutierrez, S.L.; Gomez-Cansino, R.; Garcia-Zebadua, J.C.; Jimenez-Perez, N.C.; Reyes-Chilpa, R. Antidepressant activity of *Litsea glaucescens* essential oil: Identification of beta-pinene and linalool as active principles. *J. Ethnopharmacol.* **2012**, *143*, 673–679. [CrossRef]
80. Guzman-Gutierrez, S.L.; Bollina-Jaime, H.; Gomez-Cansino, R.; Reyes-Chilpa, R. Linalool and β–pinene exert their antidepressant-like activity through the monoaminergic pathway. *Life Sci.* **2015**, *128*, 24–29. [CrossRef]
81. Huynh, Q.; Phan, T.D.; Thieu, V.Q.Q.; Tran, S.T.; Do, S.H. Extraction and refining of essential oil from Australian tea tree, Melaleuca alterfornia, and the antimicrobial activity in cosmetic products. *J. Phys. Conf. Ser.* **2012**, *352*, 012053. [CrossRef]
82. Yang, Z.; Xiao, Z.; Ji, H. Solid inclusion complex of terpinen-4-ol/β-cyclodextrin: Kinetic release, mechanism and its antibacterial activity. *Flavour Fragr. J.* **2014**, *30*, 179–187. [CrossRef]
83. Tighe, S.; Gao, Y.Y.; Tseng, S.C.G. Terpinen-4-ol is the Most Active Ingredient of Tea Tree Oil to KillDemodexMites. *Transl. Vis. Sci. Technol.* **2013**, *2*, 2. [CrossRef] [PubMed]
84. Cavaleiro, C.; Pinto, E.; Goncalves, M.J.; Salgueiro, L. Antifungal activity of *Juniperus* essential oils against dermatophyte, Aspergillus and Candida strains. *J. Appl. Microbiol.* **2006**, *100*, 1333–1338. [CrossRef]
85. Pirila, V.; Siltanen, E. On the Eczematous Agent in Oil of Turpentine. In Proceedings of the International Congress on Occupational Health, Helsinki, Finland, 6–7 January 1957; 3, p. 400.
86. Miguel, M.G. Antioxidant and Anti-Inflammatory Activities of Essential Oils: A Short Review. *Molecules* **2010**, *15*, 9252–9287. [CrossRef]
87. Moeini, R.; Memariani, Z.; Asadi, F.; Bozorgi, M.; Gorji, N. *Pistacia* Genus as a Potential Source of Neuroprotective Natural Products. *Planta Med.* **2019**, *85*, 1326–1350. [CrossRef]
88. Api, A.M.; Belsito, D.; Bruze, M.; Cadby, P.; Calow, P.; Dagli, M.L.; Dekant, W.; Ellis, G.; Fryer, A.D.; Fukayama, M.; et al. Criteria for the Research Institute for fragrance materials, Inc. (RIFM) safety evaluation process for fragrance ingredients. *Food Chem. Toxicol.* **2015**, *82*, S1–S19. [CrossRef]
89. Api, A.M.; Belsito, D.; Biserta, S.; Botelho, D.; Bruze, M.; Burton, G.A., Jr.; Buschmann, J.; Cancellieri, M.A.; Dagli, M.L.; Date, M.; et al. RIFM fragrance ingredient safety assessment, p-cymene, CAS Registry Number 99-87-6. *Food Chem. Toxicol.* **2021**, *149*, 112051. [CrossRef]
90. Kaneda, N.; Pezzuto, J.M.; Kinghorn, A.D.; Farnsworth, N.R.; Santisuk, T.; Tuchinda, P.; Udchachon, J.; Reutrakul, V. Plant anticancer agents, L. cytotoxic triterpenes from *Sandoricum koetjape* stems. *J. Nat. Prod.* **1992**, *55*, 654–659. [CrossRef]
91. Whittaker, A.A. Newman. *Chemistry of Terpenes and Terpenoids*; Academic Press: London, UK, 1972; p. 11.
92. Tiwari, M.; Kakkar, P. Plant derived antioxidants–geraniol and camphene protect rat alveolar macrophages against t-BHP induced oxidative stress. *Toxicol. Vitr.* **2009**, *23*, 295–301. [CrossRef]
93. Wang, C.Y.; Chen, Y.W.; Hou, C.Y. Antioxidant and antibacterial activity of seven predominant Terpenoids. *Int. J. Food Prop.* **2019**, *22*, 229–237. [CrossRef]
94. Pandur, E.; Balatinácz, A.; Micalizzi, G.; Mondello, L.; Horváth, A.; Sipos, K.; Horváth, G. Anti-inflammatory effect of lavender (*Lavandula angustifolia* Mill.) essential oil prepared during different plant phenophases on THP-1 macrophages. *BMC Complement. Med. Ther.* **2021**, *21*, 287. [CrossRef] [PubMed]

95. Hajjaj, G.; Chakour, R.; Bahlouli, A.; Tajani, M.; Cherrah, Y.; Zellou, A. Evaluation of CNS activity and anti-inflammatory effect of *Pistacia atlantica* desf. essential oil from Morocco. *Pharm. Chem. J.* **2018**, *5*, 86–94.
96. Minaiyan, M.; Karimi, F.; Ghannadi, A. Anti-inflammatory effect of *Pistacia atlantica* subsp. *kurdica* volatile oil and gum on acetic acid-induced acute colitis in rat. *Res. J. Pharmacogn.* **2015**, *2*, 1–12.
97. Haghdoost, F.; Baradaran Mahdavi, M.M.; Zandifar, A.; Sanei, M.H.; Zolfaghari, B.; Javanmard, S.H. *Pistacia atlantica* Resin Has a Dose-Dependent Effect on Angiogenesis and Skin Burn Wound Healing in Rat. *Evid. Based Complement. Altern. Med.* **2013**, *2013*, 893425. [CrossRef]
98. Peivastegan, M.; Rajabi, M.; Zaferani Arani, H.; Olya, M.; Atashi, H.A.; Abolghasemi, S. Comparing the Effects of Oleoresin of *Pistacia atlantica* Tree and Diclofenac Gel on the Knee Osteoarthritis Improvement. *Shiraz E-Med. J.* **2020**, *21*, e98293. [CrossRef]
99. El Zerey-Belaskri, A.; Ribeiro, T.; Alcaraz, M.L.; El Zerey, W.; Castro, S.; Loureiro, J.; Benhassaini, H.; Hormaza, J.I. Molecular characterization of *Pistacia atlantica* Desf. subsp. *atlantica* (Anacardiaceae) in Algeria: Genome size determination, chromosome count and genetic diversity analysis using SSR markers. *Sci. Hortic.* **2018**, *227*, 278–287. [CrossRef]
100. Bichatildo, H.; Borg-Karlson, A.; Araújo, J.; Mustaparta, H. Five types of olfactory receptor neurons in the strawberry blossom weevil *Anthonomus rubi* selective responses to inducible host–plant volatiles. *Chem. Sens.* **2005**, *30*, 153–170.
101. Pino, J.A.; Marbot, R.; Fuentes, V. Essential Oil of *Aloysia virgata* Juss. from Cuba. *J. Essent. Oil Res.* **2004**, *16*, 44–45. [CrossRef]
102. Montanari, R.M.; Barbosa, L.C.A.; Demuner, A.J.; Silva, C.J.; Andrade, N.J.; Ismail, F.M.D.; Barbosa, M.C.A. Exposure to *Anacardiaceae* Volatile Oils and Their Constituents Induces Lipid Peroxidation within Food-Borne Bacteria Cells. *Molecules* **2012**, *17*, 9728–9740. [CrossRef]
103. Opdyke, D.L.J. Monographs on Fragrance Raw Materials. *Food Cosmet. Toxicol.* **1973**, *11*, 1059. [CrossRef]
104. Skold, M.; Karlberg, A.T.; Matura, M.; Borje, A. The fragrance chemical β-Caryophyllene-air oxidation and skin sensitization. *Food Chem. Toxicol.* **2006**, *44*, 538–545. [CrossRef] [PubMed]
105. Bhatia, S.P.; Letizia, C.S.; Api, A.M. Fragrance material review on β-caryophyllene alcohol. *Food Chem. Toxicol.* **2008**, *46*, S95–S96. [CrossRef] [PubMed]
106. Ghelardini, C.; Galeotti, N.; Di Cesare Mannelli, L.; Mazzanti, G.; Bartolini, A. Local anaesthetic activity of β-caryophyllene. *Farmaco* **2001**, *56*, 387–389. [CrossRef]
107. Fernandes, E.S.; Passos, G.F.; Medeiros, R.D.A.; Cunha, F.M.; Ferreira, J.; Campos, M.M.; Pianowski, L.F.; Calixto, J.B. Anti-inflammatory effects of compounds alpha-humulene and (−)-trans-caryophyllene isolated from the essential oil of Cordia verbenacea. *Eur. J. Pharm.* **2007**, *569*, 228–236. [CrossRef]
108. Michielin, E.; Rosso, S.; Franceschi, E.; Borges, G.; Corazza, M.; Oliveira, J.; Ferreira, S. High-pressure phase equilibrium data for systems with carbon dioxide, α-humulene and trans-caryophyllene. *J. Chem. Thermod.* **2009**, *41*, 130–137. [CrossRef]
109. Hernandez-Leon, A.; González-Trujano, M.E.; Narváez-González, F.; Pérez-Ortega, G.; Rivero-Cruz, F.; Aguilar, M.I. Role of β-caryophyllene in the antinociceptive and anti-inflammatory effects of Tagetes lucida Cav. Essential oil. *Molecules* **2020**, *25*, 675. [CrossRef]
110. Meffo, S.C.D.; Njateng, G.S.S.; Tamokou, J.D.D.; Tane, P.; Kuiate, J.R. Essential Oils from Seeds of *Aframomum citratum* (C. Pereira) K. Schum, *Aframomum daniellii* (Hook. F.) K. Schum, *Piper capense* (Lin. F) and *Monodora myristica* (Gaertn.) Dunal NL and their Antioxidant Capacity in a Cosmetic Cream. *J. Essent. Oil Bear. Plants* **2019**, *22*, 324–334. [CrossRef]
111. Labdelli, A.; Zemour, K.; Simon, V.; Cerny, M.; Adda, A.; Merah, O. *Pistacia atlantica* Desf., a Source of Healthy Vegetable Oil. *Appl. Sci.* **2019**, *9*, 2552. [CrossRef]
112. Mehdi, S.; Asghari, A.; Ghobadian, B.; Dehghani Soufi, M. Conversion of *Pistacia atlantica* mutica oil to trimethylolpropane fatty acid triester as a sustainable lubricant. *Biomass Convers Biorefinery* **2020**, *10*, 139–148. [CrossRef]
113. Zemour, K.; Adda, A.; Labdelli, A.; Dellal, A.; Cerny, M.; Merah, O. Effects of Genotype and Climatic Conditions on the Oil Content and Its Fatty Acids Composition of *Carthamus tinctorius* L. Seeds. *Agronomy* **2021**, *11*, 2048. [CrossRef]
114. Liu, J.; Zhu, X.Y.; Deng, L.B.; Liu, H.F.; Li, J.; Zhou, X.R.; Wang, H.Z.; Hua, W. Nitric oxide affects seed oil accumulation and fatty acid composition through protein S-nitrosation. *J. Exp. Bot.* **2021**, *72*, 385–397. [CrossRef] [PubMed]
115. Salhi, M.; Gharsallaoui, M.; Gabsi, S. Tunisian *Pistacia atlantica* Desf. Extraction Process: Impact on Chemical and Nutritional Characteristics. *Eur. J. Lipid. Sci. Technol.* **2021**, *123*, 2100013. [CrossRef]
116. Acheheb, H.; Aliouane, R.; Ferradji, A. Optimization of Oil Extraction from *Pistacia atlantica* Desf. Seeds Using Hydraulic Press. *Asian J. Agric. Res.* **2012**, *6*, 73–82. [CrossRef]
117. Kim, J.; Kim, D.N.; Lee, S.H.; Yoo, S.H.; Lee, S. Correlation of fatty acid composition of vegetable oils with rheological behavior and oil uptake. *Food Chem.* **2010**, *118*, 398–402. [CrossRef]
118. Ouily, J.T.; Bazongo, P.; Bougma, A.; Kaboré, N.; Lykke, A.M.; Ouédraogo, M.; Nestor Bassolé, I.H. Chemical Composition, Physicochemical Characteristics, and Nutritional Value of Lannea kerstingii Seeds and Seed Oil. *J. Anal. Methods Chem.* **2017**, *2017*, 2840718. [CrossRef]
119. Firestone, D. (Ed.) *Official Methods Recommended Practices of the American Oil Chemistry Society*, 4th ed.; AOCS Press: Champaign, IL, USA, 2013.
120. Kandji, N. Etude de la Composition Chimique et de la Qualite D'huiles Vegetales Artisanales Consommees au Senegal. Ph.D. Thesis, Universite Cheik Anta Diop (UCAD) de Dakar, de Dakar, Senegal, 2001.
121. Djerrou, Z. Anti-hypercholesterolemic effect of *Pistacia lentiscus* fatty oil in egg yolk-fed rabbits: A comparative study with simvastatin. *Chin. J. Nat. Med.* **2014**, *12*, 561–566. [CrossRef]

22. Ziyad, B.E.; Yousfi, M.; Vander Heyden, Y. Effects of growing region and maturity stages on oil yield, fatty acid profile and tocopherols of *Pistacia atlantica* Desf. fruit and their implications on resulting biodiesel. *Renew. Energy* **2022**, *181*, 167–181. [CrossRef]
23. Hazrati, S.; Govahi, M.; Ebadi, M.T.; Habibzadeh, F. Comparison and Evaluation of Oil Content, Composition and Antioxidant Properties of *Pistacia atlantica* and *Pistacia khinjuk* Grown as Wild. *Int. J. Hortic. Sci. Technol.* **2020**, *7*, 165–174.
24. Bentireche, F.; Guenane, H.; Yousfi, M. Fatty Acids, the Unsaponifiable Matter, and Polyphenols as Criteria to Distinguish *Pistacia atlantica* Unripe Fruit Oil. *J. Am. Oil Chem. Soc.* **2019**, *96*, 903–910. [CrossRef]
25. Mohammadi, B.; Maboud, H.E.; Seyedi, S.M. Nutritional value and antioxidant properties of hull and kernel in *Pistacia atlantica* and *Pistacia khinjuk* fruits. *J. Food Sci. Technol.* **2019**, *56*, 3571–3578. [CrossRef] [PubMed]
26. Gharsallaoui, M.; Azouzi, H.; Chelli-Chaabouni, A.; Ghrab, M.; Condoret, J.S.; Ayadi, M.; Gabsi, S. Extraction methods of seed oil and oil quality of *Pistacia atlantica* grown in dry land. In *XVI GREMPA Meeting on Almonds and Pistachios*; Options Méditerranéennes. Series A: Mediterranean Seminars; CIHEAM-IAMZ: Zaragoza, Spain, 2016.
27. Guenane, H.; Bombarda, I.; Bombarda, I.; Didi OuldElhadj, M.; Yousfi, M. Effect of Maturation Degree on Composition of Fatty acids and Tocopherols of Fruit Oil from *Pistacia atlantica* Growing Wild in Algeria. *Nat. Prod. Commun.* **2015**, *10*, 1723–1728. [CrossRef] [PubMed]
28. Saber-Tehrani, M.; Givianrad, M.H.; Aberoomand-Azar, P.; Waqif-Husain, S.; Jafari Mohammadi, S.A. Chemical Composition of Iran's *Pistacia atlantica* Cold-Pressed Oil. *J. Chem.* **2013**, *2013*, 1–6. [CrossRef]
29. Ghalem, B.R.; Benhassaini, H. Etude des phytosterols et des acides gras de *Pistacia atlantica*. *Afr. Sci.* **2007**, *3*, 405–412.
30. Arena, E.; Campisi, S.; Fallico, B.; Maccarone, E. Distribution of fatty acids and phytosterols as a criterion to discriminate geographic origin of pistachio seeds. *Food Chem.* **2007**, *104*, 403–408. [CrossRef]
31. Sena-Moreno, E.; Pardo, J.E.; Catalán, L.; Alvarez-Orti, M. Drying temperature and extraction method influence physicochemical and sensory characteristics of pistachio oils: Influence of drying temperature of pistachio nuts. *Eur. J. Lipid Sci. Technol.* **2015**, *117*, 684–691. [CrossRef]
32. Esteki, M.; Ahmadi, P.; Heyden, Y.V.; Simal-Gandara, J. Fatty Acids-Based Quality Index to Differentiate Worldwide Commercial Pistachio Cultivars. *Molecules* **2019**, *24*, 58. [CrossRef]
33. Chelghoum, M.; Guenane, H.; Harrat, M.; Yousfi, M. Total Tocopherols, Carotenoids, and Fatty acids Contents Variation of *Pistacia atlantica* Desf. Different Organs Crude Oils and their Antioxidant Activity during Development Stages. *Chem. Biodivers* **2020**, *17*, 1–16.
34. Zarei Jelyani, A.; Tavakoli, J.; Lashkari, H.; Aminlari, M. Different effect of chemical refining process on Baneh (*Pistacia atlantica* var. *mutica*) kernel oil: Regeneration of tocopherols. *Food Sci. Nutr.* **2021**, *9*, 5557–5566. [CrossRef] [PubMed]
35. Fernandes, P.; Cabral, J.M.S. Phytosterols: Applications and recovery methods. *Bioresour. Technol.* **2007**, *98*, 2335–2350. [CrossRef]
36. Bai, G.; Ma, C.; Chen, X. Phytosterols in edible oil: Distribution, analysis and variation during processing. *Grain Oil Sci. Technol.* **2021**, *4*, 33–44. [CrossRef]
37. Givianrad, M.H.; Saber-Tehrani, M.; Jafari Mohammadi, S.A. Chemical composition of oils from wild almond (*Prunus scoparia*) and wild pistachio (*Pistacia atlantica*). *Grasas Y Aceites* **2013**, *64*, 77–84. [CrossRef]
38. Shahidi, F.; Costa de Camargo, A. Tocopherols and Tocotrienols in Common and Emerging Dietary Sources: Occurrence, Applications, and Health Benefits. *Int. J. Mol. Sci.* **2016**, *17*, 1745. [CrossRef] [PubMed]
39. Shahidi, F.; Shukla, V.K.S. Non-Triacylglycerol constituents of fats, oils. *Inf. Int. News Fats. Oils Relat. Mater.* **1996**, *7*, 1227–1232.
40. Zemour, K.; Labdelli, A.; Adda, A.; Dellal, A.; Talou, T.; Merah, O. Phenol Content and Antioxidant and Antiaging Activity of Safflower Seed Oil (*Carthamus Tinctorius* L.). *Cosmetics* **2019**, *6*, 55. [CrossRef]
41. Ahmad, J. Lipid Nanoparticles Based Cosmetics with Potential Application in Alleviating Skin Disorders. *Cosmetics* **2021**, *8*, 84. [CrossRef]
42. Azzi, A. Tocopherols, tocotrienols and tocomonoenols: Many similar molecules but only one vitamin E. *Redox Biol.* **2019**, *26*, 101259. [CrossRef]
43. Guenane, H. Activités biologiques des extraits lipidiques des fruits du Pistachier de l'Atlas (*Pistacia atlantica* Desf.). Ph.D. Thesis, Université Kasdi Merbah, Ouargla, Algérie, 2017.
44. Baran, M.; Miziak, P.; Bonio, K. Characteristics of carotenoids and their use in the cosmetics industry. *J. Educ. Health Sport* **2020**, *10*, 192–196. [CrossRef]
45. İnanç, A.L. Chlorophyll: Structural Properties, Health Benefits and Its Occurrence in Virgin Olive Oils. *Akad. Gıda* **2011**, *9*, 26–32.
46. Pucci, C.; Martinelli, C.; Degl'Innocenti, A.; Desii, A.; De Pasquale, D.; Ciofan, G. Light-Activated Biomedical Applications of Chlrophyll Derivatives. *Macromol. Biosci.* **2021**, *21*, 2100181. [CrossRef]
47. Farhoosh, R.; Tavakoli, J.; Hossein, M.; Khodaparast, H. Chemical Composition and Oxidative Stability of Kernel Oils from Two Current Subspecies of *Pistacia atlantica* in Iran. *J. Am. Oil Chem. Soc.* **2008**, *85*, 723–729. [CrossRef]
48. Petropoulos, S.A.; Fernandes, Â.; Calhelha, R.C.; Rouphael, Y.; Petrović, J.; Soković, M.; Ferreira, I.C.F.R.; Barros, L. Antimicrobial Properties, Cytotoxic Effects, and Fatty Acids Composition of Vegetable Oils from Purslane, Linseed, Luffa, and Pumpkin Seeds. *Appl. Sci.* **2021**, *11*, 5738. [CrossRef]
49. Mezni, F.; Aouadhi, C.; Khouja, M.L.; Khaldi, A.; Maaroufi, A. In vitro antimicrobial activity of *Pistacia lentiscus* L.edible oil and phenolic extract. *Nat. Prod. Res.* **2015**, *29*, 565–570. [CrossRef] [PubMed]
50. Dilika, F.; Bremner, P.D.; MMeyer, J.J. Antibacterial activity of linoleic and oleic acids isolated from *Helichrysum pedunculatum*: A plant used during circumcision rites. *Fitoterapia* **2000**, *71*, 450–452. [CrossRef]

151. Benmahieddine, A.; Belyagoubi-Benhammou, N.; Belyagoubi, L.; El Zerey-Belaskri, A.; Gismondi, A.; Di Marco, G.; Canini, A.; Bechlaghem, N.; Atik Bekkara, F.; Djebli, N. Influence of plant and environment parameters on phytochemical composition and biological properties of *Pistacia atlantica* Desf. *Biochem. Syst. Ecol.* **2021**, *95*, 104231. [CrossRef]
152. Mirmohammadsadegh, N.; Shakoori, M.; Moghaddam, H.N.; Farhadi, R.; Reza Shahverdi, A.; Amin, M. Wound healing and anti-inflammatory effects of bacterial cellulose coated with *Pistacia atlantica* fruit oil. *Daru J. Pharm. Sci.* **2021**, *30*, 1–10. [CrossRef]
153. Tanideh, N.; Masoumi, S.; Hosseinzadeh, M.; Reza Safarpour, A.; Erjaee, H.; Koohi-Hosseinabadi, O.; Rahimikazerooni, S. Healing Effect of *Pistacia atlantica* Fruit Oil Extract in Acetic Acid-Induced Colitis in Rats. *Iran. J. Med. Sci.* **2014**, *39*, 522–528.
154. Nazifi, S.; Saeb, M.; Sepehrimanesh, M.; Poorgonabadi, S. The effects of wild pistachio oil on serum leptin, thyroid hormones, and lipid profile in female rats with experimental hypothyroidism. *Comp. Clin. Pathol.* **2012**, *21*, 851–857. [CrossRef]
155. Hamidi, S.A.; Tabatabaei Naeini, A.; Oryan, A.; Tabandeh, M.R.; Tanideh, N.; Nazifi, S. Cutaneous Wound Healing after Topical Application of Pistacia atlantica Gel Formulation in Rats. *Turk. J. Pharm. Sci.* **2017**, *14*, 65–74. [CrossRef]
156. Jamshidi, S.; Hejazi, N.; Golmakani, M.T.; Tanideh, N. Wild pistachio (*Pistacia atlantica mutica*) oil improve metabolic syndrome features in rats with high fructose ingestion. *Iran. J. Basic Med. Sci.* **2018**, *2*, 1255–1261.
157. Yuan, C.; Zhang, X.; Long, X.; Jin, J.; Jin, R. Effect of β-sitosterol self-microemulsion and β-sitosterol ester with linoleic acid on lipid-lowering in hyperlipidemic mice. *Lipids Health Dis.* **2019**, *18*, 157. [CrossRef] [PubMed]
158. Shahouzehi, B.; Shabani, M.; Shahrokhi, N.; Sadeghiyan, S.; Masoumi –Ardakani, Y. Effects of *Pistacia atlantica* resin oil on the level of VEGF, hydroxyproline, antioxidant and wound healing activity in STZ-induced diabetic rats. *Ukr. Biochem. J.* **2018**, *90*, 34–41. [CrossRef]
159. Pacheco, B.; dos Santos, M.D.; Schultze, E.; Martins, R.M.; Lund, R.; Seixas, F.; Colepicolo, P.; Collares, T.; Paula, F.R.; De Pereira Claudio, M.P. Cytotoxic activity of fatty acids from antarctic macroalgae on the growth of human breast cancer cells. *Front. Bioeng. Biotechnol.* **2018**, *6*, 185. [CrossRef] [PubMed]
160. Elaasser, M.M.; Morsi, M.K.S.; Galal, S.M.; Abd El-Rahman, M.K.; Katry, M.A. Antioxidant, anti-inflammatory and cytotoxic activities of the unsaponifiable fraction of extra virgin olive oil. *Grasas Aceites* **2020**, *71*, e386. [CrossRef]
161. Hassan, S.B.; Gali-Muhtasib, H.; Göransson, H.; Larsson, R. Alpha terpineol: A potential anticancer agent which acts through suppressing NF-kappaB signalling. *Anticancer Res* **2010**, *30*, 1911–1919.
162. Novotny, L.; Abdel-Hamid, M.E.; Hunakova, L. Anticancer potential of β-Sitosterol. *Int. J. Clin. Pharmacol. Pharmacother.* **2017**, *2*, 129. [CrossRef]
163. Zarogoulidis, P.; Cheva, A.; Zarampouka, K.; Huang, H.; Li, C.; Huang, Y.; Katsikogiannis, N.; Zarogoulidis, K. Tocopherols and tocotrienols as anticancer treatment for lung cancer: Future nutrition. *J. Thorac. Dis.* **2013**, *5*, 349–352.
164. Naqvi, S.A.R.; Sherazi, T.A.; Zahid, M.; Mansha, A.; El Zerey-Belaskri, A. Nanotechnology: A smart translation of ingredients in the agriculture industry. In *Micro and Nano Technologies, Aquananotechnology*; Abd-Elsalam, A., Zahid, M., Eds.; Elsevier: Amsterdam, The Netherlands, 2021; pp. 47–65.
165. Sadeghi, B.; Rostami, A.; Momeni, S.S. Facile green synthesis of silver nanoparticles using seed aqueous extract of *Pistacia atlantica* and its antibacterial activity. *Spectrochim. Acta Part A Mol. Biomol. Spectrosc.* **2015**, *134*, 326–332. [CrossRef]
166. Fagionato Masiero, J.; Barbosa, E.J.; de Oliveira Macedo, L.; de Souza, A.; Yukuyama, M.N.; Arantes, G.J.; Bou-Chacra, N.A. Vegetable oils in pharmaceutical and cosmetic lipid-based nanocarriers preparations. *Ind. Crops Prod.* **2021**, *170*, 113838. [CrossRef]
167. Ahmad, A.; Ahsan, H. Lipid-based formulations in cosmeceuticals and biopharmaceuticals. *Biomed. Dermatol.* **2020**, *4*, 12. [CrossRef]
168. Balić, A.; Vlašić, D.; Žužul, K.; Marinović, B.; Bukvić Mokos, Z. Omega-3 Versus Omega-6 Polyunsaturated Fatty Acids in the Prevention and Treatment of Inflammatory Skin Diseases. *Int. J. Mol. Sci.* **2020**, *21*, 741. [CrossRef] [PubMed]
169. Sifi, I.; Dzoyem, J.P.; Ouinten, M.; Yousfi, M.; McGaw, L.J.; Eloff, J.N. Antimycobacterial, antioxidant and cytotoxic activities of essential oil of gall of *Pistacia atlantica* Desf. From Algeria. *Afr. J. Tradit. Complement. Altern. Med.* **2015**, *12*, 150–155. [CrossRef]
170. Koppel, C.; Tenczer, J.; Tonnesmann, U.; Schirop, T.; Ibe, K. Acute poisoning with pine oil-metabolism of monoterpenes. *Arch. Toxicol.* **1981**, *49*, 73–78. [CrossRef] [PubMed]

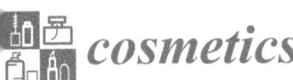

Review

Plant and Herbal Extracts as Ingredients of Topical Agents in the Prevention and Treatment Radiodermatitis: A Systematic Literature Review

Agnieszka Kulawik-Pióro * and Weronika Joanna Goździcka

Department of Organic Chemistry and Technology, Faculty of Chemical Engineering and Technology, Cracow University of Technology, Warszawska 24, 31-155 Kraków, Poland; weronikagozdzicka@windowslive.com
* Correspondence: agnieszka.kulawik-pioro@pk.edu.pl; Tel.: +48-12-628-27-59

Abstract: Background: The use of herbal extracts as the source of antioxidant substances capable of neutralizing free radicals and providing protection from ionizing radiation appears to be an alternative therapy for radiodermatitis. As concerns the prevention and treatment of side effects, a lot of recommendations are based on proper experience of radiotherapy centers. We summarize recent research aiming at reducing radiation-induced skin injuries by use of proper skin care, using topical preparations with herbal extracts including onco-cosmetics. Methods: This article is limited to a critical analysis of scientific and professional literature. It concerns preparations in different physicochemical forms, e.g., gels, emulsions, ointments. We stress the connection between the type of applied skin care (type of preparation, its composition, the dose), the properties of the herbal extract and the evaluation of its efficiency in preventing and treating radiation reaction on skin. Conclusions: Herbal extracts can be added to recipes because they are part of a category of cosmeceutical supplements and can be introduced into preparations without prescription. The effectiveness evaluation for herbal extracts in radiotherapy is not an easy task since there are no strict guidelines. Studies should be preceded by the analysis of herbal extracts and recipe in terms of physicochemical, dermatological and performance characteristics.

Keywords: herbal medicine; onco-cosmetics; plant extracts in skin care; radiodermatitis; radiotherapy treatment

Citation: Kulawik-Pióro, A.; Goździcka, W.J. Plant and Herbal Extracts as Ingredients of Topical Agents in the Prevention and Treatment Radiodermatitis: A Systematic Literature Review. *Cosmetics* 2022, 9, 63. https://doi.org/10.3390/cosmetics9030063

Academic Editor: Othmane Merah

Received: 25 May 2022
Accepted: 11 June 2022
Published: 14 June 2022

Publisher's Note: MDPI stays neutral with regard to jurisdictional claims in published maps and institutional affiliations.

Copyright: © 2022 by the authors. Licensee MDPI, Basel, Switzerland. This article is an open access article distributed under the terms and conditions of the Creative Commons Attribution (CC BY) license (https://creativecommons.org/licenses/by/4.0/).

1. Introduction

Radiotherapy is a treatment method using ionizing radiation (most frequently X rays) applied in oncology for treatment of tumors and for relieving the pain related to the disseminated tumor process [1]. Its purpose is to stop the growth of the tumor tissue while at the same time preserving the healthy tissue surrounding the tumor. High frequency waves used during treatment cause the electron to be knocked out of the atom orbit which in turn leads to tissues' ionization. Moreover, free electrons lead to the creation of free radicals and peroxides causing negative changes in the DNA, proteins and cellular membranes [2,3]. As concerns free electrons, the damage occurs as a consequence of direct effect, whereas we talk about indirect effect when the damage to the DNA structure is caused by free radicals. Most of the damages occur as indirect effect. In any case, for 6–8 h after the radiation, the enzymes can repair part of the damages [4,5]. The necessity of repeating the radiation sessions leads to the damage of the defensive systems responsible for removing free radicals. In case of large damage, repair may not be successfully completed and cells die by apoptosis. Even if the normal cell function is restored, their incomplete reconstruction causes permanent changes or mutations leading to cells dysfunction [4,6,7].

Among general side effects of radiotherapy, the following examples can be mentioned: general weakness, lack of appetite, decline in activity, changes in bold parameters, post-radiation skin reaction, hair loss, mucosal reactions in the mouth, throat, larynx and nasal cavities, reaction of respiratory tract, the heart, the intestines and the bladder. Complications and secondary effects observed by patients can occur in early stages or later [8]. The early complications concern constantly multiplying cells of marrow, epithelium—including skin, digestive track or urinary tract [2,6,7,9]. Mostly those do not cause serious consequences for patients. The second group of complications appears several months or even years after the radiation. It concerns slowly proliferating tissues like lungs, kidneys, liver, blood vessels and central nervous system [4,6,7]. The importance of secondary effects of the radiation depends on the part of the body it was applied to, the irradiation dose, and the degree of irradiation cumulated by the cells [4,6,7,9–11].

In this article, we focused only on secondary effects occurring on the skin, their prevention and treatment, and the possibility of using herbal extracts applied topically on skin.

1.1. Skin Reactions following Radiotherapy

Radiodermatitis (or radiation dermatitis, radiation induced skin reactions or radiation injury, radiation tissue damage) is a significant secondary effect of the ionizing radiation applied to the skin during a cancer treatment but also being a result of nuclear attacks or disasters [8,12]. Radiation skin damages or injuries relate to morphological and functional changes that occur in non-cancerous tissue as a direct result of ionizing radiation [6,13]. The most vulnerable parts of the skin are those at the junction of two skin surfaces like breasts and crotch, those with thin and smooth epidermis (crotch, face, armpits), but also zones with already damaged skin layers (burns, postoperative wounds, skin scales) [14]. Tissue reaction during radiotherapy also depends on the preexisting conditions, age, malnutrition, smoking, medication, chemotherapy, and skin color [9].

Among the first side effects observed by patients are skin dryness, pigmentation disorder, hair loss and erythema [4,11,12,15]. Those symptoms are caused by the damage to sebaceous and sweat glands, to hair follicles and an overstimulation of the pigmentation cells but also an increased pro-inflammatory cytokine release like interleukin 1 and 6 TNF-α, TGF-β [4,8]. Sequentially, following the damage of keratinocytes of the basal layer of the epidermis, there is dry desquamation and moist desquamation accompanied by serous effusion. This leads to the destruction of all the cells in the basal layers of epidermis and the exposure of the dermis [8,12]. Dry desquamation causes a frequent and very nagging symptom, namely itching. In case of a heavy radiation dermatitis, exposure to further fractional doses prevents cell repopulation and hence healing [16].

Late radiation reaction usually appears a few months after the completion of the therapy. It is the fibroblasts' reaction to the radiation. The decrease in fibroblast population (fibroblasts are cells with low proliferation index) and the resorption of collagen fibers lead to atrophy-like changes causing the skin to lose its elasticity and the appearance of thickening and fibrosis, telangiectasia, atrophy of the sebaceous and sweat glands as well as of hair follicles, and can even lead to skin necrosis [4]. The changes can occur immediately and last up to several months, or become permanent [8,15]. The skin response time to radiotherapy includes hemostasis (immediate), inflammation (day 0–4), granulation tissue formation (day 3–3 weeks), matrix deposition and remodeling (week 3–2 years) [6,17].

Accurate assessment and classification of radiation dermatitis is essential for appropriate treatment, management, and monitoring in clinical practice [8]. Table 1 presents the scale of the skin damage (RTOG scale) according to The Radiation Therapy Oncology Group and European Organization for Research and Treatment of Cancer.

Table 1. The Radiation Therapy Oncology Group and European Organization for Research and Treatment of Cancer acute skin toxicity scale [18].

0	I Degree	II Degree	III Degree	IV Degree	V Degree
no changes	mild erythema, dry desquamation, reduced sweating	moderate to severe erythema, intertriginous moist desquamation usually limited to skin folds and articulations, moderate edema	moist desquamation outside the skin folds and articulations, bleeding caused by minor trauma or abrasion, edematous skin	skin necrosis or ulceration across all the skin layers, spontaneous bleeding in the impacted	death

It is estimated that even 95% of patients subjected to radiation treatment experience radiodermatitis [4,6,19]. Observed post-radiation skin reactions and their complications have a severe impact on a patient's organism, and may cause countless complications including treatment delay, lowering of the quality of life (physical and psychological pain) or esthetic effects [8,15,18].

Appropriate preventive actions can be applied to improve the quality of life of patients treated for cancer. These therapeutic strategies can be divided in four categories: physical therapy, external-use dressing/cream, biological therapy and surgical reconstruction [4,11]. Properly conducted preventive actions also protect patient's skin during radiotherapy from additional injuries, irritation or UV radiation [4,16,18,20,21].

1.2. Skin Care during Radiotherapy–Preventive Measures for Radiodermatitis

Skin care during radiotherapy should be properly adapted to patient's needs. The purpose of a normal care therapy is to ensure the skin is clean, which will facilitate its healing afterwards, but also bring comfort and relief to the irritated skin, reduce pain and protect the skin against injuries, and prevent and fight infections [11,15]. Therefore, the skin care plan should include gentle cleansing, moisturizing and regeneration [11,12,22–24]. What is also important in skin care is the protection against UV radiation, appropriate clothing and appropriate diet [8,25]. There is a group of cosmetics available on the market which are dedicated to oncology patients, they are called cosmeceuticals and more precisely onco-cosmetics [11,12,22–24].

Products used for skin care and treatment during radiotherapy can be classified according to their physicochemical form (Table 2) and their purpose (Table 3).

Table 2. Physicochemical form of skin care products for oncological treatment [15,26–28].

Product Type	Physicochemical Form	Purpose	Advantages	Disadvantages
For washing	Gel, aqueous solution, foam, soap	Skin cleansing	Cleansed skin, better absorption of other care products, limited exposure to bacteriological infection	Can cause irritation, reddening or desquamation
Lotion	Aqueous solution, emulsion	Skin pH equalization, smoothing, softening	Maintaining the skin in healthy condition by providing proper moisturizing substances, supplement to self-care *	Can cause irritation, requires additional steps in skin care, i.e., application of creams, due to the water content in the composition, it requires preservatives
Serum	Emulsion, gel	Providing of active ingredients	Reinforces and intensifies daily care, increases the action of cremes, additional moisturizing, light gel texture, evaporates quickly, supplement to self-care *	High concentration of active substances can lead to skin irritation, Need to apply a second product like nourishing cream or protection cream against UV radiation

Table 2. Cont.

Product Type	Physicochemical Form	Purpose	Advantages	Disadvantages
Cream	Emulsion	Moisturization, lubrication, regeneration, nourishing	Moisturizing, soothing of side effects such as itching, burning or reddening	Need to apply several times during the day
Ointment	Emulsion, suspension	Treatment	Eliminates side effects	Greasy, heavy texture, hard to spread on skin

* Self-care: "is the ability of individuals, families and communities to promote health, prevent disease, maintain health, and to cope with illness and disability with or without the support of a health-care provider [29]".

Table 3. Classification of preparations applied to skin care during radiotherapy according to their type of action.

Type of Action	Mechanism of Operation	Types of Preparations	Advantages Disadvantages, Specific Traits	Active Substances in the Receipe	Ref.
Moisturizing	Maintain moisture, protect the skin in three ways: replacement of deficient agents (present in the product), occlusion, humectant action	Ointments, creams, pastes, foams, lotions, gels	Ointments are more penetrating that other forms such as creams or lotions, but they can be too occlusive and greasy, gels can dry on skin and cause irritation	Natural oils, ceramides, humectants, urea, sorbitol, panthenol hyaluronic acid, plant extracts	[30–32]
Emollient	Improve skin barrier function, supplement epidermal lipids, reduce itching and dermatitis	Creams, lotions, oils	Preparations based on petrolatum clog up pores, some emollients can cause hypersensitivity	Lanolin, bee wax, herbal and animal oils like: emu oil, coconut oil, olive oil, avocado oil, evening primrose, vegetable butters (i.e., shea butter), fatty alcohols	[30,33–35]
Curative: Anti-inflammatory	Reduce inflammatory skin reactions	Creams, ointments, lotions, solutions	According to MASCC directives, preventive use of steroids to be applied topically prevents and heals radiation dermatitis -there is no standard for the type of topical steroid to be used in the radiation oncology population. The concentration, frequency, and duration of steroid applications vary by institution. Long use of steroids is not indicated because of side effects. Steroid preparations are used together with emollients	Mometasone furoate, hydrocortisone	[30]
Washing (cleansing)	Help remove contaminants such as dirt, perspiration, oil, dead skin cells form the skin within the treatment area, supports cleansing, reduces potential bacterial and biological burden at the treatment site	Soaps, synthetic detergents	Because of its high pH, soap disturbs the hydro-lipid balance of the skin which might lead to irritations and bacterial overgrowth Synthetic detergents do not contain soap, they are based on surfactants, they are neutral or slightly acidic. More strongly recommended for the therapy of oncology patients	Some soaps contain additive antibacterial substances, they also contain humectants additional oils and/or lipids to prevent skin dryness Synthetic detergents also contain free fatty acids, lipids, proteins, preserving the natural epidermal barrier	[30]

Table 3. Cont.

Type of Action	Mechanism of Operation	Types of Preparations	Advantages Disadvantages, Specific Traits	Active Substances in the Receipe	Ref.
Sisnfectant and antiinfective	Cleansing aids in decreasing potential bacterial and bio burden on the treatment site (especially dry and exfoliating)	Solutions, ointments, creams, powder forms	Antibacterial and antifungal preparations for local application are active in the application zone with a minimal systemic absorption	Chlorhexidine gluconate, clotrimazole, miconazole, nystatin, bacitracin, mupirocin, silver sulfadiazine cream	[30,36,37]
Dessicants and astringent agents	They have astringent, antibacterial properties, High humidity can cause skin irritation and maceration	Solutions for compresses, powders	Powders dry out macerated skin and reduce friction by absorbing humidity. Some has tend to clump which may cause irritation. Depending on the applied substance applied, granuloma may appear but also conditions conductive to fungus development	Burrow's solution (5% aluminium sulfate tetradecahydrate) aluminum chloride solution, corn starch, talk	[30,38]
Barrier measures	Protect the skin against mechanical damage, abrasion by clothes or other parts of the skin. Reduces skin reaction severity	Cremes, ointments, liquids, protective films	Reduce injuries, keep moisture in intact skin and hence the limit potential friction and irradiated skin reactions, thereby reducing radiation injury. Reduction in frequency and duration of moist desquamation.	Create physical film barrier: polymers PVA, copolymer ethylene/acrylic acid, acrylate terpolymer, emollients: coconut oil, dimethicone, mineral oil, Because of high volume of water, liquid and creme preparations must contain preservatives.	[14,18,39]

Their composition should not include any irritating substances, preservatives or colorants. Whereas they are rich in substances rebuilding protective barrier (like free fatty acids, ceramides, squalene, phospholipids), moisturizing (like urea, niacinamide, hyaluronic acid), reducing itching (hemp oil, calendula oil, polidocanol), regenerating, oiling (squalene), soothing (allantoin, panthenol, epigallocatechin gallate) anti-inflammatory, protecting skin from oxidative stress caused by free radicals and environmental factors such as UV radiation or pollution (ascorbic acid, plant extracts or chemical substances isolated from plants: polysaccharides, anthocyanins, galantonin, polyphenols) [30,40]. Their pH is appropriate for sensitive skin. They mostly come as light lotions to prevent unpleasant viscosity and difficulty spreading [2,12].

A separate group of preparations widely applied for skin care and treatment during radiotherapy are dressings: collagen [41,42], hydrogels [43–45], based on alginate [46], silicon [47] or containing silver ions [48]. They are applied for soothing the skin friction, preventing irritations, reducing pain, improving comfort or controlling moist peeling [4,30].

1.3. Active Substances in Skin Care Preparations after Radiotherapy

In case of a strong radiation reaction, skin care alone after radiotherapy may be insufficient. In such cases patients receive treatment by topical glucocorticosteroids for their anti-inflammatory action, special dressings and antibiotics [18,30]. Despite general use of steroids and some chemical-containing ointments, e.g., trolamine and biaffine, their prolonged use may cause serious side effects [2].

The main factors that damage skin are the free radicals originating from irradiated water molecules and from granulocytes in the inflammation area ($H_2O \geq H^\bullet + {}^\bullet OH + e^- + H_3O^+ + H_2O_2 \geq e^- + O_2 \geq O_2^{\bullet -}$) [49]. Hence, the use of antioxidant substances including herbal extracts containing antioxidants, capable of neutralizing free radicals and providing protection from ionizing radiation appears as an alternative therapy for radiodermatitis [18,50]. Studies of radioprotective action of herbal extracts components are of immense use because in addition to protecting the normal tissue, they will also permit the use of higher doses of radiation to obtain better cancer control and possible cure. Unfortunately, radioprotective action of many of the substances is limited. These substances possess inadequate clinical application principally due to their inherent systemic toxicity at their optimal protective concentrations [51].

Despite this, herbal extracts are applied in skin care and treatment during radiotherapy. The first research direction concerns their application as diet supplement and as drugs administered either orally or intraperitoneally where they demonstrate radioprotective systemic action. Not only do they act as antioxidants, but they also show a range of beneficial biologic properties such as anti-inflammatory, antiemetic or antibacterial effects which contribute to improvements of patients' quality of life [52–56]. Another research concerns their introduction into medicated preparations and cosmetics in form of creams, ointments and gels. Applied topically, they act as antioxidants, they reduce irritations and redness, they help heal and protect from UV radiations.

The source of plant materials used for this purpose include crops and harvest from natural stands. As the content of active substances in plants of a given species varies and depends on many factors, they are subject to the process of standardization from processing (collection, drying, stabilization, storage) to clinical study in the process of product development. Standardization is based on the pharmacopoeia standards of a given country or on the basis of quality standards for a given raw material or preparation. The standardized raw material contains a strictly defined amount of ingredients responsible for the therapeutic effect.

Some market products containing herbal extracts for treatment of dermatosis are: My Girls™ Skin Care, RadiaGel®, RadiaPlex® Gel, Medline Remedy® Lotion, DIFINSA53 Skin Protectant Lotion, Miaderm® Radiation Relief, Pharmaceris X—Xrays Liposubtilium, AQUASTOP® Radiotherapy cream, VICCO Turmeric Skin Cream, Holoil® gel, Holoil® oil, RayGel, Capilen® cream, RadioProtect, RadioXar, Radx Oncology Therapy Cream, OnCosmetics.

Some of the above-mentioned preparations are specifically intended for skin care after radiotherapy whereas others are well known for their therapeutic actions, namely anti-inflammatory, antioxidant, and healing. The research of safe and efficient preparations containing herbal extracts is subject to R&D research and clinical trials.

2. Materials and Methods

2.1. Scope

The first attempt to gather all the information concerning the application and the role of herbal extracts in prevention and treatment of radiodermatitis was carried out by Kalekhan et al. [57] and Heydariard et al. [58]. Heydariard and co-workers [58] focused on collecting data from randomized control trials, which compared herbal compounds against a standard medication or placebo treatment or prevention of radiodermatitis. Five dimensions were evaluated: bias related to the errors in the randomization process, bias due to not receiving the desired treatment, bias due to missing data related to the outcome, bias in evaluating and measuring the outcome variables and incomplete or selective reporting outcomes. Kalekhan et al. [57] summarizes clinical observations on the prevention of radiodermatitis by plant products such as: *Adlay bran, Aloe vera, Calendula officinalis, Cucumis sativus*, honey, *Achillea millefolium, Matricaria chamomilla*, olive oil and green tea (containing epigallocatechin-3-gallate) and some of polyherbal creams.

As concerns the prevention and treatment of side effects, a lot of recommendations are based on proper experience of radiotherapy centers [23]. That is why in our literature review we summarize recent research aiming at reducing radiation-induced skin injuries by use of proper skin care, using topical preparations with herbal extracts. Our literature review concerns preparations in different physicochemical forms, e.g., gels, emulsions (creams, lotions), ointments. We stress the connection between the type of applied skin care (type of preparation, its composition, the dose), the properties of the herbal extract and the evaluation of its efficiency in preventing and treating radiation reaction on skin.

2.2. Methods

This overview article is limited to a critical analysis of scientific and professional literature (included guidelines, clinical and preclinical studies and reports of clinical trials). Patents and articles in a language other than English were excluded. Animal research and basic laboratory-based research are included. In order to prepare a literature review, search engines such as PubMed, MEDLINE, Scopus, NCBI, Google Scholar, Google Books, and ResearchGate were used. Date of access: 15 December 2021 and revisited on 20 April 2022.

Main search terms chosen were: radiodermatitis treatment; topical agents in treatment radiodermatitis; herbal in radiotherapy; topical antioxidants in radiodermatitis; skin care of patients undergoing radiotherapy; herbal creams; plant extract in prevention of radiodermatitis; *Aloe vera* extract; *Achillea millefolium* extract; *Azadirachta indica* extract; *Boswellia serrata* extract; *Calendula officinalis* extract; *Centella asiatica* extract; *Chamomilla recutita* extract; *Cucumis sativus* extract; *Glycyrrhiza glabra* extract; Green Tea extract; Silymarin extract, *Turmeric curcuma longa* extract; *Nigella sativa* extract; *Ocimum sanctum* extract; *Angelica gigas* extract; *Lithospermum* radix extract; *Annona muricata* extract; *Camellia sinensis* extract; *Hypercium perforatum* extract; *Thunbergia caurifolia*. Relevant research was systematically categorized by name of plant and appraised according to study design. To exclude risk of bias, two authors independently collected and evaluated quality of all selected data and extracted data on recipe and form product, its applications, purpose of study, subjects, methodology, and key findings. Evaluation was based on reviewers' knowledge. Reference lists of relevant articles were reviewed to identify further studies. The review was performed in accordance with PRISMA guideline. The review was not registered. The protocol was not prepared. Automation tools were not used in the process.

3. Results

The study flowchart for the selection of the relevant research is presented in Figure 1.

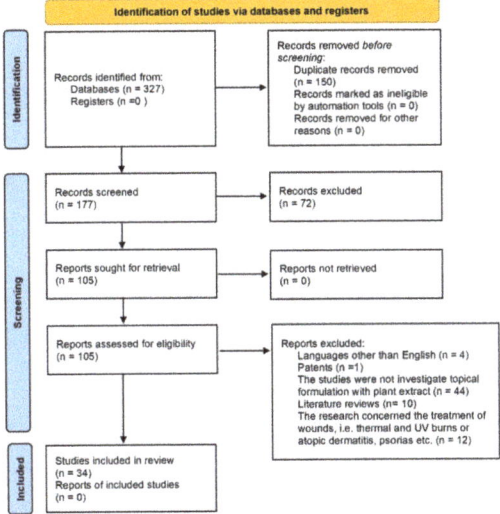

Figure 1. The study flowchart for the selection of the relevant research, e.g.,: randomized clinical trail, clinical trial, articles, clinical and preclinical studies.

A total of 327 articles were evaluated, of which 34 are included in review. Summaries of analyzed research are provided in Table 4. Plant species from which the extract was obtained were sorted in alphabetical order.

Table 4. Type of plant, form of the preparation for topical use, the recipe, study descriptions and key findings. Index of abbreviations: ARD—Acute Radiation Dermatitis; ARMSC—Acute Radiation Morbidity Scoring Criteria; ARSR—Acute Radiation Skin Reactions; Radiation-induced Acute Skin Reactions; BC—breast cancer; CT—Clinical trials; CTC—Common Toxicity Criteria; CTCAE—Common Terminology Criteria for Adverse Events; NCI-CTCAE National Cancer Institute Common Terminology for Adverse Events; PL—placebo; QLQ-C30—Core Quality of Life Questionnaire; QoL—Quality of life; RCT—Randomized Clinical Trial; RD—Radiation-induced Dermatitis; RISR—Radiation-induced Skin Reactions; RT—Radiotherapy Treatment; RTOG—Radiation Oncology Group; SARO—Scientific Association of Swiss Radiation Oncology; VAS—Visual Analogue Scale.

Plant	Form of Product	Purpose of Study. Subjects. Methodology. Product Applications	Recipe. Add. Information.	Key Findings of Effectiveness of Action	Comments	Ref.
Achillea millefolium L. (Yarrow)	cream	Assess the effect of *Glycyrrhiza glabra* L. (Licorice root) and *Achillea millefolium* (Yarrow) on preventing RD RCT. Patients with BC, who undergone mastectomy, receive RT (50 Gray in 25 fractions, over five weeks) Patients were divided into 3 groups: 1 group received Glycyrrhiza glabra cream, 2 group placebo (vanishing cream base), 3 group Achillea millefolium cream. The rate and grade of radiation dermatitis were recorded at baseline, at the end of third week and at the end of treatment using (RTOG) grading tool. Time of application was of five weeks during RT. Preparations were applied daily. Patients were instructed do not to apply other topical skin care products.	The extract of *Achillea millefolium* L. and *Glycyrrhiza glabra* Root were incorporated into a vanishing cream base. Dry Extract constituted 0.6%. Vanishing cream ingredients: Stearic Acid 15%, Cetostearyl Alcohol 2%, Mineral Oil 2%, Borax 1%, Ammonium Hydroxide 28% 1%, Preservative 0.2%, Water 71.2%, Propylene Glycol 4%, Glycerin 3%.	At the end of the third week, the group receiving Achillea millefolium cream showed milder skin complications than other groups. At the end of treatment, rate of skin complications in groups receiving herbal drugs was lower than placebo group but it was not statistically significant. The results of this study did not present a significant difference between *Glycyrrhiza glabra*, *Achillea millefolium* L. and placebo on preventing RD.	According to Author, this is the first study that has evaluated the possible protective effect of these herbal drugs against radiotherapy induced skin dermatitis. *Achillea millefolium* L., especially at lower doses of radiation, might decrease radiation induced dermatitis. There were observed only two cases with grade 1 dermatitis at the end of third week in this group, so more research is required to verify this finding.	[59]

Table 4. Cont.

Plant	Form of Product	Purpose of Study. Subjects. Methodology. Product Applications	Recipe. Add. Information.	Key Findings of Effectiveness of Action	Comments	Ref.
Aloe vera L. Burman	gel ointment	To determine: whether a gel with acemannan extracted from aloe leaves affects the severity of ARSR if so, whether other commercially products (personal lubricating jelly and healing ointment) have similar effect and when the gel with extract should be applied for maximum effect. Male C3H mice received graded single doses of gamma radiation ranging from 30 to 47.5 Gy to the right leg. Groups of mice (gel treated, untreated, jelly-treated, ointment-treated) The right inner thigh of each mouse was scored on a scale of 0 to 3.5 for severity of radiation reaction from the seventh to the 35th day after irradiation. ED_{50} values, and 95% confidence limits were also obtained. The gel was applied daily to the irradiated area beginning immediately after irradiation. To determine timing of application for best effect, gel was applied beginning on day -7, 0, or $+7$ relative to the day of irradiation (day 0) and continuing for 1, 2, 3, 4, or 5 weeks.	Wound dressing gel: Purified water, Povidone, Panthenol, Carbomer 940, Triethanolamine, Allantoin, Glutamic acid, Sodium chloride, Methylparaben, Imidazolidinyl urea, Sodium Benzoate, Potassium Sorbate, Acemannan hydrogel, Citric acid, Sodium metabisulfite. Personal lubricating jelly (water soluble hydrogel, similar in solubility and consistency to the accemannan gel): Chlorhexidine gluconate, Gluconodelta lactone, Glycerin, Hydroxyethylcellulose, Methylparaben, Purified water, Sodium hydroxide. Healing ointment: Petrolatum, Mineral oil, Mineral wax, Wool wax Alcohol, Panthenol, Glycerin, Bisabolol (Chamomile essence)	The average peak skin reactions of gel-treated mice were lower than those of the untreated mice at all radiation doses tested. The ED_{50} values for skin reactions of 2.0–2.75 were approximately 7 Gy higher in the wound dressing gel-treated mice. The average peak skin reactions and the ED_{50} values for mice treated with personal lubricating jelly or healing ointment were similar to irradiated control values. Reduction in the percentage of mice with skin reactions of 2.5 or more was greatest in the groups that received gel for at least 2 weeks beginning immediately after irradiation.	In this case, *Aloe vera* leaves were the raw material for extraction of Acemannan. Healing ointment contained the essence of chamomile. The authors of the study tried to define the time for starting the application of the preparation.	[60]

Table 4. *Cont.*

Plant	Form of Product	Purpose of Study. Subjects. Methodology. Product Applications	Recipe. Add. Information.	Key Findings of Effectiveness of Action	Comments	Ref.
Aloe vera L. Burman	gel	To determine effectiveness aloe vera gel for radiation-induced skin reactions. BC patients undergoing RT to breast and/or chest wall, minimum field 10 × 10 cm and minimum dose 50c Gy. RCT. Two groups: aloe vera gel or PL gel—first phase of trial, aloe vera gel or no treatment—second phase of trial. State of the skin was evaluated—patients self-graded skin reactions and clinical assessment by physician. Rated: severity, time of occurrence and duration of severe dermatitis. The evaluation was carried out once a week. Gel (aloe vera or placebo) was applied to the chest wall by the patient twice a day, starting 3 days within of radiation initiation. Usual skin-care (soap) advice were recommended.	No detailed information available concerning the products recipe and their quality control. Aloe vera gel—98% aloe gel plus 2% inert gel for consistency.	Aloe vera gel was not effective. The dermatitis was less severe than expected. Allergic reactions were observed among patients both in groups using aloe vera gel and placebo gel.		[11–61]
Aloe vera L. Burman	gel cream	To determine if aloe vera gel is beneficial in reducing skin side-effects of RT when compared with aqueous cream. Women with BC undergoing RT post-lumpectomy or partial mastectomy. RCT. Two group: aloe vera gel and topical aqueous cream. Evaluation of the skin by nurse—limitation of side-effects such as erythema, pain, itching, dry desquamation, moist desquamation. Standard care was recommended on top of preparations application. Topical products were applied by patients three times a day after treatment and for 2 weeks after completing care. Weekly skin assessments were performed by nursing staff.	No information available concerning the products recipe and their quality control.	Aqueous cream was significantly better than aloe vera gel in reducing dry desquamation and treatment-related pain. Allergic reactions were observed in patients using both gel and cream.	No information available to objectively evaluate the efficiency of the study (including the dose of radiation administered to patients).	[11–62]

Table 4. Cont.

Plant	Form of Product	Purpose of Study. Subjects. Methodology. Product Applications	Recipe. Add. Information.	Key Findings of Effectiveness of Action	Comments	Ref.
Aloe vera L. Burman	gel cream	Compare effectiveness of an anionic polar phospholipid (APP)-based cream and an aloe vera-based gel in preventing and treating RD. Pediatric patients with various diagnoses (RT with at least 23.4 Gy dose). Subject's skin comfort, dermatologic assessment, and CTC were evaluated. The study was carried out before, during and after completion of treatment (4–6 weeks). APP cream and aloe vera gel were symmetrically applied within the irradiated field after each treatment.	Aloe vera (market product) contain: D-panthenol, Triethanoloamine, Carbomer 943P, Hyaluronic acid, Potassium Sorbate, Diazolidinyl Urea, Methylparaben, Propylparaben. APP skin cream (Ocular Research of Boston) is an oil-in-water emulsion, not commercially available. Include: triglycerides and phospholipids, Benzyl Alcohol, Methylparaben, Propyl paraben, Diaxolipinyl urea.	APP cream improves skin comfort variables such as: dry, soft, feels good, rough, smooth and dermatologic variables: dryness, erythema and peely as compared with aloe vera gel (statistically significant differences). APP cream is more effective in prevention and treatment of RD. Grouped CTC scores were supportive of APP cream. In comparing the first and last assessments, two dermatologic variables, dryness and peely, favored APP cream.	Results in concordance with Boosley's study [63]	[64]

Table 4. Cont.

Plant	Form of Product	Purpose of Study. Subjects. Methodology. Product Applications	Recipe. Add. Information.	Key Findings of Effectiveness of Action	Comments	Ref.
Aloe vera L. Burman	cream powder	Test the efficacy of quality-tested Aloe vera extract in reducing the severity of radiation-induced skin injury. Examine the effect of a moist cream versus a dry powder skin care regimen. RCT. Patients with BC, previous mastectomy or segmental resection. RT (45–50 Gy). Acute skin toxicity was scored weekly and after treatment at weeks 1, 2, and 4 using a modified 10-point Catterall scale. The patients scored their symptom severity using a 6-point Likert scale and kept an acute phase diary. Standard radiation skin care guidelines were complied. The patients apply nonmetallic baby powder or cornstarch to the irradiated intact skin during the treatment course followed by 1 month of Glaxal base cream twice daily. If they developed moist desquamation, they were advised to discontinue the powder. Patients apply approximately 2.5 cm³ of cream to the irradiated skin, 3 times daily (avoid application within 3 h of radiation) throughout the course of radiation and for 1 month after radiation. Treatment of moist desquamation and other skin reactions, such as infection, was according to each physician's pattern of practice. Any prescribed treatment was to be applied 30 min before the use of the study creams.	Placebo cream contain: Aquatrix II, Lexamul 56, Methylparaben, Dimethicone, Isopropyl Myristate, Propylene Glycol, Cetyl Alcohol, Stearic acid, triethanolamine. The aloe cream formulation was 30 mg of the processed aloe (1000–5000 MW fraction) per 100 cm³ of placebo cream. This represents the highest concentration possible without causing cream demulsification and is relatively equivalent to 50 mg of the 1000 to 5000 MW fraction of unprocessed fresh leaf gel extract.	The aloe formulation did not reduce acute skin toxicity or symptom severity. Study speaks in favor of dry care instead of introducing herbal extracts into creams or applying creams only.	Were excluded from the study people with confirmed allergy to Aloe vera. Placebo cream was chosen for its ability to penetrate the outermost skin layers and therefore to theoretically enable absorption of the aloe elemental components. The study included also the analysis of the extract itself introduced into the recipe of the cream. Such as: murine bioassay testing under the supervision of 1 of us (F.S.). The assay testing was conducted to determine whether the aloe oligosaccharides that prevent ultraviolet B (UVB)-induced immune suppression of T-cell-mediated immune responses were active in this study. The mechanism of aloe skin protection is unknown, and this element might be necessary for aloe extract to be effective in reducing RSR severity.	[65]

Table 4. *Cont.*

Plant	Form of Product	Purpose of Study. Subjects. Methodology. Product Applications	Recipe. Add. Information.	Key Findings of Effectiveness of Action	Comments	Ref.
Aloe vera L. Burman	lotion	Evaluation of aloe vera lotion for prevention of RD. CT. Patients with a prescription of RT to a minimum dose of 40 Gy, were treatment area could be divided into two symmetrical halves. The grade of dermatitis in each half was recorded (according to RTOG) weekly until 4 weeks after the end of radiotherapy. In the case of symptomatic dermatitis, topical corticosteroids were prescribed to the patients to use on the entire treatment area. Lotion were use twice daily from the beginning of treatment until 2 weeks after the end of RT, with no medication to be used on the other half.	Market product. The recipe contains: Lanolin oil, Glyceryl Stearate, Diluted Collagen, Tocopherol, Allantoin, and paraben.	Age and radiation field size had a significant effect on the grade of dermatitis. The prophylactic use of *Aloe vera* reduces the intensity of radiation induced dermatitis. The effect was more evident in patients undergoing radiotherapy with larger treatment field and higher doses of radiation.	The study verified the quantity (dose) of the lotion used.	[66]
Aloe vera L. Burman	gel soap	Determine whether the use of mild soap and aloe vera gel versus mild soap alone would decrease the incidence of skin reactions in patients undergoing RT. RCT. Oncological patients qualified for the RT. Group of patients applying mild soap and additional aloe vera gel and second group—control treatment used only soap. RTOG Acute Radiation Morbidity scale assessed weekly by physician or nurse. Unscented soap plus aloe vera gel or soap was applied liberally to the affected area daily after the RT in case of gel reapplied through day. Gel was washed off before RT. Standard care was recommended.	No information available concerning the composition, the quality assessment of the products. Gel without other active components	Aloe vera gel seemed to offer a protective effect over soap alone when the cumulative dose increased over time. At low cumulative dose levels no difference existed in the effect of adding aloe to soap regimen.	Soap is not a typical product to compare. Besides, the differences in treatment depended on the radiation doses applied and those were different for the control group and for the group using gel with aloe and soap which leads to conflicting results.	[67]

Table 4. Cont.

Plant	Form of Product	Purpose of Study. Subjects. Methodology. Product Applications	Recipe. Add. Information.	Key Findings of Effectiveness of Action	Comments	Ref.
Aloe vera L. Burman	gel cream	Compare a anionic phospholipid-based (APP) cream and an aloe vera-based gel in the prevention and treatment of radiation dermatitis RCT. Pediatric patients treated by radiotherapy (dose of 23.4 Gy). Control group use APP cream. Subject skin comfort and dermatologic assessments were conducted before and weekly during treatment. Photography was performed at each evaluation time point and patients were seen 4–6 weeks after the completion of RT. CTC was used. Aloe vera-based gel or APP cream were applied symmetrically, once a day by nurse daily next to the radiation area after RT.	No information available concerning the composition and the quality assessment of the products.	APP-based cream showed a statistically significant advantage over aloe vera gel for skin comfort and dermatological assessment variables. Cream reduced dryness, redness, desquamation. No changes in CTC score before and after the treatment.	Complete data unavailable for objective evaluation of the study.	[11, 63]
Aloe vera L. Burman	cream oil	To evaluate the efficacy of topical application of an aloe vera-based cream (AVC) for the prevention of ionizing RD. Clinical study. Head and neck cancer patients requiring therapeutic radiation treatment (dose >62 Gy). Patients were treated with AVC or Johnson Baby Oil (JBO). Acute skin reaction was monitored and classified according to RTOG four-point rating scale on a weekly basis. The preparation was applied 5 times per day at defined timespans after RT. During the study it was recommended not to use other preparations. When moist desquamation occurred, the topical application of JBO or ACV was discontinued topically and continued on the remaining skin area.	AVC and JBO are is market products Composition unavailable. Application: 5 cm^3 JBO and 5 g AVC.	There was a statistically significant delay in the incidence of dermatitis at week three in the AVC application group. Application of AVC reduced the incidence of Grade 1, 2, and 3 dermatitis at subsequent time points, while Grade 4 dermatitis was not seen in either cohort. Continued application of AVC two weeks after the completion of RT was effective in reducing the average grade of dermatitis and was statistically significant.	This research and research with [67] indicate the usefulness of *Aloe vera* in delaying and mitigating dermatitis and promoting recovery. The action of this preparation is linked to the antioxidant properties of the *Aloe vera*. Plants from the aloe vera family decrease UVB-induced nociception, leukocyte infiltration, inflammation, and edema. Additionally, are effective in scavenging reactive oxygen and protecting DNA [68–70].	[71]

Table 4. *Cont.*

Plant	Form of Product	Purpose of Study. Subjects. Methodology. Product Applications	Recipe. Add. Information.	Key Findings of Effectiveness of Action	Comments	Ref.
Aloe vera L. Burman	gel lotion	A non-blinded three armed study of the effect of aloe vera gel, Essex lotion and no lotion on erythema was performed. BC patients who had undergone total mastectomy. Treatment with high-energy electrons (total dose 50 Gy). For measuring the erythema Near Infrared Spectroscopy, Laser Doppler Imaging and Digital Colour Photography were applied. Measurements were performed before the start of RT and there after once a week during the course of treatment. Aloe vera gel and Essex lotion were applied twice every radiation day in selected sites.	Aloe vera gel: *Aloe barbadensis* 97%, Aqua, Carbomer, Sodium Hydroxide, Phenoxyethanol, Methylparben, Butylparben, Ethylparben, Propylparben. Essex lotion consists of: Aqua, Petrolatum, Glycerin, Methyl Glucose Sesquistearate, Dimethicone, PEG-20, Palmitic acid, Steric acid, Cetyl Alcohol, Xanthan Gum, Magnesium Aluminum Silicate, Carbomer, Sodium Hydroxide.	The extent of erythema developed differed between patients. Some of them developed more severe erythema; however, no one had to stop their radiation treatment because of severe skin reactions. No significant median differences were observed between the pairs no lotion-Essex, no lotion-Aloe vera and Essex-Aloe vera for any of the techniques tested.	As indicated in manuscript Essex lotion is a commonly used lotion that is not registered as a medical product and therefore there are no specific recommendations for its use.	[72]
Aloe vera L. Burman	gel	Whether the adjunctive use of aloe vera gel might reduce the prevalence and/or severity of radiotherapy induced dermatitis. Randomized study patients with newly diagnosed BC (total dose 50 Gy). One group received aloe vera gel. Second group no treatment during RT. The patients were examined weekly by 2 physicians and dermatitis grade was registered (according ARMSC). In case of patients with second or higher degree dermatitis, additional local or systemic treatment such as antibiotics, corticosteroid or analgesics were applied. Aloe vera gel was applied twice a day in at least six hour intervals with a thickness of 1–2 mm on the radiation therapy field.	Aloe vera gel contain 1% additive such as: pectin, vitamin C and Natamycin	After 2 weeks first dermatitis was found among patients of both groups. Comparing the time of occurrence of dermatitis and their degree, no significant statistic difference were observed in both groups. Aloe vera gel did not show positive effect on prevalence or severity of radiation dermatitis in this study.		[73]

Table 4. Cont.

Plant	Form of Product	Purpose of Study. Subjects. Methodology. Product Applications	Recipe. Add. Information.	Key Findings of Effectiveness of Action	Comments	Ref.
Aloe vera L. Burman Turmeric curcuma longa L. Valeton Azadirachta indica A. Juss. Ocimum sanctum Linn	paste	Evaluation of efficacy and safety herbal paste compared to Beblomethasone cream in prevention radiation induced skin injury. CT. Patients of head and neck carcinoma. First group—patients received Beclomethasone cream. Second group received herbal paste. To assess radiation-induced reaction RTOG score were applied and group I versus group II compered. EORTC QLC-C30 was used for QoL assessment. Preparations were topically applied from the day-1 of radiotherapy till 4-weeks after completion of RT.	Paste was properly mixed with 100 g of Aloe vera juice and fresh Ocimum sanctum leaves, Azadirachta indica leaves (50 g each) and Curcuma longa roots (5 g). Herbal plants have been grounded up before mixing.	During the timespans of the study, i.e., after the 4th, 5th, 7th week and also after 6 months, skin reactions were less severe within the group using herbal preparation. On evaluating EORTC QLC-C30, on functional scale, physical, emotional, cognitive and role functioning deteriorated in Group 1 patients (except social functioning), while in Group patients all these modalities showed improvement at 6 months post-treatment. Evaluation on symptom scale revealed that fatigue, pain, dyspnea, appetite loss and insomnia got worsened in Beclomethasone group, except for diarrhea, constipation and nausea or vomiting, while in herbal pasta group patients, all 9 symptoms showed improvement 6 months after of completion of treatment.	Aloe vera was the basis for the powdered plants. Patients known to be allergic to ingredients of herbal paste or with allergy to steroids were excluded from study. No information available on the Gy dose applied to patients.	[74, 75]

Table 4. *Cont.*

Plant	Form of Product	Purpose of Study. Subjects. Methodology. Product Applications	Recipe. Add. Information.	Key Findings of Effectiveness of Action	Comments	Ref.
Angelica gigas Nakai *Lithospermum erythrorhizon* Siebold and Zucc.	ointment	Efficiency and security evaluation of adjuvant application of Jaungo (JUG) for RD in comparison with general supportive care (GSC). RTC. Women with unilateral BC, after breast conservation surgery, undergoing RT, (total dose >45 Gy). Both groups will be subjected to GSC, but only the JUG group participants will apply adjuvant JUG ointment on the irradiated skin, twice a day (not applied within 4 h of daily RT). Treatment started at onset of RT and continued until 4 weeks after RT was completed or until radiation dermatitis subsided. Assessment of incidence rate of RD using the RTOG for toxicity gradation of 2 or more. Onset and duration of RD, and maximum pain score were also evaluated. GSC—skin clean and dry by gentle washing with neutral pH soap and patting with soft towel. No prophylactic creams or lotions for radiation dermatitis were allowed to either group.	Jaungo is a herbal ointment consisting of *Angelica gigas* radix (60.6 mg/g) and *Lithospermum* radix (72.7 mg/g). Carriers: Sesame Seed Oil, Beeswax, Swine Oil. Bioactive constituents shikonin 0.07 mg/g, decursin 3.6 mg/g.	JUG reduced the incidence of grade >2 and grade >3 RD in comparison with GSC. Delayed the onset of time onset of grade 2 dermatitis in terms of time onset of grade 3 and duration dermatitis and maximum pain score showed results comparable to those achieved with GSC, no adverse effect was observed.	Because of a low number of patients (29), the authors recommended further studies with a bigger sample of people. Those studies are currently ongoing [76] and [77]. In this article market product (composition unavailable) was compared with emulsion w/o (X-derm)—composition unavailable.	[78]

Table 4. *Cont.*

Plant	Form of Product	Purpose of Study. Subjects. Methodology. Product Applications	Recipe. Add. Information.	Key Findings of Effectiveness of Action	Comments	Ref.
Angelica gigas Nakai *Lithospermum erythrorhizon* Siebold and Zucc.	ointment	Estimate clinical application of Shiunko for reducing complications related to cancer treatment such as RD and hand foot syndrome induced by molecular target drugs. Various groups of patients took part in the research: 1st group patients with simple scalp dermatitis induced by RT for brain tumors. 2nd group: severe dermatitis from concurrent treatment with chemotherapy and RT for cancers including nasopharyngeal cancer. 3th group patients with dermal complications caused by molecular target drugs including hand-foot syndrome. Shiunko was applied in the same manner as in the treatment with standard ointment. The efficiency was assessed by defining the improvement degree—excellent (more than 80%), good (more than 50%), fair (less than 50%), and no effect (less than 30%). In comparison people were treated by corticosteroid.	Recipe unavailable.	Ointment is effective in treatment of scalp dermatitis caused by radiation and dermal complications induced by molecular target drugs since favorable therapeutic effects were observed in all group of patients. Shiunko showed prominent analgesic effect in all cases which were not achieved in corticosteroid treatment but also promoted healing in areas eroded by radiations.	Ointment Shiunko is the JUG ointment JUG, the same as in the study [78]. In our document we only showed cases treated with this ointment and its positive effect. No information available on the group using placebo.	[79]

Table 4. *Cont.*

Plant	Form of Product	Purpose of Study. Subjects. Methodology. Product Applications	Recipe. Add. Information.	Key Findings of Effectiveness of Action	Comments	Ref.
Annona muricata L.	cream	Investigate the protective effects of *Annona muricata* leaf polysaccharide (ALP) on radiation induced skin injuries by using in vitro and in vivo models. Normal human epidermal keratinocytes (NHEKs) irradiated cell using ^{137}Cs source in a Gammacell 40 Exactor. The dose rate used was 1 Gy/min. Performed cell viability, terminal deoxynucleotidyl transferase-mediated dUTP nic-end labeling assay and annexin V/propidium iodide (PI) staining to detect apoptosis. Pro-inflammatory cytokines (level of TNF-IL-6, and IL-1β in the cell culture supernatants) were measured using ELISA. The mice were divided into five groups: (1) Normal group; (2) Irradiation + vehicle cream group; (3) Irradiation + 0.04% ALP (w/v) cream; (4) Irradiation + 0.2% ALP cream. The skin on the back was topically treated with 100 μL of vehicle or ALP cream for 7 days before and after irradiation. After treatment, mouse's skin was under histopathological observation.	Vehicle cream: Water, Butyl Hydroxyl Toluene (0.001%), Dibasic Potassium Phosphate (0.2%), Cetyl Alcohol (0.5%), polyglyceryl-3-methylglucose distearate (5%). ALP extract was added to the vehicle cream at concentrations of 0.04 or 0.2%.	In normal human epidermal keratinocytes (NHEKs), ALP treatments reduced irradiation-induced apoptosis by increasing antioxidant enzymes activities, including (SOD) and catalase. Furthermore, ALP treatments decreased levels of interleukin-1β, nucleotide-binding domain and leucine-rich-repeat-containing family pyrin 3 (NLRP3), and cleavage of caspase-1 and caspase-3. The topical application of the ALP cream showed protective efficacy against irradiation exposure, including the reduction of epidermal thickening, as well as an increase in the number of apoptotic cells and antioxidant enzyme (SOD and catalase) activities in skin tissue. ALP can be potentially used to treat radiation-induced skin injuries.	To determine whether ALP protects gamma irradiation-induced cell death by regulating antioxidant enzymes and inflammasome complexes, Authors analyzed the intracellular antioxidant enzymes activity and levels of pro inflammator cytokines. Hence, they are ones of the first studies of antioxidant action. Defines the mechanism of action of polysaccharides isolated from the extract and, based on that, the action of the cream, not only clinical studies or skin observation.	[2]

Table 4. Cont.

Plant	Form of Product	Purpose of Study. Subjects. Methodology. Product Applications	Recipe. Add. Information.	Key Findings of Effectiveness of Action	Comments	Ref.
Boswellia serrata Roxb. ex Colebr.	cream	The cream was evaluated in terms of its safety, efficiency for the prevention and relief of radiation induced adverse effects. Clinical study. Patients adjuvant RT after surgery for mammary carcinoma. All measures, including photographic evaluations, were performed after the patients received a dose/breast of 50 Gy, usually reached in 5 weeks of irradiation, 5 doses weekly. Skin reactions were evaluated clinically using visual intensity and computer assisted skin color analysis whereas the toxicity was assessed according to RTOG scale. Visual grading scale: slight (slight redness, spotty, and diffuse), moderate (moderate and uniform redness), intense (intense redness). Cream was applied twice daily: immediately after RT and before bed-time in radiation therapy days, in the morning and at night in days with no radiotherapy administration.	Boswellia cream (2%, Bosexil) and placebo cream composition is unavailable. However, based on a cosmeceutical formulation based on Boswellic acids for the treatment of erythematous eczema and psoriasis [80] Bosexil contains: Aqua, Glycerin; Lecithin, Boswellia Serrata Resin Extract; Disodium Ethylenediaminotetraacetic Acid, Imidazolidinyl Urea, Polyacrylamide, C13-C14 Isoparaffin, Laureth-7, Hydrogenated polydecane, Carpylic/Capric Trigliceryde, Lecithin, Tocopherol, Ascorbyl Palmitate, Citric Acid, Phenoxyethanol.	Those studies indicate that applying cream with *Bosvellia S.* is efficient for limiting the use of topical corticosteroids and can reduce the erythema and external dermal symptoms. The degree of reduction depended on the intensity of changes. The results in terms of visual intensity revealed that erythema was recorded as intense in a higher number of patients treated with base cream, compared with patients treated with boswellia cream (49.0% vs. 22.0%). Slight and moderate intensity of erythema were scored more frequently in the boswellia cream group than in base cream group: 36.4% vs. 20.3% and 41.8% vs. 30.5%, respectively. The mode values of the intensity of erythema for these samples were: intense (70.7%) for the base cream group and slight (62.5%) for the boswellia cream group.	It is not clear if 2% is the concentration of the extract in the recipe or the concentration of boswellic acids extracted from *Bosvellia serrata*—those acids have anti-inflammatory properties. *B. serrata* extract reduces skin reddening and irritation, they even out the color and sooth the skin. According to the authors, further studies are necessary to compare with other topical preparations.	[81]

Table 4. Cont.

Plant	Form of Product	Purpose of Study. Subjects. Methodology. Product Applications	Recipe. Add. Information.	Key Findings of Effectiveness of Action	Comments	Ref.
Calendula officinalis L.	ointment	Compare the effectiveness of calendula ointment with trolamine. Patients operated on for BC, received postoperative RT (2 Gy per session, five session per week). RTC. Two groups: 1st applied trolamine, 2nd calendula on the irradiated fields after each session. Occurrence of acute dermatitis of grade 2 or higher, occurrence of pain, the quantity of topical agent used, and patient satisfaction were investigated. Prognostic factors, including treatment modalities and patient characteristics, were also examined. Preparations were applied twice a day or more, depending on the occurrence of dermatitis and pain, until completion radiotherapy (not to use the agent 2 h or less before an irradiation session or before the treatment evaluation). Acute dermal toxicity was evaluated according to the RTOG scale at each irradiated volume. Pain was assessed each week on a 10-cm visual analog scale (VAS). No other prophylactic creams, lotions, or gels were allowed. Physicians can treat established dermatitis of grade 2 or higher and/or allergy as they considered appropriate.	Calendula ointment (market product) fabricated from a plant of the marigold family, *Calendula officinalis*. The digest is obtained by incubation at 75 °C in petroleum jelly to extract the liposoluble components of the plant.	The occurrence of acute dermatitis of grade 2 or higher was significantly lower (41% vs. 63%) with the use of calendula ointment than with trolamine. Patients receiving calendula has less frequent interruption of RT and significantly reduced radiation induced pain.	Trolamine is considered in many medical institutions as reference topical agent, Calendula ointment was more difficult to apply, but self-assessed satisfaction was greater.	[82, 83]

Table 4. Cont.

Plant	Form of Product	Purpose of Study. Subjects. Methodology. Product Applications	Recipe. Add. Information.	Key Findings of Effectiveness of Action	Comments	Ref.
Calendula officinalis L.	cream	Compare Calendula Weleda cream versus Essex cream in reducing the risk of serve ARSR. RCT. Patients with BC (2 Gy five day a week, total dose 50 Gy). ARSR was assessed by the nurse based on the RTOG score. Cream was applied twice a day, starting at the onset of RT and continuing until two weeks after final RT session or until ARSR was healed. Application topical agent include whole treatment area. Patients do not apply the cream within two hours of their RT. Daily washing with perfume-free soap and tap water were advised.	Calendula Weleda cream (market product) contains extract of *Marigold Plants Officinalis* 10%, Wool fat and Sesame Oil. Detailed composition not available. Essex cream probably contains: Water, Petrolatum, Liquid Paraffin. Both products contain no perfume nor coloring agent.	No differences in ARSR between calendula cream and aqueous cream and in patient reported symptoms (pain, burning, itching, pulling, tenderness) from the treatment area at any of the evaluation points. Thus, there is no reason to recommend one of the studied skin care product over the other.	Patients describe the calendula cream to be more difficult in application and absorption when compared to the Essex cream. Probably because it contains Wool fat. Essex patients were strongly advised to refrain from using other topical agents in the irradiated area. Calendula cream used in this study was not the same market product as the one used in Pommier [82] study (however, both contained 10% extract), besides, possible differences in efficiency can result from the reference sample, in this case Essex cream.	[83,84]
Calendula officinalis L.	lotion cream	Compare Calendula topical lotion efficacy versus standard of care sorbolene in reducing the prevalence of RD. RCT. Women undergoing BC RT, treatment phase up to 6 weeks Evaluate a prevalence of acute radiation-induced dermatitis (RTOG grade 2+) assessed at multiple skin sites. Participants were encouraged to begin applying their treatment 2–3 days prior to commencement of radiation therapy.	Calendula lotion (<5% v/v): Calendula tincture and extract, Lecithin, Glycerine, Ethanol, Xanthan Gum, Distilates (Rose, Chamomile, with hazel, extracts (Citrus, Gum, Rosemary), Rice Bran Oil, Ascorbic acid, Wheatgerm Oil, Arrowroot, Guar Gum, Sodium Hyaluronate, Lactacid acid. Sorbolene: 10% glycerin in cetomacrogol cream other ingredients: Ceteareth-20, Cetearyl Alcohol, Glycerin, Mineral oil, p-chloro-m-cresol, Petrolatum, Aqua.	No detectable difference in prevalence of radiation-induced dermatitis grade 2+ between Calendula and Sorbolene groups.	Study carried out on a small group of people. People with allergy to Marigold, salicylate, or taking aspirin were excluded from study.	[85]

Table 4. Cont.

Plant	Form of Product	Purpose of Study. Subjects. Methodology. Product Applications	Recipe. Add. Information.	Key Findings of Effectiveness of Action	Comments	Ref.
Calendula officinalis L.	oil	Efficiency evaluation of Calendula officinalis in relation to Essential Fatty Acids (EFA) for prevention and treatment of RD. RCT: Patients with head and neck cancer, received RT. Two groups: control applied EFA and experimental used Calendula oil. Radiodermatitis were assessed by the toxicity grade, according to the criteria RTOG. The participant's skin in the irradiation field was evaluated in the first radiotherapy session, every five sessions and 30 days after the end of treatment. The evaluation of skin toxicity was performed by a team of trained researchers. Participants applied EFA or calendula topically. Research protocol: mode of application—application to the skin with a gauze soaked with the product of research in all treatment field every 12 h (twice/day), from the first to the last day of RT session; first application—hospital: conducted by the research collaborator—average of 10 cm^3/application; during application, study participant and/or family member.	EFA: Sunflower Oil, 1% Vitamin A, 0.2% Vitamin E and 5% Caprylic acid. Calendula oil: 4% Calendula Oil, 1% Vitamin A and Liquid vaseline.	Statistically significant evidence that the proportion of radiodermatitis grade 2 in EFA group is higher than Calendula group. Lower risk of developing radiodermatitis grade 1, form experimental group, it makes the usage of Calendula oil more effective.	Excluded patients with allergic reaction in the use of one of the research products (EFA or Calendula officinalis). Due to the physicochemical form of the products, they were applied to gauze.	[86]

Table 4. *Cont.*

Plant	Form of Product	Purpose of Study. Subjects. Methodology. Product Applications	Recipe. Add. Information.	Key Findings of Effectiveness of Action	Comments	Ref.
Calendula officinalis L.	ointment	Evaluation of anti-inflammatory action and of the impact on ionizing radiation induced skin toxicity of the extract from *Calendula officinalis* (CO) and Ching Wan Hung (CWH)—ointment. SKH-hr1 hairless mice (10 Gy/day for 4 days). Skin toxicity and inflammatory factors (Serum interleukin (IL)-1α monocyte, chemotactic protein-1 (MCP1), keratinocyte-derived chemokine (KC), and granulocyte colony-stimulating factor (G-CSF)) were evaluated at multiple time points up to 15 days post-radiation. Mice were evaluated every 2 days following IR with and without topical treatment of CO and CWH. IR-induced skin reactions, erythema, blood vessel dilation, and crust/scaling were noted. Gross assessment of early radiation dermatitis, erythema, edema, dyspigmentation, desquamation, exudation, and ulceration, was conducted using the dermatoscope. Skin toxicity was evaluated and scored as either 0 (no visible lesion), 1 (moderate lesion), or 2 (severe lesion), for both erythema and blood vessel dilation.	CWH is a Chinese herbal ointment which is sold as an over-counter soothing lotion for burns. Some of the active ingredients include: lobelia (27.5%), myrrh (17.5%), tangkuei (12%), borneol (12%), sanguisorba (8.5%), chaenomeles (8.5%), frankincense (8.5%), carthamus (8.5%), and pistacia (8.5%). CO extract to ointment available with the trade name Pommade au Calendula Par Digestion. Contains the extract in 4% concentration.	Both CO and CWH significantly inhibited IR-induced MCP1 KC and G-CSF. IR-induced erythema and blood vessel dilation were significantly reduced by CWH but not by CO at day 10 post-IR. Both agents inhibited IR-induced IL-1α, MCP1 and vascular endothelial growth factor. There were continuous inhibitory effects of CWH on IR-induced skin toxicities and inflammation. In contrast, CO treatment resulted in skin reactions compared to IR alone both CO and CWH reduce IR-induced inflammation and CWH reduced IR-induced erythema.	Looking at the composition, it is not surprising that the preparation with higher quantity of active substances showed better result. The same market product as in Pommier study [82].	[87]

Table 4. Cont.

Plant	Form of Product	Purpose of Study. Subjects. Methodology. Product Applications	Recipe. Add. Information.	Key Findings of Effectiveness of Action	Comments	Ref.
Centella asiatica L.	cream	Attempted to determine whether prophylactic treatment with herbal creams as well as a commercial moisturizing cream could reduce acute skin reaction RCT. BC patients undergoing RT (total physical dose 40-5-Gy). 5 different groups: 1—no treatment (standard care, no creams or substances). Other groups using creams containing respectively extracts from *Centella asiatica* L., *Cucumis sativus* L., *Thunbergia laurifolia* or using moisturizing market product (Johnson and Johnson). Participants' skin was evaluated by an oncologist-radiologist weekly up to one month after the irradiation in order to identify all kinds of dermatologic reaction (according to RTOG score). Satisfaction with the preparation was also evaluated (scale 1–5 with 5 being mostly satisfied and 1 being least). Creams were applied once a day after the first session of radiotherapy up to one month after the irradiation.	*Centella asiatica* 7% (w/w) Information on other components unavailable. They do not contain fragrance. Market creams available in Thailand.	Topical application of all herbal cream or the moisturizing cream could neither reduce the severity nor delay onset of dermatitis compared with no treatment group. *Cucumis sativus* cream was shown to help with skin recovery post-irradiation. Study authors advise to prophylactically use moisturizing preparations on the irradiated area of skin.	One clinical study which evaluated three plants *Centella asiatica* L., *Cucumis sativus* L., *Thunbergia laurifolia*. Before the study allergic tests were made for unwanted reaction to the extracts and the moisturizing cream.	[88]

Table 4. Cont.

Plant	Form of Product	Purpose of Study. Subjects. Methodology. Product Applications	Recipe. Add. Information.	Key Findings of Effectiveness of Action	Comments	Ref.
Chamomilla recutita L. Rauschert (*Matricaria chamomilla* L.)	gel cream	Assessed safety and potential efficacy of a chamomile gel compared with urea cream to prevent and delay acute RD. Before starting the comparative clinical study chamomile gel in various concentrations was analyzed: 2.5%, 5.00% and 8.35%. Considering the effectiveness and the safety, the concentration of 8.35% was chosen for the clinical study. Safety assessment was based on the presence or absence of skin toxicity according to RTOG score and time to development of erythema, measured as number of sessions of radiation therapy before erythema development. RCT. Patients with head and neck cancer receiving RT with or without concomitant CT. Group chamomile gel comparing with urea cream group. Nurse was evaluated the person's skin weekly (skin toxicity according RTOG score) until the end of treatment. Photographs of the regions of the participant's head and neck on a weekly basis were taken. During the study, it was recommended to use skin care with a moisturizing soap (Dove™) and not to apply any products to the irradiated area to avoid undesirable bolus effects. Product were applied topically 3 times a day (morning, afternoon and night) on the skin of the irradiated area for the entire period of the RT (5 day week for 6–8 week).	Data about composition not available. Both product's validity was 3 months.	The gel containing 8.35% chamomile was still safe when compared to concentrations of 2.5% and 5.0% used by participants receiving RT for head and neck cancer. Increasing concentrations tended to delay the development of erythema in those participants. Formulation of 8.35% chamomile gel was not statistically different from urea cream in the delay the development of grades 1 (2.08 to 2.2 weeks) and 2 (5.1 weeks to 4.5 weeks) RD, though the effect size of delay of Grade 2 was of moderate size. No statistical differences over time were seen between the groups on adverse events. Itching, burning and hyperpigmentation were more frequently reported in the urea group.	According to the Brazilian Health Surveillance Agency (Agencia de Vigilância Sanitária—ANVISA), products made of *Chamomile recutita* do not require proof of safety because chamomile is already registered at the Brazilian Simplified Registry of Traditional Phytotherapic Products. The study in which the concentration of the active substance was defined before starting the comparative study.	[89, 90]

Table 4. Cont.

Plant	Form of Product	Purpose of Study. Subjects. Methodology. Product Applications	Recipe. Add. Information.	Key Findings of Effectiveness of Action	Comments	Ref.
Cucumis sativus L.	cream	the same as in *Centella asiatica* L. research [88]	*Cucumis sativus* L. 20% (w/w). No information available on remaining components. They do not contain fragrance. Market creams available in Thailand	Topical application of all herbal cream or the moisturizing cream could neither reduce the severity nor delay onset of dermatitis compared with no treatment group. *Cucumis sativus* cream was shown to help with skin recovery post-irradiation. It is related to the high content of water and soothing properties reducing irritations and skin oedema in cucumber. Cucumber cream proved efficient in regeneration of irradiated skin which most probably is also linked to the presence of tannins and flavonoids.	One clinical study analyzing three plants: *Centella asiatica* L., *Cucumis sativus* L., *Thunbergia laurifolia*. Before the study there were allergic tests made to check on side effects of the extracts and moisturizing creams. Cucumber has protective effects against both reactive oxygen species and reactive carbonyl species by free radical scavenging activity.	[88]
Glycyrrhiza glabra Torr. (Licorice root)	cream	The same as in *Achillea milefolium* L. research [59]	The same as in *Achillea milefolium* L. research [59]	The same as in *Achillea milefolium* L. research [59]	The same as in *Achillea milefolium* L. research	[59]

Table 4. Cont.

Plant	Form of Product	Purpose of Study. Subjects. Methodology. Product Applications	Recipe. Add. Information.	Key Findings of Effectiveness of Action	Comments	Ref.
Green tee Black tee	cream compress of aqueous tea extracts	To explore the effect of topically-applied tea extracts on the duration of radiation-induced skin toxicity. Patients with head, neck or pelvis area cancer undergoing RT (daily fractions of 1.8–2.0 Gy). During the study, patients used standard skin care program which consisted of once-daily treatment with moisturizing creme. In case of erythema, the cream was applied 2–3 times and stopped with occurence of moist desquamation. Green or black tea extracts were applied to the irradiated skin area with lesions of 2nd degree and higher (RTOG score) 3 times per day for 10 min from the occurrence of moist desquamation. Dermal toxicity was evaluated daily by the qualified medical personnel before each extract application. The disappearance of moist desquamation was considered as the end of the study. Tea extracts were compared for their ability to modulate IL-1β, IL-6, IL-8, TNFα and PGE2 release from human monocytes. Effects of tea extracts on 26S proteasome function were also assessed and NF-κβ activity was monitored by EMSAs. Viability and radiation response of macrophages after exposure to tea extracts was measured by MTT assays.	Moisturizing cream—market preparation containing 3% of urea.	Tea extracts are effective for treatment of patients suffering from acute dermal toxicity caused by irradiation. Tea extracts supported the restitution of skin integrity, inhibited proteasome function and suppressed cytokine release. NF-κβ activity was altered by tea extracts in a complex, caspase dependent manner, which differed from the effects of epigallocatechin gallate. Analyzed tea extracts, as well as epigallocatechin-gallate, slightly protected macrophages from ionizing radiation. The molecular mechanisms underlying the beneficial effects are complex, and most likely not exclusively dependent on effects of tea polyphenols such as epigallocatechin-gallate. No difference between green and black tea in duration of grade 2+ skin reactions in patients treated for cancer of the head and neck region.	There is no information, if without the application of moisturizing cream the extracts effect on skin would be the same.	[91]

Table 4. *Cont.*

Plant	Form of Product	Purpose of Study. Subjects. Methodology. Product Applications	Recipe. Add. Information.	Key Findings of Effectiveness of Action	Comments	Ref.
Camellia sinensis L. Kuntze (Chinese tea)	gel lotion cream	Evaluation of the effectiveness for the preparations with *Camellia Sinesis* Nonfermentatum extract (CSNF) (NPE®) in prevention and recovery of ARSR and skin care during postoperative whole breast RT. Open label Pilot-study. 20 patients received adapted post-operatory radiotherapy (45 Gy/20 fraction boost: 10–15 Gy/4–6 fractions or ± whole breast: 40 Gy/15 fractions). Data from these study were compared with 100 retrospectively collected matched data sets derived from hospital records. These routine medical care patients were treated according to the hospital treatment guidelines and recommendations of the SASRO. The assessments of ARSR Grades 1, 2, 3, and 4 were performed according to CTCAE. Lotion (0.4% CSNF) was applied 2× per day 7 days before RT—during RT on irradiated zones (but not directly before the RT), 4–8 weeks after RT if necessary. CSNF prophylactic gel (2.5%) was applied 1–2 h before each RT session on the day of irradiation. Irradiated zones were: thoracic and supraclavicular zones, front and back.	Composition unavailable. The only information available concerns the % of extract in the given form of preparation and that the extract is proprietary. Comparative preparations were various market preparations such as Excipial® hydrolotion (oil-in-water emulsion containing urea), Bepanthol® body lotion or Bepanthen® cream (preparations contained dexpanthenol and sodium hyaluronate or sodium hyaluronate and silver sulfadiazine.	The study showed that combined use of gel and CSNF balsam retarded the occurrence of ARSR ≥ G2 and can reduce the risk of moist desquamation of irradiated skin by 50%. The proportion of patients requiring rescue treatment during RT and follow-up was markedly higher in the control compared to the CSNF group (1% to 51% vs. 0% to 15%). CSNF gel and lotion were well tolerated both during and after RT. Camellia Sinensis Nonfermentatum Extract is potentially effective in healing skin irritation in women with breast cancer.	Comparative studies with the data from hospital files. The first study in which two types of skin care preparations were used, they contained the extract from a given plant but there was no comparison with the placebo group. According to Authors, preparations containing oils cannot be used directly before the RT because they can increase the risk of skin irritation following radiation concentration in tissues. The CSNF extract reduces oxidative stress and DNA damage, downregulates numerous factors related to apoptosis, inflammation, and carcinogenesis in experimental studies, and showed a similar protective effect for skin of healthy volunteers exposed to UV-light.	[92]

143

Table 4. Cont.

Plant	Form of Product	Purpose of Study. Subjects. Methodology. Product Applications	Recipe. Add. Information.	Key Findings of Effectiveness of Action	Comments	Ref.
Hypericum perforatum L.	ointment (gel) oil	Effectiveness of Holoil® series in treatment of acute skin toxicity (G2 acute). Sigle-arm, prospective observational study. Patients undergoing RTor chemo radiotherapy for head and neck cancer (70 Gy/35 fractions (2 Gy daily). Medical evaluation consisted of a weekly clinical evaluation with a visual examination of the neck region skin performed by the physician in charge of the patient and a consequent physician-rated score of acute skin toxicity up to 90 day after end of treatment (according to RTOG/EORTC toxicity scale). Holoil® product series treatment were started whenever bright erythema, moderate oedema or patchy moist desquamation were observed. For erythema and/or oedema gel preparation was employed. For patchy moist desquamation the oil preparation was administered. Holoil® was used during all RT course and during follow up time, until acute skin toxicity recovery. Before the lesions appeared, patients received moisturizing cream. Holoil® was applied on the bilateral neck 2–3 times a day, at least 3 h before treatment session. Other creams or cosmetic products in the irradiated area were prohibited.	No information available on the product composition (market products). Carrier for *Hypericum perforatum* L. was neem oil. According to [93]: Holoil® gel: Ingredients: Melia Azadirachta Seed Oil; Olea Europaea Oil; Hypericum Perforatum Flower Extract. Excipients: Aqua; Propylene Glycol; Ciclodextrin; Carbomer; Triethanolamine; Phenoxyethanol; Benzoic Acid; Dehydroacetic Acid; Sodium Dehydroacetate; Ethylhexylglycerin; Aroma. Holoil® oil: Ingredients: Melia Azadirachta Seed Oil; Olea Europaea Oil; Hypericum Perforatum Flower Extract.	The maximum detected acute skin toxicity was Grade 1 in 7% of patients, Grade 2 in 68%, Grade 3 in 25%, while at the end of RT was Grade 0 in 3.5%, Grade 1 in 32%, Grade 2 in 61%, Grade 3 in 3.5%. G2 acute skin toxicity mainly started at weeks 4–5; G3 begun during weeks 5–6. Median times spent with G2 or G3 toxicity were 17.5 and 11 days. Time between maximum acute skin toxicity and complete skin recovery after RT was 27 days.	Various physicochemical forms were used in the studies, depending on the radiodermatitis type: Holoil® as gel (erythema and oedema) or oil formulation (moist desquamation). Patient's compliance was consistent, with no particular complaints or difficulties. Carrier neem oil itself has anti-inflammatory, antioxidant and regenerating properties. No information available on the concentration of *Hypericum perforatum* L. in products. According to Authors Holoil® proved to be a safe and active option in the management of acute skin toxicity. A prophylactic effect in the prevention of moist desquamation may be hypothesized for hypericum and neem oil and need to be tested within a prospective controlled study.	[94]

Table 4. *Cont.*

Plant	Form of Product	Purpose of Study. Subjects. Methodology. Product Applications	Recipe. Add. Information.	Key Findings of Effectiveness of Action	Comments	Ref.
Nigela sativa L.	gel	Evaluate the effectiveness of *Nigella sativa* L. extract on preventing the incidence of ARD. RCT. BC patients undergoing RT after breast surgery (minimum total prescribed dose, 50 Gy). 2 group: placebo and *N. sativa* 5% gel. The severity of ARD, the incidence of moist desquamation, worst experienced pain, and skin-related quality of life (SRQOL) scores were assessed weekly during RT. Preparations application: twice daily during RT period at least two hours before and after RT. After applying the gel, patients were asked to wait for at least 10 min before dressing and not to wash the affected area for at least 2 h.	*N. sativa* dried extract (5% *w/w*), Glycerol (5%), Carbopol®940 (1%), Triethanolamine (0.09%), Methylparaben (0.18%), propylparaben (0.02%), water up to 100% Placebo gel contain all of these ingredients except the *N. sativa* extract.	Group of patients treated with the *N. sativa* gel developed ARD significantly less frequently compared to those who used the placebo. The incidence time of grade 2 and 3 dermatitis was prolonged significantly with *N. sativa* gel as compared to placebo (35 vs. 29 days and 42 vs. 40 days, respectively). Also occurrence of moist desquamation was delayed 37 vs. 33 days for *N. sativa* gel vs. placebo respectively. At week 3 the mean score of the worst pain that patients experienced in *N. sativa* gel was significantly lower than in placebo group. No significant effect on the SRQOL after application of *N. sativa* gel was observed.	Both extract and gels were obtained by the authors. Active substance in the isolated extract was Thymoquinone the concentration of which in gel was 0.01% Gels were also studied with respect to their microbiological purity and stability. Participants with known allergy or hypersensitivity to *N. sativa* or any ingredients of the gel were excluded from the study.	[95]
Silybum marianum (L.) Gaertner	gel	Investigate the efficacy of silymarin gel in prevention of RD. RCT. Patients with BC received placebo or silymarin gel on chest walk skin following modified radical mastectomy (total radiation dose of 50 Gy). RD severity was assessed weekly based on RTOG and NCI-CTCAE criteria radiodermatitis grading scale for 5 weeks. Preparations (half fingertip unit) applied daily starting at the first day of RT for 5 weeks.	1% silymarin gel Used in the recipe dry extract contain 80% active ingredient based on silymarin flavonolignans (including silybin, silychristin, silydianin, 2,3-dehydrosilybin, and 2,3-dihydrosilychristin). No information available on the remaining components for both placebo gel and silymarin gel	The median NCI-CTCAE and RTOG scores were significantly lower in silymarin group at the end of the third to fifth weeks. The scores increased significantly in both placebo and silymarin groups during RT but there was a delay in RD development and progression in silymarin group. Prophylactic administration of silymarin gel could significantly reduce the severity of RD and delay its occurrence after 5 weeks of application (80% patients in this group remained asymptomatic). None of patients in silymarin group experienced grades higher than 1 during RT in contrast to placebo group were was patients with grade 2 and grade 3.	Were excluded from the study people with history of allergy to silymarin, history of autoimmune and connective tissue diseases, concomitant use of nonsteroidal anti-inflammatory drugs, corticosteroids, and other immunosuppressive or antioxidant medications. Because Silymarin could reduce the severity of radiodermatitis the silymarin gel should be prescribe before the beginning of the RT. The authors of the study suggest that the silymarin 1% gel, and increasing the silymarin content of the gel may increase its efficacy in RD prevention.	[96]

Table 4. Cont.

Plant	Form of Product	Purpose of Study. Subjects. Methodology. Product Applications	Recipe. Add. Information.	Key Findings of Effectiveness of Action	Comments	Ref.
Silybum marianum (L.) Gaertner	cream	Silymarin-based cream (Leviaderm®) was tested in efficacy in prevention of RD comparison to standard of care (SOC). Patients with histologically documented diagnosis of BC were evaluated after breast-conserving surgery followed by RT with 50.4 Gy plus boost 9–16 Gy. Participants were documented consecutively before, during, and 4 weeks after the scheduled end of RT. The occurrence of side effects and adverse drug reactions were recorded unblinded by the medical staff of the department during the weekly clinical examinations. One group of patients were treated with the silymarin based cream, second group were documented receiving a panthenol-containing cream interventionally, if local skin lesions occurred. The acute skin reactions were classified according to the RTOG and VASscores. SOC treatment consisting out of 5% dexpanthenol containing cream, which was applied as an interventional treatment to the affected breast skin after occurrence of the first signs of skin alterations (e.g., erythema) every day during RT and, thereafter, until skin recovered to normal. Silymarin-based cream was applied to the skin three times a day, 2 weeks before beginning RT, during RT, and 2 weeks afterwards. During RT, silymarin-based cream was applied daily at least 2 h before radiation. Silymarin-based cream was not applied to open wounds.	Leviaderm® market product, patented. It is mainly based on silymarin (Silybum marianum, content 0.25%), Adelmidrol®, vitamin E, bisabolol, and extracts from *Vitis vinifera*, *Epilobium angustifolium*, and *Hordeum vulgare*. The reference cream was the cream used in standard care. No detailed recipe for the product (contains 5% dexpanthenol)	The median time to toxicity was prolonged significantly with silymarin-based cream (45 vs. 29 days (SOC). Only 9.8% of patients using silymarin-based cream showed grade 2 toxicity in week 5 of RT in comparison to 52% with SOC. At the end of RT, 23.5% of patients in the silymarin-based study group developed no skin reactions vs. 2% with SOC, while grade 3 toxicity occurred only in 2% in the silymarin-based arm compared to 28% (SOC). These results reaching statistical significance for RTOG are in line with those determined for subjective toxicity (VAS). Silymarin-based cream was well tolerated and can, thus, be used over several weeks.	Patients with allergies to the product were excluded from study. According to Authors Leviaderm® represents a new concept of cream by combining prevention and therapy of RD. It may induce antioxidative actions when skin is exposed to irradiation because silymarin, protect against free radical-induced inflammation. Additonaly Adelmidrol®, or N,N-bis (hydroxyethyl)-nonandiamide, here used in a subclinical concentration of 0.5%, belongs to a family of lipidic molecules collectively defined as ALIAmides, which in preclinical and clinical testing using therapeutical concentrations (at least 2%) have been reported to restore skin reactivity by down regulating mast cell hyperactivity. To confirm the results of this nonrandomized, observational trial, this product should be tested in larger multicenter studies in this setting.	[97]

Table 4. Cont.

Plant	Form of Product	Purpose of Study. Subjects. Methodology. Product Applications	Recipe. Add. Information.	Key Findings of Effectiveness of Action	Comments	Ref.
Thunbergia laurifolia Lindl.	cream	The same as *Centella asiatica* research [88]	*Thunbergia laurifolia* 5% (w/w) No information available concerning the remaining components. They do not contain fragrance. Market creams available in Thailand.	Topical application of all herbal cream or the moisturizing cream could neither reduce the severity nor delay onset of dermatitis compared with no treatment group. *Cucumis sativus* cream wash shown to help with skin recovery post-irradiation. Authors recommend prophylactic application of moisturizing preparations on irradiated area of skin.	One clinical study in which three plants were analyzed: *Centella asiatica* L., *Cucumis sativus* L., *Thunbergia laurifolia*. Before the study, allergy tests were carried out to prevent side effects of extracts and moisturizing cream.	[88]
Turmeric curcuma longa L.	cream oil	Assess effectiveness of Vicco turmeric cream (VTC) on radiodermatitis. RCT. Patients with head and neck cancer scheduled to receive chemoradiotherapy or RT (dose 60 Gy). Two groups of patients first received topical Johnson's baby oil (JBO), second group received VTC. Acute skin reactions were assessed twice weekly (according to RTOG scores) by an investigator who was unaware of the details. Time of application: 2 weeks after the end of the RT, starting on day 1, preparations were applied 5 times per day on the irradiated area.	VTC contain: extracts of *Turmeric curcuma longa* (16% w/w), Sandalwood Oil in a non-greasy base Oil—petroleum oil Oil and VTC cream both are market preparations.	Cream based on *Curcuma longa* and Sandalwood oil was effective against post-radiation dermatitis. Significant reduction in grades of dermatitis was seen at all time points, including 2 weeks post RT. The occurrence of grade 3 dermatitis was lower in the cohorts using VTC and was statistically significant. No adverse effects (allergic reactions) were found in the groups, indicating that Curcuma cream is safe for patients with head and neck cancer.	VTC was shown to be effective in preventing radiodermatitis and needs to be validated in larger double-blind trials.	[98]
Turmeric Curcuma longa L.	cream oil	To ascertain the benefit of Vicco turmeric Ayurvedic cream (VTC) in preventing radiodermatitis. Investigator-blinded randomized trial (double blind). Women receiving breast radiation therapy (50 Gy in 2 Gy fractions daily for 5 weeks). Two groups of patients first received topical Johnson's baby oil (JBO) second group received VTC. To assess the delay in the appearance and the degree of severity (RTG score) of dermatitis throughout the study period. Application of products 5 times a day.	Market preparations. No information on composition available. VTC contain: extracts of *Turmeric Curcuma longa* (16% w/w), Sandalwood Oil in a non-greasy base.	Topical application of VTC delayed and mitigated the radiodermatitis. Compared to the JBO significant decrease in the incidence of 1 grade was seen at two week, and also in grade 2 and 3 at week 3 and 4 respectively in the VCT cohort. VCT cream significantly reduced radiation dermatitis.	Studies extended with regards to Pallaty [98]. Studies carried out with Johnson&Johnson company. Cream dose 5 g at each application and 5 cm^3 for the oil. The authors tend to attribute the effectiveness to the curcuma and oil properties such as: anti-inflammatory, antioxidant, modulating cytokines and enhancing wound healing process. All of it contributes to the mechanism giving protective effects.	[99]

Table 4. Cont.

Plant	Form of Product	Purpose of Study. Subjects. Methodology. Product Applications	Recipe. Add. Information.	Key Findings of Effectiveness of Action	Comments	Ref.
Turmeric Curcuma longa L. Valeton	gel lotion	The assessment of the prophylactical application of topical means in preventing or reducing RD and associated pain. RCT. BC patients, scheduled to receive conventional fractionated RT (total dose 44 to 66 Gy). Market preparations: Psoria Gold Curcumin gel (containing Curcumin extract), HPR Plus and placebo gel were applied. For pain assessment Skin Pain Inventory form was used. The evaluation of RDS (radiation dermatitis severity) was done by the physician or by qualified personnel. Preparations were applied on irradiated areas three times daily starting the first day of RT until 1 week after treatment completion. Standard self-care was recommended.	Psoria Gold Curcumin gel: Water Aloe Vera Leaf Juice Powder, Curcumin Extract, Hydroxypropyl Methylcellulose, Isopropyl Alcohol, Glycerin, Niacinamide (Vitamin B3) Acrylates/C10-30 Alkyl Acrylate Crosspolymer, Aminomethyl Propanol, Caprylhydroxamic Acid, Glyceryl Caprylate, Citric Acid. HPR Plus (lotion): Sodium Magnesium Fluorosilicate, Cyclomethicone, Phosphoric Acid, Sodium Chloride, Sodium Bicarbonate, Hypochlorus Acid, Water. Placebo gel (Psoria Gold)—composition unavailable	Mean RDS scores did not significantly differ between study arms. Additionally, no differences were detected in self-reported skin problems or pain ratings between the treatment groups in the total study sample. Exploratory subgroup analysis suggests that prophylactic treatment with topical curcumin may be effective for minimizing skin reactions and pain for patients with high breast separation who may have the worst skin reactions.	In the recipe including curcumin there's also aloe vera extract.	[100]
Turmeric Curcuma longa L. Valeton	gel	Determining the effect of topical curcumin treatment on radiation burns Mini-pig model. Histological and clinical changes (ulceration, erythema, moist desquamation, dry desquamation) were observed five weeks after radiation exposure (total dose 50 Gy). Curcumin gel with ethanolic extract applied twice a day for 35 days. First application just after radiation. The reference sample was vehicle cream. The preparation dose was 200 mg/cm^2 of skin.	Curcumin gel: Carbopol 934P, Water, Methanol, Ethanol, Triethanoloamine Dose of curcumin 200 mg/2 cm^3 ethanol on 200 mg carbomer. Vehicle cream (hydrogel): the same ingredients as curcumin gel but without active ingredients such as curcumin extract.	Decreased the epithelial desquamation after radiation group treated with curcumin—showed reduced expression of cyclooxygenase-2 and nuclear factor-kappaB. Curcumin treatment stimulated wound healing.	The authors obtained the gel with the extract themselves. They also refer to the results of study [101] which demonstrated that the gel showed the highest permeability of curcumin without skin irritation or anti-inflammatory effects. Physicochemical study of the preparation was not presented. Besides, in the study the authors use the terminology vehicle cream whereas it is a gel (hydrogel) with no active substance (curcumin) added.	[102]

4. Discussion

In this literature review we quoted the results of 34 studies (between 1996 and 2021), three of which concern preparations containing more than one herbal extract (paste with a mixture of *Aloe vera* L., Turmeric curcuma longa, Azadirachta indica and Ocimum sanctum [74,75], ointment Jaungo containing Angelica gigas, Lithospermum radix [78,79]). In addition, in two presented studies, two or more preparations were analyzed in parallel: specifically, preparations containing Achillea millefolium or Glycyrrhiza glabra [59], or the preparations containing respectively Centella asiatica, Cucumis sativus or Thunbergia laurifolia [88]. In the study by Franco et al. [94] the carrier of Hypericum perforatum extract was neem oil with curative properties.

In total, 36.4%, which is the highest fraction of the quoted studies, used *Aloe vera* L. (12 studies). This is due to the fact that *Aloe vera* L. is the most used plant with soothing properties. The most important therapeutic effects described after applying *Aloe vera* L. are: the reduction of dermatitis, reduction of skin colonization by bacteria and healing acceleration. Second place is occupied by studies concerning Calendula officinalis (15.2%, 5 studies). In total, 4 studies (12.1%) concern the application of Turmeric curcuma longa, and 2 (6%) Silybum marianum.

Plant materials are one the best remedies for the treatment of wide variety of persistent diseases due to the presence of large number of bioactive natural products with potential biological properties. The plants used to carry out the study were characterized by various actions and indications in skin care after radiotherapy following due to presence of compounds such as flavonoids, saponin, polyphenols, polysaccharides, phytosterols, tannins, etc. (Table 5).

The dominant actions among the plants presented in the table are: anti-inflammatory, antioxidant and antimicrobial. This is linked to the mechanism of formation and healing of radiodermatitis but also to the physician's actions aiming at preventing and treating inflammation, pain or skin damage and bleeding which are prone to bacterial superinfection. Some of the plants used in the study prove efficient in skin smoothing and moisturizing because dry skin with a pathological basis caused by dermatosis requires the same care as dry non-pathological skin [23]. Works of Hoopfer et al. [65], Byun et al. [2], Pajonk et al. [91] were the only ones including the analysis of the herbal extract as such. The main purpose of these studies was to discover skin protection mechanisms for the given extract and to link it to the effectiveness in reducing radiation skin reaction severity.

For a cosmeceutical to be effective, its recipe is essential. Recipe assumptions concern not only the esthetic aspect such as application, scent, sensation on the skin (which are certainly important for oncological patients), but they also allow for the maximum action during regular application [103]. Therefore, the recipe is an integral part of the system for providing active substance aiming at maximum action and visible effect for the consumer, meaning the cosmetic is effective. The effectiveness concerns immediate effects, short term effects and effects occurring after 30–60 days. Besides, the process of healing for the skin takes 4–5 weeks. Hence, the studies evaluated the skin condition weekly, after various time lapses until, on average, 2–6 and even 8 weeks after the end of the radiotherapy. They allowed us to demonstrate the preparation's long-term effectiveness. The longest study of preparation impact on the skin was analyzed in [74,75] and lasted 6 months. To determine the timing of application resulting in the best effect, in studies [60,97], cosmeceutical was applied beginning on day −7, 0, +7 relative to the day of irradiation (day 0) and continued for 5 weeks and applied beginning on day −14, 0 +14 respectively.

For a full assessment of the cosmetic's impact on skin after radiotherapy, a threefold approach should be considered: instrumental measurement of skin condition, expert's evaluation, and self-evaluation by the participants to the study group. A double-blind testing with control group using placebo or positive control of the prescribed product carried out by independent experts using a statistically significant number of participants are also acceptable sources of information. In total, 83.5% of the studies presented by us were randomized clinical studies and clinical studies. Studies on animals included 11.76%

of the quoted studies. In most discussed clinical studies, the assessment was done by a team of experts or the members of the study group. To do this, the assessment tools were: the scale (guidelines) RTOG/EORTC [59,66,67,71,74,75,78,81–86,88–90,94,96–99], Acute Radiation Morbidity Scoring Criteria [73], Common Toxicity Criteria [63,64], modified 10-point Catterall scale [65], Common Terminology Criteria for Adverse Events [92] or National Cancer Institute Common Terminology for Adverse Events [96]. Photographs of skin were taken in studies [11,63,72,81,89,90]. To measure erythema Near Infrared Spectroscopy, Laser Doppler Imaging and Digital Colour Photography were applied [72]. A subject's skin comfort [64] and skin-related quality of life (SRQOL) [95] was also evaluated, mostly using QLQ-C30 questionnaire [74,75]. The effectiveness was also evaluated by defining the degree of improvement of skin lesions [69].

Table 5. Selected plants with confirmed therapeutic and care effect, applied in preparations for radiotherapy.

Action	Plant Species	Chemical Compounds	Indications
Anti-inflammatory	*Achiellea millefolium* L.	flavonoids	skin irritation sensitive skin dry skin
	Aloe vera L. Burman	polysaccharides, mucilage	
	Annona muricata L.	flavonols, sesquiterpene lactones, acetogenins	
	Azadriachta indica A. Juss	isoprenoids, catechins, tannins,	
	Boswellia serrata Roxb. ex Colebr.	boswelin acids	
	Calendula officinalis L.	saponins, flavonoids, polysaccharides	
	Centella asiatica L.	triterpene saponins	
	Chamomilla recutita Rauschert	flavonoids	
	Cucumis sativus L.	cucurbitacins, phytosterole, unsaturated fatty acids	
	Glycyrrhiza glabra Torr.	triterpene saponins, flavanones	
	Green tea	polyphenols	
	Hypericum perforatum L.	flavonoids, oligomeric proanthocyanindines, xanthones, acylfluoroglucinols, derivatives of caffeic acid	
	Lithospermum erythrorhizon Siebold and Zucc.	naftochinony	
	Nigela sativa L.	flavonoids, alkaloids, unsaturated fatty acids	
	Ocimum santum Linn	terpenes, unsaturated fatty acids, saponins	
	Silybum mariannum L. Gaerther	unsaturated fatty acids, flavonolignans	
	Thunbergia laurifolia Lindl.	iridoid glucosides, rosmarinic acid	
	Turmeric curcuma longa L. Valeton	curcuminoids	

Table 5. Cont.

Action	Plant Species	Chemical Compounds	Indications
accelerating skin healing and regeneration	*Aloe vera* L. Burman	glycoprotein, mukopolysaccharides, amino acids, hydroxyquinone glycosides, minerals	wounds burns scars sensitive skin
	Hypericum perforatum L.	hyperforin, flavonoids	
	Annona muricata L.	lactones, acetogenins	
	Lithospermum erythrorhizon Siebold and Zucc.	naphthoquinones	
	Cucumis sativus L.	phytosterols, tannins,	
	Calendula officinalis L.	saponins, flavonoids	
	Azadirachta indica A. Juss	tanins	
	Centella asiatica L.	triterpenes, flavonoids	
antimicrobial (bacteria, fungi)	*Achiellea millefolium* L.	polyacetylenes, flavonoids, sesquiterpene lactones, tannins	skin infections protection of the skin against infection
	Angelica gigas Nakai	tannins, tannins, aliphatic acids	
	Azadirachta indica A. Juss	isoprenoids, tannins, polyphenols	
	Calendula officinalis L.	aliphatic acids, polysaccharides, saponins, flavonoids	
	Camellia sinesis L. Kuntze	catechins	
	Centella asiatica L.	triterpene saponins	
	Chamomilla recutita L. Rauschert	cyclic ethers, sesquiterpene alcohols	
	Glycyrrhiza glabra Torr.	flavonoids, triterpene saponins	
	Lithospermum erythrorhizon Siebold and Zucc.	naphthoquinones	
	Nigela sativa L.	alkaloids, triterpene saponins	
	Ocimum santum Linn	phenols, triterpenoids, tannins	
	Turmeric curcuma longa Valeton	curcuminoids	
moisturizing	*Aloe vera* L. Burman	polysaccharides, glycoprotein	dry skin sensitive skin
	Azadirachta indica A. Juss	polysaccharides, proteins	
	Cucumis sativus L.	amino acids, minerals, pectins,	
antioxidant	*Annona muricata* L.	phenolic compounds, vitamins, carotenoids, enzymes	neutralization of free radicals, protection of DNA strands and support of collagen and elastin production delay in lipid oxidation regeneration of primary antioxidants
	Azadirachta indica A. Juss	polyphenols, limonoids	
	Camellia sinesis L. Kuntze	polyphenols, flavonoids, phenolic acids, vitamins	
	Centella asiatica L.	flavonoids, triterpenes	
	Chamomilla recutita L. Rauschert	flavonoids, phenolic compound	
	Cucumis sativus L.	phenolic compounds, vitamins,	
	Glycyrrhiza glabra Torr.	flavonoids	
	Green tea	Catechins	
	Lithospermum erythrorhizon Siebold and Zucc.	naphthoquinones	
	Nigela sativa L.	tannins, vitamins, flavonols	
	Silybum marianum L. Gaertner	flavonolignans, phenolic compound	
	Thunbergia laurifolia Lindl.	flavonoids, polyphenols,	
	Turmeric curcuma longa Valeton	feluric acids, polyphenols	

Table 5. Cont.

Action	Plant Species	Chemical Compounds	Indications
antiseptic—disinfecting	*Angelica gigas* Nakai	tannins, alifactic acids,	cleansing of skin and wounds
	Azadirachta indica A. Juss	isoprenoids, polyphenols	
analgesic anesthetics	*Achillea millefolium* L.	flavonoids, alkaloids	local analgesic effect
	Boswellia serrata Roxb. ex Colebr.	boswellic acids	
	Ocimum santum Linn.	triterpenoids	
antipruritic	*Ocimum santum* Linn.	terpenes, tanins	itch
anti-edematous	*Cucumis sativus* L.	tanins	swelling

The availability and the effectiveness of the given component can be modified depending on the phase in which it was added to the preparation during production. The type of the solvent used for extraction is hence essential. The effectiveness can be increased by using a proper substrate and carrier system. Known ways of delivery of herbal extract in topical therapy are: creams and water-based liquids, ointments based on oils and waxes, powders and pastes, masks from freshly cut herbs, warming compresses or compresses from warm soaked herbs [104]. Among the analyzed physicochemical forms including extracts, 42.9% were gels (15 studies), 28.6% were creams (10 studies), 11.4% ointments (4 studies). Rarely used substances were (5.8%): lotions and oils (2 studies each), but also pastes and solutions (single studies, 2.8%). One work among presented studies analyzed more than one physicochemical form of the preparation [94]. A gel preparation gives a refreshing sensation, and it is oil-free, which is a more appropriate formulation to apply in skin exposed to radiation therapy, avoiding a bolus-like effect and making it easier to remove before the next radiation therapy session.

In terms of products' effectiveness assessment, it should be emphasized that in case of radiation reaction, its characteristics should be analyzed, and appropriate treatment and care should be adopted for the given degree. In the case of dry desquamation, treatments aim mainly at moisturizing the skin and reducing the skin discomfort linked to burning and itching. Hence, hydrophilic preparation (mostly gels) with neutral pH are most appropriate. They are often combined with the topical application of corticosteroids. Corticosteroids however have a lot of side effects. In works [74,75] the effectiveness of the paste with herbal extracts was compared to Beclomethasone cream. The evaluation of paste effectiveness as compared to corticosteroids was analyzed in [79]. In case of moist desquamation, the principle of treating the moist with the moist is applied; hence, the best option seems to be hydrocolloid dressings.

Most of the quoted studies aimed at preventing dermatitis. Hence, the studied preparation was applied throughout the whole treatment. Possible changes in treatment were linked to allergy or to development of dermatitis of second degree or higher, which required the introduction of corticosteroids, antibiotics or analgesics. In the case of moist desquamation, individual works [71,88] stopped the application of the preparation in the area of occurrence. Only the studies carried out by the team Franco et al. [94] included the application of two forms of preparations depending on the type of radiodermatitis observed. Thus, for erythema and/or oedema, gel preparation was employed. For patchy moist desquamation, the oil preparation was administered.

In the works quoted, multiple forms of preparations were compared simultaneously during the study; for example, cream and oil or powder [65,71,98,99], creams with water infusion [88], gels with creams [11,62–64,72,89,90,100], gels with soap [67], gels with ointments [60], gels with oils [94]. We know currently that the skin barrier layer should not only be moisturized but also rebuilt, which cannot be done with preparations such as soap. Besides, in studies [11,61,67,78,83,84,100] standard care was recommended or moisturizing preparations were applied together with the analyzed one [88,92]. The study results presented in [65] speak in favor of dry skin care instead of applying moisturizing creams enriched with herbal extracts.

In some of the clinical studies [60,64,66,71,72,82–84,88,91,92,94,97–100] generally available, market products were applied (they were not registered as medical products hence they did not have any specific use recommendations). They had no antioxidant, moisturizing or redness reducing action, which should characterize preparations after radiotherapy. Market preparations played a role of placebo [60,72,83,84,87,92], or extract carrier [59], but were also a well-known preparation containing active substances of plant origin like Juango ointment [78,79] or Vicco Turmeric cream [98,99]. Besides, some of the placebo preparations contained active substances [60]. One of the certain defects of the presented works [11,61–63,67,71,79,84,88–92,96,99] is the lack of composition for evaluated products.

From a scientific but also from practical point of view, the time of application of cosmeceuticals and the dosage are important. As shown in [60], there was no effect if the gel was applied only before irradiation or beginning 1 week after irradiation. According to [97], the minimal application time is two weeks before the beginning of radiotherapy, while a significant part of the works concerned studies in which the preparation application started at the same time as the irradiation. Studies [73,79,102] mentioned the doses of applied products.

5. Conclusions

In the current review paper, the literature data have been systematically reviewed and we discussed the connection between the type of applied skin care (type of preparation, its composition, the dose), the properties of the herbal extract, and the evaluation of its efficiency in preventing and treating radiation reaction on skin.

From this research, the following conclusions can be drawn:

1. The application of herbal extracts in preparations preventing radiodermatitis is important and still up-to-date (most recent publications about ongoing clinical studies are from 2021). Moreover, many herbal extracts such as Dilenia idica, and the Lamicale Family show potential in treating dermatitis but have not been introduced in the recipes of ointments, creams or gels.
2. Herbal extracts obtained from plants can be added to recipes because they are part of a category of cosmeceutical supplements which are not subject to regulations and can be introduced into preparations without prescription. Herbal extracts can be a raw material from which active substances are isolated. For example, tea is a source of epigallocate-hin-3-gallatechin. Polysaccharides can be obtained from Annona muricata L. Both have potential in the treatment of dermatitis.
3. The dominant actions among the plants are: anti-inflammatory, antioxidant and antimicrobial. This is linked to the mechanism of formation and healing of radiodermatitis but also to the physician's actions aiming at preventing and treating inflammation, pain or skin damage and bleeding which are prone to bacterial superinfection. Some of the plants used in the study prove efficient in skin smoothing and moisturizing because dry skin with a pathological basis caused by dermatosis requires the same care as dry non-pathological skin.
4. In the available study results there is conflicting information concerning the effectiveness in treatment and prevention of radiodermatitis by the products containing herbal extracts in their recipe (e.g., *Aloe vera*). There are also works mentioning that preparations such as ointments are poorly tolerated and appreciated by patients, and that some preparations cause allergies. Hence there are premises indicating that there is a need to widen the preparations offer for radiotherapy patients, the recipe of which is projected already at the evaluation stage of herbal extracts.
5. The effectiveness evaluation for herbal extracts in radiotherapy is not an easy task since there are no strict guidelines. Studies should include both apparatus analyses of the skin condition and clinical studies including patients. They should also be

preceded by the analysis of herbal extracts and recipe in terms of physicochemical, dermatological, and performance characteristics.

Author Contributions: Conceptualization, A.K.-P.; writing—original draft preparation, review and editing A.K.-P., W.J.G. All authors have read and agreed to the published version of the manuscript.

Funding: This research received no external funding.

Institutional Review Board Statement: Not applicable.

Informed Consent Statement: Not applicable.

Data Availability Statement: Not applicable.

Acknowledgments: Authors would like to thank Anna Riondet for providing language help.

Conflicts of Interest: The authors declare no conflict of interest.

References

1. Jaffray, D.A.; Gospodarowicz, M.K. Chapter 14—Radiation Therapy for Cancer. In *Cancer: Disease Control Priorities*, 3rd ed.; Gelband, H., Jha, P., Sankaranarayanan, R., Horton, S., Eds.; The International Bank for Reconstruction and Development/The World Bank: Washington, DC, USA, 2015; Volume 3, pp. 1–16.
2. Byun, E.B.; Song, H.Y.; Sik Kim, W. Polysaccharides from Annona muricata leaves protect normal human epidermal keratinocytes and mice skin from radiation-induced injuries. *Radiat. Phys. Chem.* **2020**, *170*, 198672. [CrossRef]
3. Wei, J.; Meng, L.; Hou, X.; Qu, C.; Wang, B.; Xin, Y.; Jiang, X. Radiation-induced skin reactions mechanism and treatment. *Cancer Manag. Res.* **2019**, *11*, 1670177. [CrossRef] [PubMed]
4. Wang, Y.; Tu, W.; Tang, Y.; Zhang, S. Prevention and treatment for radiation-induced skin injury during radiotherapy. *Radiat. Med. Prot.* **2020**, *1*, 60–68. [CrossRef]
5. What Is Cancer Radiotherapy? Available online: https://www.zwrotnikraka.pl/na-czym-polega-radioterapia/ (accessed on 18 May 2022).
6. Robson, V. Using honey to treat skin damaged by radiotherapy. *Wounds* **2009**, *5*, 51–57.
7. Porock, D.; Kristjanosn, L. Skin reactions during radiotherapy for breast cancer: The use and impact of topical agents and dressings. *Eur. J. Cancer Care* **1999**, *8*, 143–153. [CrossRef] [PubMed]
8. Singh, M.; Alavi, A.; Wong, R.; Akita, S. Radiodermatitis: A Review of Our Current Understanding. *Am. J. Clin. Dermatol.* **2016**, *17*, 277–292. [CrossRef]
9. Hogl, W.P. Chapter 1—Overview of Skin Issues Related to the Oncology Patient. In *Principles of Skin Care and the Oncology Patient*; Haas, M.L., Moore-Higgs, G.J., Eds.; Oncology Nursing Society: Pittsburgh, PA, USA, 2011; pp. 1–32.
10. Stone, H.B.; Coleman, C.N.; Anscher, M.; McBride, W.H. Effects of radiation on normal tissue: Consequences and mechanisms. *Lancet Oncol.* **2003**, *4*, 529–536. [CrossRef]
11. Richardson, J.; Smith, J.; McIntyre, M.; Thomas, R.; Pilkington, K. Aloe Vera for Preventing Radiation-induced Skin Reactions: A Systematic Literature Review. *Clin. Oncol.* **2005**, *17*, 478–484. [CrossRef]
12. Bensadoun, R.J.; Humbert, P.; Krutmann, J.; Luger, T.; Triller, R.; Rougier, A.; Seité, S.; Dreno, B. Daily baseline skin care in the prevention, treatment, and supportive care of skin toxicity in oncology patients: Recommendations from a multinational expert panel. *Cancer Manag. Res.* **2013**, *5*, 401–408. [CrossRef]
13. Mendelsohn, F.A.; Divino, C.M.; Reis, E.D.; Kerstein, M.D. Wound Care After Radiation Therapy. *Adv. Ski. Wound Care* **2002**, *15*, 216–224. [CrossRef]
14. McQuestion, M. Evidence-based skin care management in radiation therapy. *Semin. Oncol. Nurs.* **2006**, *23*, 163–173. [CrossRef] [PubMed]
15. Seité, S.; Bensadoun, R.-J.; Mazer, J.-M. Prevention and treatment of acute and chronic radiodermatitis. *Breast Cancer Targets Ther.* **2017**, *9*, 551–557. [CrossRef] [PubMed]
16. Wiśniewski, M.; Graczyk, M.; Szpinda, M.; Brzozowska-Mańkowska, S. Popromienne zapalenie skóry—Zasady postępowania. *Med. Paliatywna W Prakt.* **2013**, *7*, 41–45.
17. Dormand, E.-L.; Banwell, P.E.; Goodacre, T.E. Radiotherapy and wound healing. *Int. Wound J.* **2005**, *2*, 112–127. [CrossRef] [PubMed]
18. Kodiyan, J.; Amber, K.T. Topical antioxidants in radiodermatitis: A clinical review. *Int. J. Palliat. Nurs.* **2015**, *21*, 446–452. [CrossRef]
19. De Conno, F.; Ventafridda, V.; Saita, L. Skin problems in advanced and terminal cancer patients. *J. Pain Symptom Manag.* **1991**, *6*, 247–256. [CrossRef]
20. Haley, A.C.; Calahan, C.; Gandhi, M.; West, D.P.; Rademaker, A.; Lacouture, M.E. Skin care management in cancer patients: An evaluation of quality of life and tolerability. *Support. Care Cancer* **2010**, *19*, 545–554. [CrossRef]

21. Michalewska, J. Odczyny popromienne w radioterapii oraz popromienne zapalenie skóry. *Lett. Oncol. Sci.* **2017**, *14*, 104–109. [CrossRef]
22. Skin Care Guidelines for Patients Receiving Radiotherapy. Available online: https://www.uhb.nhs.uk/Downloads/pdf/PiSkinCareGuideRadiotherapy.pdf (accessed on 17 October 2021).
23. Stryczyńska, G. Assessment of the effectiveness and results of application research of soft cream Aquastop® Radioterapia (Ziołolek sp. z o.o.) in patients with dry and irritated skin, receiving radiotherapy. *Contemp. Oncol.* **2011**, *15*, 59–65.
24. Topczewska-Bruns, J.; Filipowski, T.; Demska, M. Pielęgnacja i ochrona skóry w trakcie i po radioterapii. *Opieka Onkol.* **2014**, *2*, 56–58.
25. Sauder, M.B.; Addona, M.; Andreiessen, A.; Butler, M.; Claveau, J.; Feugas, N.; Hijal, T.; Iannattone, L.; Kalia, S.; Teauge, L.; et al. The Role of Skin Care in Oncology Patients. *Ski. Ther. Lett.* **2020**, 2–12.
26. Draelos, Z.D. The science behind skin care: Moisturizers. *J. Cosmet. Dermatol.* **2018**, *17*, 138–144. [CrossRef] [PubMed]
27. Purnamawati, S.; Indrastuti, N.; Danarti, R.; Saefudin, T. The Role of Moisturizers in Addressing Various Kinds of Dermatitis: A Review. *Clin. Med. Res.* **2017**, *15*, 75–87. [CrossRef] [PubMed]
28. Werschler, W.P.; Trookman, N.S.; Rizer, R.L.; Ho, E.T.; Mehta, R. Enhanced efficacy of a facial hydrating serum in subjects with normal or self-perceived dry skin. *J. Clin. Aesthetic Dermatol.* **2011**, *4*, 51–55.
29. Narasimhan, M.; Allotey, P.; Hardon, A. Self care interventions to advance health and wellbeing: A conceptual framework to inform normative guidance. *BMJ* **2019**, *365*, l688. [CrossRef]
30. Yuen, F.; Arron, S. Chapter 4—Skin Care Products Used During Radiation Therapy. In *Skin Care in Radiation Oncology: A Practical Guide*, 1st ed.; Fowble, B., Yom, S.S., Yuen, F., Arron, S., Eds.; Springer: Berlin/Heidelberg, Germany, 2016; pp. 31–45. [CrossRef]
31. Lodén, M. Role of Topical Emollients and Moisturizers in the Treatment of Dry Skin Barrier Disorders. *Am. J. Clin. Dermatol.* **2003**, *4*, 771–788. [CrossRef]
32. Kraft, J.N.; Lynde, C.W. Moisturizers: What they are and a practical approach to product selection. *Ski. Ther. Lett.* **2005**, *10*, 1–8.
33. DebMandal, M.; Mandal, S. Coconut (Cocos nucifera L.: Arecaceae): In health promotion and disease prevention. *Asian Pac. J. Trop. Med.* **2011**, *4*, 241–247. [CrossRef]
34. Danby, S.G.; AlEnzi, T.; Sultan, A.; Lavender, T.; Chittock, J.; Brown, K.; Cork, M.J. Effect of olive and sunflover seed oil on the adult skin barrier: Implications for neonatal skin care. *Pediatr. Dermatol.* **2013**, *30*, 42. [CrossRef]
35. Nayak, B.; Raju, S.; Rao, A.C. Wound healing activity of *Persea americana* (avocado) fruit: A preclinical study on rats. *J. Wound Care* **2008**, *17*, 123–125. [CrossRef]
36. Muangman, P.; Pundee, C.; Opasanon, S.; Muangman, S. A prospective, randomized trial of silver containing hydrofiber dressing versus 1% silver sulfadiazine for the treatment of partial thickness burns. *Int. Wound J.* **2010**, *7*, 271–276. [CrossRef] [PubMed]
37. Black, J.S.; Drake, D.B. A prospective randomized trial comparing silver sulfadiazine cream with watersoluble polyantimicrobial gel in partial-thickness burn wounds. *Plast. Surg. Nurs.* **2015**, *35*, 46–49. [CrossRef] [PubMed]
38. Kerri, J.E. Principles of Topical Dermatologic Therapy. Available online: https://www.msdmanuals.com/professional/dermatologic-disorders/principles-of-topical-dermatologic-therapy/principles-of-topical-dermatologic-therapy (accessed on 18 May 2022).
39. McQuestion, M. Evidence-Based Skin Care Management in Radiation Therapy: Clinical Update. *Semin. Oncol. Nurs.* **2011**, *27*, e1–e17. [CrossRef] [PubMed]
40. Reszke, R.; Szepietowski, J. Special dermatological vehicles in concomitant therapy of chronic dermatoses. *Forum Dermatol.* **2016**, *2*, 48943. Available online: https://journals.viamedica.pl/forum_dermatologicum/article/view/48943/37310 (accessed on 18 May 2022).
41. Elgharably, H.; Ganesh, K.; Dickerson, J.; Khanna, S.; Abas, M.; Das Ghatak, P.; Dixit, S.; Bergdall, V.; Roy, S.; Sen, C.K. A modified collagen gel dressing promotes angiogenesis in a preclinical swine model of chronic ischemic wounds. *Wound Repair Regen.* **2014**, *22*, 720–729. [CrossRef]
42. Brett, D. A Review of Collagen and Collagen-based Wound Dressings. *Wounds* **2008**, *20*, 347–356.
43. Macmillan, M.S.; Wells, M.; MacBride, S.; Raab, G.M.; Munro, A.; MacDougall, H. Randomized Comparison of Dry Dressings Versus Hydrogel in Management of Radiation-Induced Moist Desquamation. *Int. J. Radiat. Oncol.* **2007**, *68*, 864–872. [CrossRef]
44. Gollins, S.; Gaffney, C.; Slade, S.; Swindell, R. RCT on gentian violet versus a hydrogel dressing for radiotherapy-induced moist skin desquamation. *J. Wound Care* **2008**, *17*, 268–275. [CrossRef]
45. Sopata, M.; Szewczyk, M.T.; Zaporowska-Stachowiak, I.; Mościcka, P.; Jawień, A. Zastosowanie opatrunku w żelu w leczeniu ran przewlekłych. *Leczenie Ran* **2021**, *18*, 123–130. [CrossRef]
46. Aderibigbe, B.A.; Buyana, B. Alginate in Wound Dressings. *Pharmaceutics* **2018**, *10*, 42. [CrossRef]
47. Herst, P.M.; Bennett, N.C.; Sutherland, A.E.; Peszynski, R.I.; Paterson, D.B.; Jasperse, M.L. Prophylactic use of Mepitel Film prevents radiation-induced moist desquamation in an intra-patient randomised controlled clinical trial of 78 breast cancer patients. *Radiother. Oncol.* **2014**, *110*, 137–143. [CrossRef] [PubMed]
48. Fong, J.; Wood, F. Nanocrystaline silver dressings in wound management: A review. *Int. J. Nanomed.* **2006**, *1*, 441–449. [CrossRef] [PubMed]
49. Skalska-Kamińska, A.; Woźniak, A.; Paduch, R.; Kocjan, R.; Rejdak, R. Herbal preparation extract for skin after radiotherapy treatment. Part One—Preclinical tests. *Acta Pol. Pharm. Drug Res.* **2014**, *71*, 781–788.

50. Griñan-Lison, C.; Blaya-Cánovas, J.L.; López-Tejada, A.; Ávalos-Moreno, M.; Navarro-Ocón, A.; Cara, F.E.; González-González, A.; Lorente, J.A.; Marchal, J.A.; Granados-Principal, S. Antioxidants for the Treatment of Breast Cancer: Are We There Yet? *Antioxidants* **2021**, *10*, 205. [CrossRef]
51. Baliga, M.S.; Rao, S.; Rai, M.P.; D'souza, P. Radio protective effects of the Ayurvedic medicinal plant Ocimum santum Linn. (Holy Basil): A memoir. *J. Cancer Res. Ther.* **2016**, *12*, 20. [CrossRef]
52. Szejk, M.; Kołodziejczyk-Czepas, J.; Żbikowska, H.M. Radioprotectors in radiotherapy—advances in the potential application of phytochemicals. *Postepy Hig. Med. Dosw.* **2016**, *70*, 722–734. [CrossRef]
53. Unlu, A.; Nayir, E.; Kalenderoglu, M.D.; Kirca, O.; Ozdogan, M. Curcumin (Turmeric) and cancer. *JBUON* **2016**, *21*, 1050–1060.
54. Ryan, J.L.; Heckler, C.E.; Ling, M.; Katz, A.; Williams, J.P.; Pentland, A.P.; Morrow, G.R. Curcumin for Radiation Dermatitis: A Randomized, Double-Blind, Placebo-Controlled Clinical Trial of Thirty Breast Cancer Patients. *Radiat. Res.* **2013**, *180*, 34–43. [CrossRef]
55. Aqil, F.; Munagala, R.; Agrawal, A.K.; Gupta, R. Chapter 10—Anticancer Phytocompounds: Experimental and Clinical Updates. In *New Look to Phytomedicine Advancements in Herbal Products as Novel Drug Leads*; Ahmad Khan, M.S., Ahmad, I., Chattophadhyay, D., Eds.; Academic Press: Cambridge, MA, USA, 2018; pp. 237–272. [CrossRef]
56. Yahyapour, R.; Shabeeb, D.; Cheki, M.; Musa, A.E.; Farhood, B.; Rezaeyan, A.; Amini, P.; Fallah, H.; Najafi, M. Radiation Protection and Mitigation by Natural Antioxidants and Flavonoids: Implications to Radiotherapy and Radiation Disasters. *Curr. Mol. Pharmacol.* **2018**, *11*, 285–304. [CrossRef]
57. Kalekhan, F.; Kudva, A.K.; Raghu, S.V.; Rao, S.; Hegde, S.K.; Simon, P.; Baliga, M.S. Traditionally Used Natural Products in Preventing Ionizing Radiation-Induced Dermatitis: First Review on the Clinial Study. *Anti-Cancer Agents Med. Chem.* **2022**, *22*, 64–82. [CrossRef]
58. Heydarirad, G.; Ahadi, B.; Vardanjani, H.M.; Cramer, H.; Mirzaei, H.R.; Pasalar, M. Herbal Medicines for Treatment of Radiodermatitis: A Systematic Review and Meta-Analysis. *J. Altern. Complement. Med.* **2021**, *27*, 1098–1104. [CrossRef] [PubMed]
59. Malekzadeh, M.; Sandoughdaran, S.; Shandiz, F.H.; Honary, S. The Efficacy of Licorice Root (Glycyrrhiza glabra) and Yarrow (Achillea millefolium) in Preventing Radiation Dermatitis in Patients with Breast Cancer: A Randomized, Double-Blinded, Placebo-Controlled Clinical Trial. *Asian Pac. J. Cancer Care* **2016**, *1*, 9–13. [CrossRef]
60. Roberts, D.B.; Travis, E.L. Acemannan-containing wound dressing gel reduces radiation-induced skin reactions in C3H mice. *Int. J. Radiat. Oncol.* **1995**, *32*, 1047–1052. [CrossRef]
61. Williams, M.S.; Burk, M.; Loprinzi, C.L.; Hill, M.; Schomberg, P.J.; Nearhood, K.; O'Fallon, J.R.; Laurie, J.A.; Shanahan, T.G.; Moore, R.L.; et al. Phase III double-blind evaluation of an aloe vera gel as a prophylactic agent for radiation-induced skin toxicity. *Int. J. Radiat. Oncol. Biol. Phys.* **1996**, *36*, 345–349. [CrossRef]
62. Heggie, S.; Bryant, G.P.; Tripcony, L.; Keller, J.; Rose, P.; Glendenning, M.; Heath, J. A Phase III Study on the Efficacy of Topical Aloe Vera Gel on Irradiated Breast Tissue. *Cancer Nurs.* **2002**, *25*, 442–451. [CrossRef] [PubMed]
63. Bosley, C.; Smith, J.; Baratti, P.; Pritchard, D.; Xiong, X.; Li, C.; Merchant, T. A phase III trial comparing an anionic phospholipid-based (APP) cream and aloe vera-based gel in the prevention and treatment of radiation dermatitis. *Int. J. Radiat. Oncol.* **2003**, *57*, S438. [CrossRef]
64. Merchant, T.E.; Bosley, C.; Smith, J.; Baratti, P.; Pritchard, D.; Davis, T.; Li, C.; Xiong, X. A phase III trial comparing an anionic phospholipid-based cream and aloe vera-based gel in the prevention of radiation dermatitis in pediatric patients. *Radiat. Oncol.* **2007**, *2*, 45–48. [CrossRef]
65. Hoopfer, D.; Holloway, C.; Gabos, Z.; Alidrisi, M.; Chafe, S.; Krause, B.; Lees, A.; Mehta, N.; Tankel, K.; Strickland, F.; et al. Three-Arm Randomized Phase III Trial: Quality Aloe and Placebo Cream Versus Powder as Skin Treatment During Breast Cancer Radiation Therapy. *Clin. Breast Cancer* **2015**, *15*, 181–190.e4. [CrossRef]
66. Haddad, P.; Amouzgar-Hashemi, F.; Samsami, S.; Chinichian, S.; Oghabian, M.A. Aloe vera for prevention of radiation-induced dermatitis: A self-controlled clinical trial. *Curr. Oncol.* **2013**, *20*, e345–e348. [CrossRef]
67. Olsen, D.L.; Raub, W., Jr.; Bradley, C.; Johnson, M.; Macias, J.L.; Love, V.; Markoe, A. The effect of aloe vera gel/mild soap versus mild soap alone in preventing skin reactions inpatients undergoing radiation therapy. *Oncol. Nurs. Forum* **2001**, *28*, 543–547.
68. Goyal, P.K.; Gehlot, P. Radioprotective Effects of Aloe Vera Leaf Extract on Swiss Albino Mice against Whole-Body Gamma Irradiation. *J. Environ. Pathol. Toxicol. Oncol.* **2009**, *28*, 53–61. [CrossRef] [PubMed]
69. Shimpo, K.; Ida, C.; Chihara, T.; Beppu, H.; Kaneko, T.; Kuzuya, H. Aloe arborescens extract inhibits TPA-induced ear oedema, putrescine increase and tumour promotion in mouse skin. *Phytother. Res.* **2002**, *16*, 491–493. [CrossRef] [PubMed]
70. Silva, M.A.; Trevisan, G.; Hoffmeister, C.; Rossato, M.F.; Boligon, A.; Walker, C.; Klafke, J.Z.; Oliveira, S.M.; Silva, C.R.; Athayde, M.L.; et al. Anti-inflammatory and antioxidant effects of Aloe saponaria Haw in a model of UVB-induced paw sunburn in rats. *J. Photochem. Photobiol. B Biol.* **2014**, *133*, 47–54. [CrossRef] [PubMed]
71. Rao, S.; Hegde, S.K.; Baliga-Rao, M.P.; Palatty, P.L.; George, T.; Baliga, M.S. An Aloe Vera-Based Cosmeceutical Cream Delays and Mitigates Ionizing Radiation-Induced Dermatitis in Head and Neck Cancer Patients Undergoing Curative Radiotherapy: A Clinical Study. *Medicines* **2017**, *4*, 44. [CrossRef] [PubMed]
72. Nyström, J.; Svensk, A.-C.; Lindholm-Sethson, B.; Geladi, P.; Larson, J.; Franzén, L. Comparison of three instrumental methods for the objective evaluation of radiotherapy induced erythema in breast cancer patients and a study of the effect of skin lotions. *Acta Oncol.* **2007**, *46*, 893–899. [CrossRef] [PubMed]

73. Ahmadloo, N.; Kadkhodaei, B.; Omidvari, S.; Mosalaei, A.; Ansari, M.; Nasrolahi, H.; Hamedi, S.H.; Mohammadianpanah, M. Lack of Prophylactic Effects of Aloe Vera Gel on Radiation Induced Dermatitis in Breast Cancer Patients. *Asian Pac. J. Cancer Prev.* **2017**, *18*, 1139–1143. [CrossRef]
74. Sharma, S.; Sharma, V.; Gupta, M.C.; Verma, Y. Comparative Evaluation of Efficacy and Safety of Herbal Preparation vis-à-vis Beclomethasone Cream on Radiation Induced Skin Injury in Head and Neck Carcinoma Patients Receiving Radiotherapy or Chemoradiation in Oncology Department at a Tertiary Care Hospital. *Int. J. Med. Res. Prof.* **2019**, *5*, 14–18.
75. Sharma, S.; Sharma, V.; Gupta, M.C.; Verma, Y. Comparative Evaluation of Quality of Life in Patients of Head and Neck Carcinoma with Radiation Induced Skin-injury in Oncology Department at Tertiary Care Hospital. *Int. J. Interdiscip. Multidiscip. Stud.* **2019**, *6*, 65–79.
76. Shin, S.; Jang, B.-H.; Suh, H.S.; Park, S.-H.; Lee, J.-W.; Yoon, S.W.; Kong, M.; Lim, Y.J.; Hwang, D.-S. Effectiveness, safety, and economic evaluation of topical application of a herbal ointment, Jaungo, for radiation dermatitis after breast conserving surgery in patients with breast cancer (GREEN study): Study protocol for a randomized controlled trial. *Medicine* **2019**, *98*, e15174. [CrossRef]
77. Kim, E.H.; Yoon, J.-H.; Bin Park, S.; Lee, J.Y.; Chung, W.K.; Yoon, S.W. Comparative Efficacy of Jaungo, A Traditional Herbal Ointment, and the Water-in-Oil Type Non-Steroidal Moisturizer for Radiation-Induced Dermatitis in Patients With Breast Cancer: A Study Protocol for a Prospective, Randomized, Single-Blinded, Pilot Study. *Front. Pharmacol.* **2021**, *12*, 751812. [CrossRef]
78. Kong, M.; Hwang, D.-S.; Lee, J.Y.; Yoon, S.W. The Efficacy and Safety of Jaungo, a Traditional Medicinal Ointment, in Preventing Radiation Dermatitis in Patients with Breast Cancer: A Prospective, Single-Blinded, Randomized Pilot Study. *Evid. Based Complement. Altern. Med.* **2016**, *2016*, 9481413. [CrossRef] [PubMed]
79. Hayashi, A. Clinical application of shinuko. *J. Trad. Med.* **2013**, *30*, 27–30.
80. Maramaldi, G.; Togni, S.; Di Pierro, F.; Biondi, M. A cosmeceutical formulation based on boswellic acids for the treatment of erythematous eczema and psoriasis. *Clin. Cosmet. Investig. Dermatol.* **2014**, *7*, 321–327. [CrossRef] [PubMed]
81. Togni, S.; Maramaldi, G.; Bonetta, A.; Giacomelli, L.; Di Pierro, F. Clinical evaluation of safety and efficacy of Boswellia-based cream for prevention of adjuvant radiotherapy skin damage in mammary carcinoma: A randomized placebo controlled trial. *Eur. Rev. Med. Pharmacol. Sci.* **2015**, *19*, 1338–1344.
82. Pommier, P.; Gomez, F.; Sunyach, M.; D'Hombres, A.; Carrie, C.; Montbarbon, X. Phase III Randomized Trial of Calendula Officinalis Compared With Trolamine for the Prevention of Acute Dermatitis During Irradiation for Breast Cancer. *J. Clin. Oncol.* **2004**, *22*, 1447–1453. [CrossRef]
83. Kodiyan, J.; Amber, K.T. A Review of the Use of Topical Calendula in the Prevention and Treatment of Radiotherapy-Induced Skin Reactions. *Antioxidants* **2015**, *4*, 293–303. [CrossRef]
84. Sharp, L.; Finnilä, K.; Johansson, H.; Abrahamsson, M.; Hatschek, T.; Bergenmar, M. No differences between Calendula cream and aqueous cream in the prevention of acute radiation skin reactions—Results from a randomised blinded trial. *Eur. J. Oncol. Nurs.* **2013**, *17*, 429–435. [CrossRef]
85. Siddiquee, S.; A McGee, M.; Vincent, A.D.; Giles, E.; Clothier, R.; Carruthers, S.; Penniment, M. Efficacy of topical Calendula officinalis on prevalence of radiation-induced dermatitis: A randomised controlled trial. *Australas. J. Dermatol.* **2021**, *62*, e35–e40. [CrossRef]
86. Schneider, F.; Danski, M.T.R.; Vayego, S.A. Usage of Calendula officinalis in the prevention and treatment of radiodermatitis: A randomized double-blind controlled clinical trial. *Rev. Esc. Enferm. USP* **2015**, *49*, 221–228. [CrossRef]
87. Hu, J.J.; Cui, T.; Rodriguez-Gil, J.L.; Allen, G.O.; Li, J.; Takita, C.; Lally, B.E. Complementary and alternative medicine in reducing radiation-induced skin toxicity. *Radiat. Environ. Biophys.* **2014**, *53*, 621–626. [CrossRef]
88. Thanthong, S.; Nanthong, R.; Kongwattanakul, S.; Laebua, K.; Trirussapanich, P.; Pitiporn, S.; Nantajit, D. Prophylaxis of Radiation-Induced Dermatitis in Patients With Breast Cancer Using Herbal Creams: A Prospective Randomized Controlled Trial. *Integr. Cancer Ther.* **2020**, *19*, 1534735420920714. [CrossRef] [PubMed]
89. Ferreira, E.B.; Ciol, M.A.; De Meneses, A.G.; Bontempo, P.D.S.M.; Hoffman, J.M.; Dos Reis, P.E.D. Chamomile Gel versus Urea Cream to Prevent Acute Radiation Dermatitis in Head and Neck Cancer Patients: Results from a Preliminary Clinical Trial. *Integr. Cancer Ther.* **2020**, *19*, 1534735420962174. [CrossRef] [PubMed]
90. Ferreira, E.B.; Ciol, M.; Vasques, C.I.; Bontempo, P.D.S.M.; Vieira, N.N.P.; Silva, L.F.O.E.; Avelino, S.R.; Dos Santos, M.A.; Dos Reis, P.E.D. Gel of chamomile vs. urea cream to prevent acute radiation dermatitis in patients with head and neck cancer: A randomized controlled trial. *J. Adv. Nurs.* **2016**, *72*, 1926–1934. [CrossRef] [PubMed]
91. Pajonk, F.; Riedisser, A.; Henke, M.; McBride, W.H.; Fiebich, B. The effects of tea extracts on proinflammatory signaling. *BMC Med.* **2006**, *4*, 28. [CrossRef] [PubMed]
92. Näf, G.; Gasser, U.E.; Holzgang, H.E.; Schafroth, S.; Oehler, C.; Zwahlen, D.R. Prevention of Acute Radiation-Induced Skin Reaction with NPE® Camellia Sinensis Nonfermentatum Extract in Female Breast Cancer Patients Undergoing Postoperative Radiotherapy: A Single Centre, Prospective, Open-Label Pilot Study. *Int. J. Breast Cancer* **2018**, *2018*, 2479274. [CrossRef] [PubMed]
93. Composition of Holoil® Series. Available online: https://www.holoil.it/site (accessed on 19 May 2022).
94. Franco, P.; Potenza, I.; Moretto, F.; Segantin, M.; Grosso, M.; Lombardo, A.; Taricco, D.; Vallario, P.; Filippi, A.R.; Rampino, M.; et al. Hypericum perforatum and neem oil for the management of acute skin toxicity in head and neck cancer patients undergoing radiation or chemo-radiation: A single-arm prospective observational study. *Radiat. Oncol.* **2014**, *9*, 297. [CrossRef]

95. Rafati, M.; Ghasemi, A.; Saeedi, M.; Habibi, E.; Salehifar, E.; Mosazadeh, M.; Maham, M. Nigella sativa L. for prevention of acute radiation dermatitis in breast cancer: A randomized, double-blind, placebo-controlled, clinical trial. *Complement. Ther. Med.* **2019**, *47*, 102205. [CrossRef]
96. Karbasforooshan, H.; Hosseini, S.; Elyasi, S.; Pakdel, A.F.; Karimi, G. Topical silymarin administration for prevention of acute radiodermatitis in breast cancer patients: A randomized, double-blind, placebo-controlled clinical trial. *Phytother. Res.* **2018**, *33*, 379–386. [CrossRef]
97. Becker-Schiebe, M.; Mengs, U.; Schaefer, M.; Bulitta, M.; Hoffmann, W. Topical use of a silymarin-based preparation to prevent radiodermatitis: Results of a prospective study in breast cancer patients. *Strahlenther. Onkol.* **2011**, *187*, 485. [CrossRef]
98. Palatty, P.L.; Azmidah, A.; Rao, S.; Jayachander, D.; Thilakchand, K.R.; Rai, M.P.; Haniadka, R.; Simon, P.; Ravi, R.; Jimmy, R.; et al. Topical application of a sandal wood oil and turmeric based cream prevents radiodermatitis in head and neck cancer patients undergoing external beam radiotherapy: A pilot study. *Br. J. Radiol.* **2014**, *87*, 20130490. [CrossRef]
99. Rao, S.; Hegde, S.K.; Baliga-Rao, M.P.; Lobo, J.; Palatty, P.L.; George, T.; Baliga, M.S. Sandalwood Oil and Turmeric-Based Cream Prevents Ionizing Radiation-Induced Dermatitis in Breast Cancer Patients: Clinical Study. *Medicines* **2017**, *4*, 43. [CrossRef] [PubMed]
100. Wolf, J.R.; Gewandter, J.S.; Bautista, J.; Heckler, C.E.; Strasser, J.; Dyk, P.; Anderson, T.; Gross, H.; Speer, T.; Dolohanty, L.; et al. Utility of topical agents for radiation dermatitis and pain: A randomized clinical trial. *Support. Care Cancer* **2019**, *28*, 3303–3311. [CrossRef] [PubMed]
101. Patel, N.A.; Patel, N.J.; Patel, R.P. Formulation and Evaluation of Curcumin Gel for Topical Application. *Pharm. Dev. Technol.* **2008**, *14*, 83–92. [CrossRef] [PubMed]
102. Kim, J.; Park, S.; Jeon, B.-S.; Jang, W.-S.; Lee, S.-J.; Son, Y.; Rhim, K.-J.; Lee, S.I.; Lee, S.-S. Therapeutic effect of topical application of curcumin during treatment of radiation burns in a mini-pig model. *J. Vet. Sci.* **2016**, *17*, 435–444. [CrossRef] [PubMed]
103. Palefsky, I. Rozdział Uwagi dotyczące wytwarzania kosmeceutyków. In *Kosmeceutyki*, 2nd ed.; Draelos, Z.D., Ed.; Elsevier Edra Urban & Partner: Wrocław, Poland, 2009; pp. 19–26.
104. Thornfeldt, C.R. Rozdział 12: Rośliny jako kosmeceutyki. In *Kosmeceutyki*, 2nd ed.; Draelos, Z.D., Ed.; część 2; Elsevier Edra Urban & Partner: Wrocław, Poland, 2009; pp. 87–98.

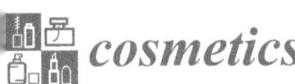

Review

Apiaceae as an Important Source of Antioxidants and Their Applications

Punniamoorthy Thiviya [1], Ashoka Gamage [2], Dinushika Piumali [1], Othmane Merah [3,4,*] and Terrence Madhujith [5,*]

1. Postgraduate Institute of Agriculture, University of Peradeniya, Peradeniya 20400, Sri Lanka; thiviya904@gmail.com (P.T.); dinushikapiumali@gmail.com (D.P.)
2. Chemical and Process Engineering, Faculty of Engineering, University of Peradeniya, Peradeniya 20400, Sri Lanka; ashogamage@gmail.com
3. Laboratoire de Chimie Agro-Industrielle (LCA), Institut National de la Recherche Agronomique, Université de Toulouse, CEDEX 4, 31030 Toulouse, France
4. Département Génie Biologique, IUT Paul Sabatier, Université Paul Sabatier, 32000 Auch, France
5. Department of Food Science and Technology, Faculty of Agriculture, University of Peradeniya, Peradeniya 20400, Sri Lanka
* Correspondence: othmane.merah@ensiacet.fr (O.M.); tmadhujith@agri.pdn.ac.lk (T.M.); Tel.: +33-53-432-3523 (O.M.); +94-71-341-2172 (T.M.)

Citation: Thiviya, P.; Gamage, A.; Piumali, D.; Merah, O.; Madhujith, T. Apiaceae as an Important Source of Antioxidants and Their Applications. *Cosmetics* **2021**, *8*, 111. https://doi.org/10.3390/cosmetics8040111

Academic Editor: Isabel Martins de Almeida

Received: 22 October 2021
Accepted: 17 November 2021
Published: 22 November 2021

Publisher's Note: MDPI stays neutral with regard to jurisdictional claims in published maps and institutional affiliations.

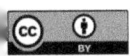

Copyright: © 2021 by the authors. Licensee MDPI, Basel, Switzerland. This article is an open access article distributed under the terms and conditions of the Creative Commons Attribution (CC BY) license (https://creativecommons.org/licenses/by/4.0/).

Abstract: The excess level of reactive oxygen species (ROS) disturbs the oxidative balance leading to oxidative stress, which, in turn, causes diabetes mellites, cancer, and cardiovascular diseases. These effects of ROS and oxidative stress can be balanced by dietary antioxidants. In recent years, there has been an increasing trend in the use of herbal products for personal and beauty care. The Apiaceae (previously Umbelliferae) family is a good source of antioxidants, predominantly phenolic compounds, therefore, widely used in the pharmaceutical, cosmetic, cosmeceutical, flavor, and perfumery industries. These natural antioxidants include polyphenolic acids, flavonoids, carotenoids, tocopherols, and ascorbic acids, and exhibit a wide range of biological effects, including anti-inflammatory, anti-aging, anti-atherosclerosis, and anticancer. This review discusses the Apiaceae family plants as an important source of antioxidants their therapeutic value and the use in cosmetics.

Keywords: antioxidants; Apiaceae; phenolic compounds

1. Introduction

The Apiaceae (previously Umbelliferae) is one of the best-known families of flowering plants (*Angiosperms*), which comprises of nearly 300–455 genera and 3000–3750 species distributed globally [1]. Apiaceae (Umbellifers) are nearly cosmopolitan whilethe Asia has the highest number of genera (289) of which most of them are endemics (177) followed by the Europe (126) and Africa (121) [2]. Celery (*Apium graveolens*), carrot (*Daucus carota*), Indian pennywort/Vallarai/Gotukola (*Centella asiatica* L. Urb), parsley (*Petroselinum crispum*), parsnip (*Pastinaca sativa*), wild celery (*Angelica archangelica*), coriander (*Coriandrum sativum*), cumin (*Cuminum cyminum*), fennel (*Foeniculum vulgare*), anise (*Pimpinella anisum*), dill (*Anethum graveolens*), and caraway (*Carum carvi*) are the economically important foods, herbs, and spice plants in the Apiaceae family [3–5]. Apiaceae plants have also been traditionally used for ethnomedicines; *Ferulago trachycarpa* [6], *Trachyspermum ammi* (Ajowain) [7], and *Capnophyllum peregrinum* [1,8]. Figure 1 shows some species from the Apiaceae family.

The comparison of global production statistics of Apiaceae crops is difficult as the data tracked by the Food and Agriculture Organization of the United Nations (FAO) is recorded under the crops belonging to other families. The only Apiaceae family crops recorded by FAO are grouped as "carrots and turnips" and "Anise, badian, fennel, coriander". Production of anise, badian, fennel, and coriander was recorded to be 1.97 million MT in

2019 with the highest quantity from Asia (87.6%) especially from India (1.4 MT). Other top five producers are Mexico, Syria, Iran, China, and Turkey. However, the production of carrots and turnips in 2019 was estimated to be 44.76 MT which is nearly 23-fold higher than that of carrots and turnips. The major production is again arising from the Asia (64.8%) especially in China while the other top five countries are Uzbekistan, the United States of America, Russia, Ukraine, and the United Kingdom [9].

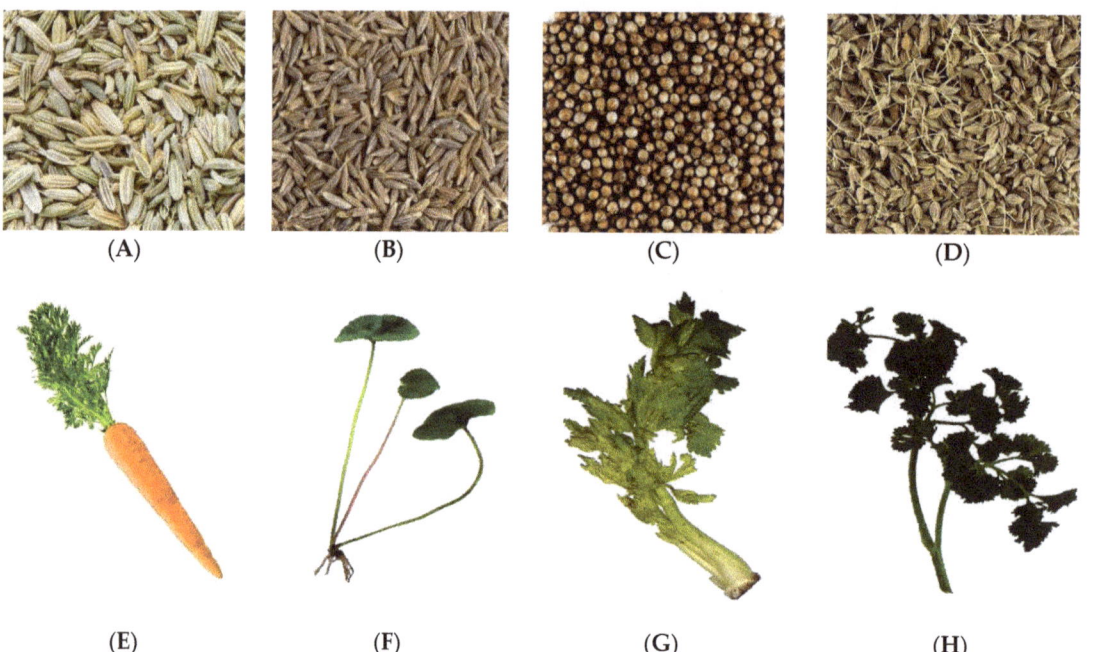

Figure 1. Different parts of selected Apiaceae family: (**A**) Fennel seeds; (**B**) Cumin seeds; (**C**) Coriander seeds; (**D**) Anise seeds; (**E**) Carrot; (**F**) Indian pennywort; (**G**) Celery plant; (**H**) Parsley (Photo courtesy of Thevin Randika).

Apiaceae family consists of economically important aromatic plants and are commonly used as food, flavors (spices, condiments), ornamental plants, for medical purposes and used in the food, perfume, pharmaceutical, cosmetic and cosmeceutical industries [5,10–12]. Some of the Apiaceae are spices, which have been used as a flavoring, seasoning, and coloring agent, and sometimes as preservatives throughout the world since ancient times, especially in India, China, and many other southeastern Asian countries [13]. Many species from Apiaceae have been used as a common household medicinal remedy for various health complications traditionally [14,15]. Many recent studies have also reported that several species in this Apiaceae family are good sources of bioactive phytochemicals with potent antioxidant, antibacterial, antibiotic or antimicrobial, and anti-inflammatory properties, antidiabetic, anticarcinogenic, cardioprotective, antihyperglycemic, hypolipidemic effects, and among others [7,15–17].

Due to health risks and toxicity, synthetic phenolic antioxidants are replaced with natural antioxidants [18–20]. The natural antioxidants from plant or spices and herbs extracts are vitamins, tocopherols, ascorbic acids, carotenoids, phenolic acid, flavonoids, tannins, stilbenes, lignans, terpenes, anthocyanins, alkaloids, components of essential oils, phospholipids, among others [13,19,21,22]. Apiaceae plants are rich source of these natural antioxidants of which phenolic compounds especially phenolic acids and flavonoids are found predominantly [7]. They are responsible for organoleptic characteristics such as bitterness, astringency, color, flavor, and odor [23].

Overproduction of the reactive oxygen species (ROS) results in oxidative stress that leads to several pathologies, such as hypertriglyceridemia, cancer, neurodegenerative diseases, diabetes, skin diseases, aging, wound healing, and cardiovascular diseases, because of its role in reducing inflammation, DNA damage changes to proteins and peroxidation of lipids [24–28]. These effects of reactive oxygen species (ROS) and oxidative stress can be balanced by antioxidant enzymes and natural dietary antioxidants [29]. Apiaceae rich in antioxidants, predominantly phenolic acids and flavonoids have many therapeutic benefits [7,30,31]. Table 1 shows the reported therapeutic effects of antioxidants from Apiaceae species.

Table 1. Therapeutic effects of antioxidants from Apiaceae species.

Apiaceae Family	Disease Condition
Anise (*Pimpinella anisum*)	Dementia [32], neurological disorder [33], Alzheimer's disease [34], depression [35], diabetes mellitus [36],
Caraway (*Carum carvi*)	Hypertriglyceridemia [30], reducing oxidative stress in diabetes mellitus [37], sepsis-induced organ failure [38], hypertension, eczema, and antiradical profile are the underlying mechanism for pharmacological properties such as antimicrobial, antidiabetic, anticarcinogenic/antimutagenic, antistress, antiulcerogenic agents [31,39]
Celery (*Apium graveolens*)	Hypertriglyceridemia [30], hyperlipidemia [40], pimples [41], antiproliferative and antiangiogenic effect on cancer [42]
Coriander (*Coriandrum sativum*)	Pimples/acne [41,43], breast cancer [43,44], hepatoprotective effect, gastric ulcers [45],
Cumin (*Cuminum cyminum*)	Antiradical profile are the underlying mechanism for pharmacological properties such as antimicrobial, antidiabetic, anticarcinogenic/antimutagenic, antistress, antiulcerogenic agents [31], neurodegeneration seen in Parkinson's disease [46]
Dill (*Anethum graveolens*)	Diabetes mellitus [15], hypertriglyceridemia [30],
Indian pennywort (*Centella asiatica* L. Urb)	Diabetes mellitus and its related complication [47], neuroprotective effect [48], skin aging, skin diseases, and damage [49], obesity [50], wound healing [51]

Furthermore, antioxidants such as vitamin A, vitamin C, vitamin E, thiols, flavonoids, and other polyphenolics have known applications in dermatology and cosmetology [49,52]. The application of these phenolic compounds in cosmetics has also proved for their anti-aging, photoprotective, antimicrobial, wound healing, and anti-inflammatory action [49,53].

Free radical scavenging and collagenase and elastase inhibitory activities of polyphenols can delay the aging process. The high antioxidant capacity of phytonutrients, especially flavonoids, and triterpenoids, involve in the stimulation of keratinocyte and fibroblast proliferation and play an important role in wound healing. Further polyphenols act as free-radical scavengers and can protect against ultraviolet (UV) damage [49,54–56]. Other than the active ingredients, antioxidants are added as protectors of other active ingredients of the cosmetics against oxidation [53,57].

Recently, natural antioxidants derived from plant sources such as spices, herbs, and the essential oil extracted from them have gained mounting interest in the application of cosmetic and pharmaceutical products [49,58]. Many studies revealed that plants from the Apiaceae family can be a good source of natural antioxidants and have the potential for pharmaceutical and cosmetic applications [1,59,60]. In this context, this review discusses the Apiaceae as an important source of antioxidants, its therapeutical benefit, anti-oxidant content, and anti-oxidant capacity of different species of Apiaceae, mechanism, and the application of antioxidants in cosmetics and cosmeceuticals.

2. Importance of Apiaceae as Food and Nutraceuticals

Different parts of the Apiaceae plants are generally consumed as vegetables or spices, such as leaves (carrot, fennel, dill, celery, parsley, and coriander), seeds (caraway, cumin, anise, dill, fennel, celery, angelica, and coriander), root (carrot, angelica), and leaf stalks (fennel) [23,61]. Aromatic spices have been traditionally used for the preparation of herbal teas, salads, and flavoring agents in stewed, boiled, grilled, or baked dishes, meat and fish dishes, and ice cream [62]. Some spices from Apiaceae are used as preservative agents in food due to the antioxidant components [13,23]. Apiaceae is largely produced for its application in foods, pharmaceuticals, perfumes, and cosmetic productions [63].

Furthermore, plants from the Apiaceae family are also a very important source of nutraceuticals and are well-known for their medicinal use since ancient times. Particularly in Asia and Africa, seeds and other plant parts of the Apiaceae have been used as a common household medicinal remedy for various health complications such as indigestion, constipation, hypertension, cardiovascular diseases, appendicitis, kidney stones, stomach ailments, abdominal pain, and acidity and to stimulates appetite, among others [14,15]. Many recent studies have reported that several species in the Apiaceae family are good sources of bioactive phytochemicals with potent antioxidant, antibacterial, antibiotic or antimicrobial, and anti-inflammatory properties, antidiabetic, anticarcinogenic, cardioprotective, antihyperglycemic, hypolipidemic effects, and among others [7,15–17].

Daucus carota Linn. (carrot) is reported to have anti-nociceptive, anti-inflammatory effects, hypoglycemic and antidiabetic activities [64]. Different parts of *Coriandrum sativum* Linn. (coriander) were reported to have antioxidant, antidiabetic, anticancer, antibacterial, antifungal, anti-inflammatory, antinociceptive, and anti-edema properties [65,66]. *Foeniculum vulgare* Mill. (fennel) has antimicrobial, antiviral, antiprotozoal, antioxidant, antitumor, anti-inflammatory, cytoprotective, hepatoprotective, hypoglycemic, and estrogenic effects [67]. Some studies showed that *Centella asiatica* (Indian pennywort) has antioxidant, antihyperglycemic, anti-inflammatory, analgesic effects, neuroprotective, memory enhancing, and skin protective activity [47,48,60,68]. In addition to that, *Centella asiatica* has also been used in treating all kinds of diseases such as gastrointestinal disease, gastric ulcer, asthma, wound healing, and eczema [60].

Essential oils of Apiaceous fruit such as cumin, caraway, and coriander have potent bactericidal activity against Gram-negative bacterial strains *E. coli* and *Bordetella bronchiseptica* [16]. Additionally, antioxidant and hepatoprotective effect has reported with essential oil extracted from caraway and coriander [69]. Essential oils extracted from plant source including Apiaceae has an effective antiviral agent that has potential to inhibit the viral spike protein and can be used as alternative therapies to manage diseases including SARS-CoV-2 [70]. Essential oil from *Coriandrum sativum* L. (coriander) has also shown antidiabetic, antioxidant, hypocholesterolemic, antihelmintic, antibacterial, hepatoprotective, anticancer, anti-inflammatory, antianxiety, and anxiolytic activities [45,58].

Angelica biserrata is a well-known medicinal plant in Chinese traditional medicine which has been broadly applied to treat inflammation, arthritis, and headache. They are also reported to have antitumor, anti-inflammatory, antioxidant, antibacterial, immunomodulatory, sedative, and analgesic effects and are being used in cosmetics [71,72]. *Ferulago* species have been used as a sedative, tonic, digestive, carminative, aphrodisiac and in the treatment of the intestinal worms and hemorrhoids [6]. Coumarin is the main phytochemical compound in *Ferulago* which has antibacterial, antifungal, anticoagulant, anti-inflammatory, anticancer, antihypertensive, antihyperglycemic, antioxidant, and anti-inflammatory [6].

3. Chemical Composition of Apiaceae Family and Their Antioxidant Activity

Antioxidants can be defined as substances that, when present at low concentrations, delay or prevent oxidation of a substrate mainly through their free radical scavenging activity [73]. The natural antioxidant capacity of plant or spices and herbs or their extract is mainly associated with the wide range of biologically active compounds that includes phenolic acid, flavonoids, alkaloids, carotenoids, vitamins, tocopherols, ascorbic acids, tannins, lignans, terpenes, components of essential oils, anthocyanins, phospholipids, among others [13,19,21,49]. Tables 2 and 3 summarize the primary antioxidant and other biologically active compounds present in the Apiaceae family.

Table 2. Chemical composition of some Apiaceae species.

Apiaceae	Plant Part Used	Uses [1]	Important Chemical Constituents	Reference
Anise (*Pimpinella anisum*)	S [2]	C [2]	Phenolic acids including anisic acid, chlorogenic acid isomers, caffeoylquinic acid, flavonoids including rutin, luteolin-7-glucoside, apigenin-7-glucoside, disorienting, other components trans-anethole, estragole, anise ketone caryophyllene, anisaldehyde, linalool, limonene, pinene, acetaldehyde, p-cresol, creosol, hydroquinine, farnasene, camphene, eugenol, acetanisole,	[21,74]
Caraway (*Carum carvi*)	R, L, S	C	Phenolic acids including chlorogenic, p-coumaric, caffeic, and ferulic acid, flavonoids including kaempferol, quercetin, 3-glucuronide, isoquercitrin, volatile compound including limonene, carvone, sesquiterpene, aromatic aldehydes, terpene esters, terpenol, terpenal, terpenon, safranal, tannins	[21,23]
Carrot (*Daucus carota*)	R, L	V	α- and β-Carotenes, ascorbic acid, tannin, phenolic acids including caffeic, chlorogenic, ferulic, 5-caffeolquinic acid, volatile terpinolene, β-caryophyllene, γ-terpinene, γ-bisabolene, myrcene, limonene, and α-pinene	[23,29,75]
Celery (*Apium graveolens*)	L, S	C, V	Phenolic acids including, p-coumaric, caffeic, ferulic, chlorogenic, and gallic acid, flavonoids included apigenin, luteolin, quercetin, rutin, and kaempferol, volatile compounds (limonene, myrcene, α-pinene, β-selinene) and other tannin, saponin, carotenoids, anthocyanins	[18,76,77]
Coriander (*Coriandrum sativum*)	L, S	C, V	Phenolic acids including p-coumaric, ferulic, vanillic, chlorogenic, caffeic, and gallic acid, flavonoids including quercetin, kaempferol, acacetin, rutin other linalool, borneol, geraniol, terpineol, cumene, pinene, γ-terpinene, limonene, myrcene, camphene, tocopherols, pyrogallol, p-cymol, n-decylaldehyde, acetic acid esters	[18,21,23]
Cumin (*Cuminum cyminum*)	S [3]	C, V [3]	Phenolic acids including quercetin, p-p-coumaric, rosmarinic, vanillic and cinnamic acids, and trans-2-dihydrocinnamic acid others cuminal, cuminaldehyde, linalool, cymene and γ-terpenoids, thymoquinone, 3-caren-10-al, γ-terpinene, p-cymene and β-pinene, pinocarveol, carotol, resorcinol, tannin	[23,78–81]
Dill (*Anethum graveolens*)	L, S	C, V	Phenolic acids: chlorogenic and benzoic acids, flavonoids: quercetin, kaempferol, myricetin, catechins, isorhamnetin, others carvone, limonene, geraniol, α-phellandrene, p-cymene	[21,23]
Fennel (*Foeniculum vulgare*)	L, S	C, V	Phenolic acids: p-coumaric acid, ferulic, quercetin, rosmarinic, tannic, caffeic, gallic, cinnamic, vanillic, ellagic, chlorogenic, and acid, flavonoids: rutin, quercetin, kaempferol, others vitamin C and E, oleoresins, β-carotene, β-sitosterol, campesterol, eugenol, carnosil, limonene, camphene, β-pinene, fenchyl alcohol, anisaldehyde, myristicin, dillapiole	[23,62,74,82]

Table 2. Cont.

Apiaceae	Plant Part Used	Uses [1]	Important Chemical Constituents	Reference
Indian pennywort (Centella asiatica L. Urb)	L	V	Flavonoids including quercetin, kaempferol, volatile pinene, terpene acetate, p-cyrnol, caryophyllene	[60]
Parsley (Petroselinum crispum)	L	C, V	Phenolic acids: chlorogenic acid, p-coumaric acid, caffeic acid, gallic acid, vanillic acid flavonoids: apigenin, luteolin, kaempferol, myricetin, rutin, quercetin	[18,21]
Wild celery (Angelica archangelica)	L, R, S [4]	C, V [4]	Phenolic acids: coumarin, other: terpenoids including α-pinene, δ-3-carene, β-phellandrene and limonene	[23]

[1] Christensen and Brandt, 2006 [61]; [2] Gülçın et al., 2003 [83]; [3] Embuscado, 2015 [78]; [4] Roslon et al., 2011 [84]; R: Root; L: Leaves; S: Seeds; C: Condiment or flavoring; V: Vegetable.

Table 3. Flavonoid content of some Apiaceae species.

Apiaceae Family	Mean Flavonoid Content (mg per 100 g)
Carrot (Daucus carota)	Kaempferol (0.24), Quercetin (0.21), Luteolin (0.11), Myricetin (0.04) (raw)
Celery (Apium graveolens)	Luteolin (762.4), apigenin (78.65) (seeds) Apigenin (19.10), Luteolin (3.50) (celery hearts, green) Apigenin (2.85), Luteolin (1.05), Quercetin (0.39), Kaempferol (0.22) (raw)
Coriander (Coriandrum sativum)	Quercetin (52.90) (leaves, raw)
Dill (Anethum graveolens)	Quercetin (55.15), isorhamnetin (43.50), kaempferol (13.33), myricetin (0.70) (fresh)
Fennel (Foeniculum vulgare)	Eriodictyo (1.08), Quercetin (0.23) (bulb) Quercetin (48.80), myricetin (19.80), isorhamnetin (9.30), kaempferol (6.50), luteolin (0.10) (leaves, raw)
Parsley (Petroselinum crispum)	Apigenin (4503.50), Isorhamnetin (331.24), Luteolin (19.75) (dried) Apigenin (215.46), Myricetin (14.84), Kaempferol (1.49), Luteolin (1.09), Quercetin (0.28) (fresh)
Parsnip (Pastinaca sativa)	Quercetin (0.99) (raw)

Source: USDA Database for flavonoid content [85].

Studies have shown that Apiaceae are excellent sources of antioxidants with a high content of phenolic compounds particularly phenolic acid and flavonoids [7]. A strong correlation between antioxidative activities and phenolic compounds was found [7,49,86]. Therefore, phenolic compounds are probably the major contributor to their antioxidant capacity.

Widely occurring phenolic compounds in plants includes flavonoids, flavanones, flavonols, and isoflavonoids, lignans, phenols, and phenolic acids, phenolic ketones, phenylpropanoids, quinonoids, stilbenoids, anthocyanins, anthochlors, benzofurans, chromones, coumarins, tannins, and xanthones [23].

4. Methods of Extraction and Identification of Antioxidant

Phenolics, flavanoids, anthocyanins stilbene, and lignan are hydro-soluble antioxidants while carotene, lycopene, lutein, and zeaxanthin are lipid-soluble antioxidants [87]. The effective extraction and proper assessment of antioxidants from food and medicinal plants are crucial to explore the potential antioxidant sources and promote the application as functional ingredients [87]. The antioxidative bioactive compounds can be extracted from fresh or dried (freeze-dried or air-dried) and treated (milling and homogenization) samples using conventional and unconventional methods [88].

Conventional methods or classical methods are generally based on the extractive potential of various solvents, using heating or mixing [54,89]. Solvents and their combination have been used for the extraction of plant phenolic compounds, often with different proportions of water [88]. Solvents are chosen based on the polarity of the compounds to be extracted [90]. Various common solvents in order of increasing polarity are hexane < ether < dichloromethane < chloroform < ethyl acetate < acetone < ethanol < methanol < water [89,90]. The combined use of water and organic solvent may facilitate the extraction of chemicals that are soluble in water and/or organic solvent [22]. Multiple solvents can be used sequentially to limit the number of analogous compounds in the desired yield [90]. Many other factors such as type and concentration of extraction solvent (sample to solvent ratio), extraction temperature, extraction time, and extraction pH, as well as the chemical composition and physical characteristics of the samples also influence the extraction efficiency [87,88].

Various classical methods include Soxhlet extraction, maceration, hydro-distillation, infusion, percolation, decoction, cold pressing or expression, and aqueous alcoholic extraction by fermentation [54]. In aqueous alcoholic extraction by fermentation, ethanol formed during fermentation enables the extraction of the active principles from the material and contributes to preserving the product's qualities [54]. These classical methods are time consuming, low efficient methods, require relatively large amounts of organic solvents, and may result in thermal degradation of compounds [87].

Non-conventional methods include ultrasound, microwave, and enzyme assisted extraction, high voltage electrical discharges, pulsed electric fields, and techniques based on the use of compressed fluids as extracting agents such as supercritical fluid extraction, subcritical water extraction, or pressurized fluid extraction [22,88,89]. These techniques are suitable to decrease volatility and thermal degradation during compounds extraction [19]. Some of them are considered to be "green techniques" [89].

The Folin–Ciocalteau method (F-C), has been widely used for the quantification of total phenolic compounds in plant material including Apiaceae [13,88,91,92]. Techniques such as gas chromatography (GC) and high performance liquid chromatography (HPLC) are used for chemical profiling and quantification of phenolic compounds [88]. Gas chromatographic (GC) techniques have been widely used especially for the separation and quantification of lipid peroxides, aldehydes, tocopherols, sterols, phenolic acids, and flavonoids [88,93]. Currently, HPLC is the most popular and reliable technique for the analysis of phenolic compounds [7,15,88,92], and several supports and mobile phases are available for the analysis of phenolics including anthocyanins, proanthocyanidins, hydrolysable tannins, flavonols, flavan-3-ols, flavanones, flavones, and phenolic acids in different plant extract and food samples [88].

5. Total Phenolic Content (TPC) and the Total Flavonoid Content (TFC) of Apiaceae

The total phenolic content (TPC) and the total flavonoid content (TFC) are varied within the Apiaceae family [7,91]. Table 4 shows the TPC and TFC content of some species of the Apiaceae family.

Other than these tabulated species, the TPC and TFC content of orange carrot in 80% methanolic extract is recorded as 179.3 mg GAE/100 g and 121.9 mg QE/100 g, respectively [96]. TPC and TFC content of aqueous extract of Indian pennywort (*Centella asiatica* (L.) Urb. was reported to be 2.86 g/100 g and 0.361 g/100 g [97].

However, the concentration of phenolic compounds in a particular species of plants varies significantly (Table 4) and depends on various factors such as variety or cultivar and its parts (seed, stem, root, etc.), geographical factors (characteristics of soil), environmental conditions such as temperature [23], climatic conditions [98], cultivation technology, and extraction parameters such as solvents used for extraction [23,99–102].

Table 4. The TPC and TFC of common plants of Apiaceae family.

Plant	TPC (F–C Assay)						TFC		
	[91] mg GAE/100 g DW (Seeds) ¹	[92] mg GAE/100 g (Essential oil)	[13] g of GAE/100 g of DW (edible parts) ²	[94] mg GAE/100 g DW (Seeds) ²	[95] mg GAE/g DW (Aerial Parts) ²	[7] mg GAE/g DW (Fruit) ³	[94] mg CE/100 g DW (Seeds) ²	[95] mg RE/g DW (Aerial Parts) ²	[7] mg RE/g DW (Fruit) ³
Coriander (*Coriandrum sativum* L.)	160	28.48	0.88	17.04	13.72	38.83	11.10	10.24	45.26
Anise (*Pimpinella anisum* L.)	310	10.89		46.17			17.43		
Caraway (*Carum carvi* L.)		28.58	0.61	25.96		35.45	11.77		12.81
Dill (*Anethum graveolens*)	340		0.98	69.87		14.64	49.10		18.16
Parsley (*Petroselinum crispum*)		40.81	0.97		21.63			15.73	
Celery (*Apium graveolens*); Fresh	490	7.32			17.39	19.44		8.14	13.24
Fennel (*Foeniculum vulgare*)	320			115.96		21.71	68.10		15.85
Cumin (*Cuminum cyminum*)			0.23			25.29			38.36

F–C: Folin–Ciocalteu; GAE: Gallic acid equivalent; CE: Catechin equivalents; RE: Rutin equivalents; ¹ 70% methanolic extract; ² 80% methanolic extract; ³ methanolic extract.

6. Antioxidant Capacity of Apiaceae

So far, there is no single appropriate method to determine the total antioxidant capacity of a particular sample because lack of a validated assay that can reliably measure the antioxidant capacity of foods and biological samples [21,103]. Thus, various tests have been used and based on the chemical reactions involved, the methods are broadly categorized into two categories: single electron transfer (ET), and hydrogen atom transfer (HAT) assays. ET-based assays include 2,2-diphenyl-1-picrylhydrazyl (DPPH) and 2,2′-azinobis-3-ethylbenzothiazoline-6-sulfonate (ABTS) also known as Trolox equivalent antioxidant capacity (TEAC), and ferric reducing antioxidant power (FRAP), while HAT-based assays include oxygen radical absorbance capacity (ORAC) and total peroxyl radical-trapping antioxidant parameter (TRAP) [104,105].

These test assays can also be categorized as organic substrate-based assays such as DPPH and ABTS/TEAC, mineral substrate-based tests such as FRAP, and biological substrate-based ones such as and 2,2,-azobis(2-amidinopropane) dihydrochloride- (AAPH-) induced hemolysis assays [18].

Free-radical trapping capacity can be estimated using DPPH and TEAC/ABTS assays. The FRAP assay is a test that measures the antioxidant power based on the reduction of Ferric (Fe^{3+}) to Ferrous ions (Fe^{2+}) [18,87]. DPPH and TEAC/ABTS assays are broadly applied in assaying food samples [49,103]. Table 5 shows the antioxidant capacity of various plant materials from the Apiaceae family.

Table 5. Antioxidant capacity of Apiaceae species.

Plant of the Apiaceae Family	Total Antioxidant Capacity										
	[91] (Seeds) [1]		[92] (Essential Oil)			[13] (Edible Parts) [2]	[94] (Seeds) [2]		[95] (Aerial Parts) [2]		[7] (Fruit) [3]
	DPPH [a]	ABTS [a]	DPPH [b]	ABTS [c]	FRAP [c]	DPPH [d]	DPPH, IC50 [e]	DPPH IC50 [f]	ABTS [g]	FRAP [h]	DPPH, IC50 [i]
Anise (*Pimpinella anisum* L.)	260	187	5.21	798.8	654.8	-	39.4	-	-	-	-
Caraway (*Carum carvi* L.)	-	-	7.72	455.9	899.8	5.50	13.9	-	-	-	0.046
Celery (*Apium graveolens*); Fresh	480	1000	10.46	85.0	472.3	-	-	-	-	252.1	0.318
Coriander (*Coriandrum sativum* L.)	160	52	8.15	599.2	956.5	7.02	9.6	77.6	103.0	185.0	0.021
Cumin (*Cuminum cyminum*)	-	-	-	-	-	6.61	-	-	-	-	0.112
Dill (*Anethum graveolens*)	500	684	-	-	-	6.36	81.5	-	-	-	0.572
Fennel (*Foeniculum vulgare*)	170	180	-	-	-	-	113.2	-	-	-	0.146
Parsley (*Petroselinum crispum*)	-	-	13.3	788.4	2104.4	-	-	-	22.8	231.5	331.8

[1] 70% methanolic extract; [2] 80% methanolic extract; [3] methanolic extract; [a] mg TEAC/100 g DW; [b] mg AAE/100 g oil; [c] mM TE/100 g oil; [d] mmol of Trolox/100 g of DW; [e] mL/L; [f] µg/mL; [g] µmol TE/g); [h] µmol TE/g; [i] mg/mL.

Furthermore, methanolic and ethyl acetate extracts of aerial parts of carrot (*Daucus carota*) showed best antioxidant activity with IC_{50} of 86.89 µg/mL and 166.79 µg/mL, respectively [106]. Essential oil from wild carrot (*Daucus carota* L. ssp. Carota) contains phenylpropanoids, monoterpenes, sesquiterpenes, phenols, and flavonoids and showed an in vitro antioxidant activity with the good results of DPPH (2.1 mg/mL) and ABTS (164 mmol $FeSO_4$/g) assay [107]. The values for antioxidant capacity highly varied between the studies. Due to lack of a standard assay, it is difficult to compare the results reported by different research groups and the food and nutraceutical industry cannot perform strict quality control for antioxidant products [103].

7. Mechanisms of Antioxidant Activity

7.1. Free Radicals and Oxidative Stress

Oxidative stress is defined as an event where a transient or permanent disturbance in the ROS balance-state generates physiological consequences within the cell, and the precise outcome depends on ROS targets and concentrations [24]. An appropriate amount of ROS serves as signaling molecules to regulate biological and physiological processes including cell protection, in contrast, increased levels of ROS are shown to modify or degenerate biological macromolecules such as nucleic acid (DNA degeneration), lipids (lipid oxidation), and proteins (membrane protein degeneration), thus inducing cell dysfunction or death [28,108]. There are different types of ROS, such as superoxide (O_2^-), hydroxyl radicals (HO·), hydrogen peroxide (H_2O_2), singlet oxygen ($^1O_2$), peroxynitrite ($OONO^{·-}$), nitric oxide (NO·), among others [24,109].

Normally, ROS are being constantly produced, and in the biological defense system, both enzymatic (superoxide dismutase, glutathione peroxidase, and catalase) and non-enzymatic (glutathione and ascorbic acid) antioxidants exist in the intracellular and extracellular environment to detoxify ROS and to maintain the oxidative balance [110]. In contrast, many factors such as diet, lifestyle, air pollution, exposure to UV radiation, chemicals, or inflammatory cytokines lead to increased intracellular ROS [28,49]. Excess ROS production, which exceeds the buffering capacity of antioxidant enzymes and antioxidants, shift the balance toward a more oxidative state [49].

7.2. Mechanisms of Antioxidant Activity

Antioxidants act as radical scavengers, hydrogen donors, electron donors, peroxide decomposers, singlet oxygen quenchers, metal-chelating agents, enzyme inhibitors, and synergists [110]. Phenolic compounds are classified as primary antioxidants and can protect from deleterious effects of oxidation in many ways, including free-radical quenching, chelating metal ions, preventing the accumulation of ROS, stimulation of in vivo antioxidative enzyme activities, and inhibiting lipid peroxidation [18,21].

Phenolic compounds are mainly free-radical scavengers which can delay or inhibit free-radical formation in the initiation step and/or interrupt the propagation step of autoxidation or lipid oxidation (Equations (1)–(7)), thus decreasing the formation of volatile decomposition products (e.g., aldehydes, ketones, alcohols, and epoxides) that cause rancidity [19,111].

Lipid autoxidation
Initiation:

$$RH \rightarrow R^\bullet + H^\bullet \text{ (by UV/singlet oxygen/metal catalysts/heat)} \quad (1)$$

Propagation:

$$R^\bullet + O_2 \rightarrow ROO^\bullet \quad (2)$$

$$ROO^\bullet + RH \rightarrow ROOH + R^\bullet \quad (3)$$

$$ROOH \rightarrow RO^\bullet + HO^\bullet \quad (4)$$

Termination:

$$R^\bullet + R^\bullet \rightarrow RR \text{ (Nonradical products)} \quad (5)$$

$$R^\bullet + ROO^\bullet \rightarrow ROOR \text{ (Nonradical products)} \quad (6)$$

$$ROO^\bullet + ROO^\bullet \rightarrow ROOR + O_2 \text{ (Nonradical products)} \quad (7)$$

Phenolic antioxidants (AH) can donate hydrogen atoms to lipid radicals and produce lipid derivatives and antioxidant radicals (Equation (8)), which are more stable and less readily available to promote autoxidation [112]. The antioxidant free radical may further interfere with the chain-propagation reactions (Equations (9) and (10)) [19,103,111,112].

$$R^\bullet/RO^\bullet/ROO^\bullet + AH \rightarrow RH/ROH/ROOH + A^\bullet \quad (8)$$

$$A^\bullet + RO^\bullet/ROO^\bullet \rightarrow ROA/ROOA \quad (9)$$

$$RH + ROO^\bullet \rightarrow ROOH + R^\bullet \quad (10)$$

Other than the phenolic antioxidants, fat-soluble vitamin E (α-tocopherol) and water-soluble vitamin C (L-ascorbic acid) also scavenges free radicals [111]. α-Tocopherol has a free-radical-scavenging activity that prevents propagation of lipid peroxidation by scavenging lipid peroxyl radicals (ROO$^\bullet$) and plays a role as singlet oxygen quenchers and chemical scavengers [19]. Ascorbic acid is also able to chelate metal ions (Fe^{2+}), quenches O_2, and acts as a reducing agent [111]. Flavoring plant extracts often have strong H-donating activity thus making them extremely effective antioxidants mainly due to their phenolic acids (gallic, protocatechuic, caffeic, and rosmarinic acids), flavonoids (quercetin, catechin, naringenin, and kaempferol), phenolic diterpenes (carnosol, carnosic acid, rosmanol, and rosmadial), and volatile oils (eugenol, carvacrol, thymol, and menthol) content. Some plant pigments such as anthocyanin and anthocyanidin can chelate metals and donate H to oxygen radicals thus slowing oxidation via two mechanisms [111].

Phenolic acid can bind and precipitate macromolecules such as proteins, carbohydrates, and digestive enzymes imparting deleterious nutritional effects and influence functional properties [113].

8. Antioxidants in Skin Health

The aging process depends on various pathophysiological processes. Free radicals and ROS are the main factors inducing the skin aging process which causes many changes in the structure and chemical composition of skin cells; oxidative damage to DNA, lipids, and proteins, and degeneration of the tissues [26,49]. As a result of the activity of free radicals, structural proteins such as collagen and elastin are damaged because of the overexpression of the collagenase and elastase enzymes [49]. Therefore, inhibition of collagenase and elastase is one of the key factors that can prevent the loss of skin elasticity and therefore delay the aging process. Plants that are rich in biologically active polyphenols such as flavonoids, phenolic acids, tocopherols, tannins, among others, may have collagenase and elastase inhibitory activity [49]. Furthermore, free radicals may also cause the oxidation of lipids and proteins that build cell membranes leading to their damage. After a cell membrane damage, free radicals may cause DNA damage, which leads to cell death [49,56]. Therefore, the use of antioxidants is an effective approach to treat skin aging and related problems [114].

Many plants have been used in traditional medicine because of their beneficial effects on wound healing. Research also suggests that phytonutrients, especially flavonoids and triterpenoids, also play an important role in wound healing due to their anti-oxidant properties [51]. In the early stages of wound healing, fibroblasts play an extremely important role, which induces the synthesis of collagen or a new extracellular matrix and thick actin myofibroblasts. High anti-oxidant capacity and free radicals scavenging effect of antioxidants may involve in the stimulation of keratinocyte and fibroblast proliferation [49,51].

The topical applications of Indian pennywort (*Centella asiatica* L.) in cosmetic formulations containing phenolic compounds can reduce the effects of skin aging (specifically for wrinkles), skin diseases, damage, and protection against type B UV damage [49,55]. Indian pennywort (*C. asiatica* L.) has also a positive effect on wound healing because of various mechanisms including inhibition of inflammation, promotion of angiogenesis, induction of vasodilatation, and reduction of oxidative stress [49,51]. Dill (*Anethum graveolens*) and coriander (*Coriandrum sativum*) are used to treat pimples, the latex of *Ferula foetida* is used for wound healing and leaves of *Pleurospermum brunonis* are used to treat skin diseases in northern Pakistan [41]. Study of supplementation with antioxidant (carotene, lutein, lycopene, and tocopherol) resulted in reduced skin roughness and scaling [115]. Carrot (*Daucus carota*) and coriander (*Coriandrum sativum*) has sun-blocking, antioxidant, and anti-inflammatory properties [116]. Furthermore, carrot (*Daucus carota*), coriander (*Coriandrum sativum*), and fennel (*Foeniculum vulgare*) extract can be used in hyperpigmentation or skin brightening [115,116].

9. Cosmetic and Cosmeceutical Applications of Antioxidants from Apiaceae

Antioxidants are widely used in the pharmaceutical, food, and cosmetic industries [49]. Vitamin C (ascorbates), vitamin E (tocopherols), carotenoids, thiols, flavonoids, and other polyphenolics are some antioxidants with known application in dermatology and cosmetology [52]. Presently, natural antioxidants are preferred over synthetic antioxidants [3]. Permitted synthetic antioxidants, such as butylated hydroxytoluene (BHT), butylated hydroxyanisole (BHA), tertiary butylhydroquinone (TBHQ), and propyl gallate (PG) are frequently questioned for their safety because of their potential toxicity and health risk [18–20].

Recently, natural antioxidants derived from plant sources particularly spices and herbs, and their essential oil, have gained increasing interest in the application of cosmetic and pharmaceutical products [49,58]. Studies indicated that the plants from the Apiaceae family can be a good source of natural antioxidants (Table 2) and have the potential for pharmaceutical and cosmetic applications [19,49,92]. The application of phenolic compounds in cosmetics has also proved for their anti-aging, photoprotective, antimicrobial, wound healing, and anti-inflammatory action [53]. In cosmetic preparations, antioxidants have two functions: (1) as the active ingredients and (2) as protectors of other ingredients against oxidation or preservatives [57].

The cosmetic and dermatological importance of polyphenolic compounds is mainly based on antioxidant action [53]. Polyphenols reduce oxidative damage, prevent premature aging, provide photoprotective action, and helps in the treatment of sensitive or sun-stressed skin by anti-inflammatory activity. Antioxidants are also applied to prevent or reduce oxidative deterioration of active constituents of cosmetics and to avoid oxidation of oily content present in the formulation [53].

9.1. Apiaceae in Cosmetic Formulation

Furthermore, antioxidants can be added to cosmetic products because of their free-radical scavenging capacity which has a beneficial effect on the protection of human skin against the oxidative damage caused by ultraviolet radiation and by free radicals [54]. Apiaceae plant extract can be used as a natural sunscreen in pharmaceutics or cosmetic formulations and as a valuable source of natural antioxidants [1]. Carrot (*Daucus carota*) and coriander (*Coriandrum sativum*) from Apiaceae family are used in sunscreen as they contain a phenolic compound, 7-hydroxycoumarin that absorbs ultraviolet light strongly at several wavelengths (300, 305, 325 nm) [116]. β-carotene a predominant constituent in carrot (*Daucus carota*) and lycopene play a role in the protection against photooxidative damage by singlet oxygen and peroxyl radical scavenging activity and can interact synergistically with other antioxidants [117]. Other phytochemical compounds such as tocopherols, tocotrienols, ascorbate, polyphenols (flavonoids), selenium compounds, polyunsaturated fatty acids (PUFAs), also have photoprotective effect on skin [118].

Oils and extracts of Apiaceae seeds are widely used in pharmaceuticals as a flavoring agent in mouthwash and as fragrance component in toothpastes, soaps, lotions, and perfumes [63]. Coriander (*Coriandrum sativum*) oils are also used in cosmetic emulsions, and have beneficial effects in cellulites, relieving of facial neuralgia, fungal infection, arthritis, broken capillaries, dandruff, eczema, muscular aches and pains, rheumatism, spasms, stiffness, and sweaty feet [63].

Essential oils are used in skin cream, lotion, ointment, and other various cosmetic and personal care products. Essential oil from Apiaceae, anise (*Pimpinella anisum*), caraway (*Carum carvi*), coriander (*Coriandrum sativum*), cumin (*Cuminum cyminum*), and fennel (*Foeniculum vulgare*) is used in cosmetic industries as they are reported to have antimicrobial, anti-oxidant, anti-inflammatory, and anticancer activities [59,119]. Indian pennywort/Gotukola (*Centella asiatica*) is also used in the ointment, cream, among others [60]. Coriander (*Coriandrum sativum*) oil is also used in cosmetics, body care products and perfumes [45]. However, the cost of natural essential oils is higher than the synthetic oil source [59].

Essential oil of Apiaceae species such as coriander, caraway, carrot, cumin, fennel, and celery are used as fragrance component in cosmetic preparations including creams, lotions, perfumes, and oral care products [120] as they contain high volatile aromatic monoterpenes including cuminaldehyde, anethole, linalool, carvone, among others [121]. In addition, linalool (coriander, 30–80%), carvone (dill, 30–60%; caraway, 76.8–80.5%), cuminaldehyde (cumin, 27–50%), trans-anethole (anise, 77–94%; fennel, 69.7–78.3%), are the main component in essential oil from various Apiaceae shows potential anti-oxidant property [63,122].

Cuminaldehyde (4-isopropyl benzaldehyde) is an aromatic monoterpenoid volatile compound, a main constituent in essential oil of cumin (*Cuminum cyminum* L.), and found in caraway (*Carum carvi*) have been commercially used in perfumes and other cosmetics [123]. Linalool, a monoterpene alcohol, is predominantly present in coriander oil (30–80%) [63] and possess antioxidant, antibacterial and antifungal properties [124]. Linalool is widely used as a fragrance component in perfumes and cosmetics and can also be used as cosmetics preservatives [124,125]. D-carvone, a monoterpene, is the main component of the essential oil extracted from caraway (*Carum carvi*) (50–76%), and dill (*Anethum graveolens*) (30–60%) seeds extensively used in the perfumery, oral care, and cosmetic applications [126]. D-carvone in dill (*Anethum graveolens*) seed oil is a volatile compound that shows strong antioxidant activity than α-tocopherol and can be used as a natural preservative and anti-oxidant to prevent lipid oxidation and rancidity [127].

Fennel (*F. vulgare*) seed oils can be used in moisturizing cream formulas without altering their rheological properties (steady-flow, thixotropy and viscoelastic properties) and the low peroxide value indicated that it is rich in antioxidants which can react with radicals and thus prevent peroxide formation [128]. Cumin (*Cuminum cyminum*) seed extracts (oil) and their by-products can be used for functional food applications as well as for cosmetic, scented, and pharmaceutical applications [129].

Antioxidants from carrot (*Daucus carota*) (carotenoid and plant extracts) are used in moisturizer for their beneficial effect of breaking chain in lipid peroxidation, decreasing UV-induced erythema, and sunburn cell formation [130]. Spices and herbs, whole, or ground or essential oil extracts are proved to have the potential of inhibiting lipid oxidation and microbial growth. Therefore, they can delay the onset of lipid oxidation and development of rancidity and reduce the formation of harmful substances such as heterocyclic amines [78].

9.2. Limitation to Be Considered

The stability of antioxidants is one of the major problems as they are susceptible to hydrolysis and photodegradation in the presence of oxygen. Therefore, the selection of antioxidants and their concentrations in cosmetic formulations must be optimized [130]. The best current approach being to combine anti-aging natural antioxidants acting in synergy [131]. Generally, plant-derived antioxidants contain a mixture of compounds, which have synergetic effects [112]. The use of natural antioxidants including tocopherols, carotenoids can inhibit oxidative rancidity thus protect the oil-based food systems from their quality degradation. Some natural antioxidants (citric acid, ascorbic acid, lecithin) are often termed synergists because of their ability to promote the action of the primary antioxidant [112].

10. Safety

Sometimes the frequent use of *Centella asiatica*, *Coriandrum sativum*, and caraway are limited as they can cause allergic contact dermatitis [69,132]. Coriander essential oil intake resulted in elevated serum alanine transaminase and aspartate transaminase that correlated with the noted noxious effect on liver function [69]. Furthermore, autoxidation of linalool (a major component in coriander oil) on exposure to air forms linalool hydroperoxides which increase the allergenicity of linalool [125].

11. Conclusions

The imbalance between oxidative stress and the antioxidant defense caused by overproduction of ROS is considered to be the key factor in the development of several pathologies, including aging and skin-related diseases. The effect of ROS can be balanced by natural dietary antioxidants.

Recently, there has been a growing interest in the use of natural antioxidants from plant sources instead of synthetic compounds. Several data have been highlighted regarding the antioxidant capacity of various Apiaceae plants. They are excellent sources of antioxidants such as phenolic acids, flavonoids, tannins, stilbenes, coumarins, lignans, carotenoids, tocopherols, and ascorbates, of which phenolic compounds particularly phenolic acid and flavonoids are the major contributors. Many researchers have also studied several therapeutic benefits of Apiaceae.

The application of phenolic compounds in cosmetics has proved for their anti-aging-aging, photoprotective, antimicrobial, and anti-inflammatory action because of their free-radical quenching, chelating metal ions, inhibiting lipid peroxidation, and stimulation of in vivo antioxidative enzyme activities.

Many studies explored the potential of Apiaceae as a natural antioxidant source in pharmaceutical and cosmetic applications. Though, only a few studies mentioned the application of Apiaceae plants as a source of antioxidants in cosmetics and cosmeceuticals. Further investigations can be focused on the incorporation of Apiaceae plant-based antioxidants in cosmetics and personal care products and their stability, and toxicity.

Author Contributions: Writing—original draft, P.T., A.G., D.P., O.M. and T.M. Writing—review and editing, P.T., A.G., D.P., O.M. and T.M. All authors have read and agreed to the published version of the manuscript.

Funding: This research received no external funding.

Institutional Review Board Statement: Not applicable.

Informed Consent Statement: Not applicable.

Conflicts of Interest: The authors declare no conflict of interest.

References

1. Lefahal, M.; Zaabat, N.; Ayad, R.; Makhloufi, E.H.; Djarri, L.; Benahmed, M.; Laouer, H.; Nieto, G.; Akkal, S. In Vitro Assessment of Total Phenolic and Flavonoid Contents, Antioxidant and Photoprotective Activities of Crude Methanolic Extract of Aerial Parts of *Capnophyllum peregrinum* (L.) Lange (Apiaceae) Growing in Algeria. *Medicines* **2018**, *5*, 26. [CrossRef]
2. Plunkett, G.M.; Pimenov, M.G.; Reduron, J.-P.; Kljuykov, E.V.; van Wyk, B.-E.; Ostroumova, T.A.; Henwood, M.J.; Tilney, P.M.; Spalik, K.; Watson, M.F.; et al. Apiaceae. In *Flowering Plants. Eudicots: Apiales, Gentianales (Except Rubiaceae)*; Kadereit, J.W., Bittrich, V., Eds.; The Families and Genera of Vascular Plants; Springer International Publishing: Cham, Switzerland, 2018; Volume 15, pp. 9–206. ISBN 978-3-319-93605-5.
3. Geoffriau, E.; Simon, P.W. *Carrots and Related Apiaceae Crops*, 2nd ed.; CABI: London, UK, 2020; Volume 33, ISBN 978-1-78924-095-5.
4. Simpson, M.G. 8-Diversity and Classification of Flowering Plants: Eudicots. In *Plant Systematics*, 2nd ed.; Simpson, M.G., Ed.; Academic Press: San Diego, CA, USA, 2010; pp. 275–448. ISBN 978-0-12-374380-0.
5. Tamokou, J.D.D.; Mbaveng, A.T.; Kuete, V. Chapter 8-Antimicrobial Activities of African Medicinal Spices and Vegetables. In *Medicinal Spices and Vegetables from Africa*; Kuete, V., Ed.; Academic Press: San Diego, CA, USA, 2017; pp. 207–237. ISBN 978-0-12-809286-6.
6. Dikpınar, T.; Süzgeç-Selçuk, S.; Çelik, B.Ö.; Uruşak, E.A. Antimicrobial activity of rhizomes of *Ferulago trachycarpa* Boiss. and bioguided isolation of active coumarin constituents. *Ind. Crops Prod.* **2018**, *123*, 762–767. [CrossRef]
7. Pandey, M.M.; Vijayakumar, M.; Rastogi, S.; Rawat, A.K.S. Phenolic Content and Antioxidant Properties of Selected Indian Spices of Apiaceae. *J. Herbs Spices Med. Plants* **2012**, *18*, 246–256. [CrossRef]
8. WFO World Flora Online. Available online: http://www.worldfloraonline.org/ (accessed on 6 September 2021).
9. FAOSTAT Crops and Livestock Products. Available online: http://www.fao.org/faostat/en/#data/QCL (accessed on 7 September 2021).
10. Ngahang Kamte, S.L.; Ranjbarian, F.; Cianfaglione, K.; Sut, S.; Dall'Acqua, S.; Bruno, M.; Afshar, F.H.; Iannarelli, R.; Benelli, G.; Cappellacci, L.; et al. Identification of highly effective antitrypanosomal compounds in essential oils from the Apiaceae family. *Ecotoxicol. Environ. Saf.* **2018**, *156*, 154–165. [CrossRef] [PubMed]
11. Önder, A.; Çinar, A.S.; Yilmaz Sarialtin, S.; İzgi, M.N.; Çoban, T. Evaluation of the Antioxidant Potency of *Seseli* L. Species (Apiaceae). *Turk. J. Pharm. Sci.* **2020**, *17*, 197–202. [CrossRef]
12. Shelef, L.A. HERBS | Herbs of the Umbelliferae. In *Encyclopedia of Food Sciences and Nutrition*, 2nd ed.; Caballero, B., Ed.; Academic Press: Oxford, UK, 2003; pp. 3090–3098, ISBN 978-0-12-227055-0.
13. Shan, B.; Cai, Y.Z.; Sun, M.; Corke, H. Antioxidant Capacity of 26 Spice Extracts and Characterization of Their Phenolic Constituents. *J. Agric. Food Chem.* **2005**, *53*, 7749–7759. [CrossRef]
14. Khare, C.P. *Indian Medicinal Plants: An Illustrated Dictionary*; Springer Science & Business Media: Berlin, Germany, 2008; ISBN 978-0-387-70637-5.
15. Saleem, F.; Sarkar, D.; Ankolekar, C.; Shetty, K. Phenolic bioactives and associated antioxidant and anti-hyperglycemic functions of select species of Apiaceae family targeting for type 2 diabetes relevant nutraceuticals. *Ind. Crops Prod.* **2017**, *107*, 518–525. [CrossRef]
16. Khalil, N.; Ashour, M.; Fikry, S.; Singab, A.N.; Salama, O. Chemical composition and antimicrobial activity of the essential oils of selected Apiaceous fruits. *Future J. Pharm. Sci.* **2018**, *4*, 88–92. [CrossRef]
17. Rathore, S.S.; Saxena, S.N.; Singh, B. Potential health benefits of major seed spices. *Int J Seed Spices* **2013**, *3*, 1–12.

18. Derouich, M.; Bouhlali, E.D.T.; Bammou, M.; Hmidani, A.; Sellam, K.; Alem, C. Bioactive Compounds and Antioxidant, Antiperoxidative, and Antihemolytic Properties Investigation of Three Apiaceae Species Grown in the Southeast of Morocco. *Scientifica* **2020**, *2020*, e3971041. [CrossRef]
19. Shahidi, F.; Ambigaipalan, P. Phenolics and polyphenolics in foods, beverages and spices: Antioxidant activity and health effects—A review. *J. Funct. Foods* **2015**, *18*, 820–897. [CrossRef]
20. Tosun, A.; Khan, S. Chapter 32—Antioxidant Actions of Spices and Their Phytochemicals on Age-Related Diseases. In *Bioactive Nutraceuticals and Dietary Supplements in Neurological and Brain Disease*; Watson, R.R., Preedy, V.R., Eds.; Academic Press: San Diego, CA, USA, 2015; pp. 311–318, ISBN 978-0-12-411462-3.
21. Yashin, A.; Yashin, Y.; Xia, X.; Nemzer, B. Antioxidant Activity of Spices and Their Impact on Human Health: A Review. *Antioxidants* **2017**, *6*, 70. [CrossRef] [PubMed]
22. Oroian, M.; Escriche, I. Antioxidants: Characterization, natural sources, extraction and analysis. *Food Res. Int.* **2015**, *74*, 10–36. [CrossRef] [PubMed]
23. Aćimović, M.G. Nutraceutical Potential of Apiaceae. In *Reference Series in Phytochemistry*; Milica, A., Ed.; Springer International Publishing: Cham, Switzerland, 2019; pp. 1311–1341. ISBN 978-3-319-78030-6.
24. Cervantes Gracia, K.; Llanas-Cornejo, D.; Husi, H. CVD and Oxidative Stress. *J. Clin. Med.* **2017**, *6*, 22. [CrossRef]
25. Poljsak, B.; Šuput, D.; Milisav, I. Achieving the Balance between ROS and Antioxidants: When to Use the Synthetic Antioxidants. *Oxid. Med. Cell. Longev.* **2013**, *2013*, e956792. [CrossRef]
26. Salehi, B.; Azzini, E.; Zucca, P.; Maria Varoni, E.; V Anil Kumar, N.; Dini, L.; Panzarini, E.; Rajkovic, J.; Valere Tsouh Fokou, P.; Peluso, I.; et al. Plant-Derived Bioactives and Oxidative Stress-Related Disorders: A Key Trend towards Healthy Aging and Longevity Promotion. *Appl. Sci.* **2020**, *10*, 947. [CrossRef]
27. Sharifi-Rad, M.; Anil Kumar, N.V.; Zucca, P.; Varoni, E.M.; Dini, L.; Panzarini, E.; Rajkovic, J.; Tsouh Fokou, P.V.; Azzini, E.; Peluso, I.; et al. Lifestyle, Oxidative Stress, and Antioxidants: Back and Forth in the Pathophysiology of Chronic Diseases. *Front. Physiol.* **2020**, *11*, 694. [CrossRef]
28. Kayama, Y.; Raaz, U.; Jagger, A.; Adam, M.; Schellinger, I.N.; Sakamoto, M.; Suzuki, H.; Toyama, K.; Spin, J.M.; Tsao, P.S. Diabetic Cardiovascular Disease Induced by Oxidative Stress. *Int. J. Mol. Sci.* **2015**, *16*, 25234–25263. [CrossRef]
29. Koley, T.K.; Singh, S.; Khemariya, P.; Sarkar, A.; Kaur, C.; Chaurasia, S.N.S.; Naik, P.S. Evaluation of bioactive properties of Indian carrot (*Daucus carota* L.): A chemometric approach. *Food Res. Int.* **2014**, *60*, 76–85. [CrossRef]
30. Mollazadeh, H.; Mahdian, D.; Hosseinzadeh, H. Medicinal plants in treatment of hypertriglyceridemia: A review based on their mechanisms and effectiveness. *Phytomedicine* **2019**, *53*, 43–52. [CrossRef]
31. Johri, R.K. Cuminum cyminum and Carum carvi: An update. *Pharmacogn. Rev.* **2011**, *5*, 63–72. [CrossRef]
32. Mushtaq, A.; Anwar, R.; Ahmad, M. Methanolic Extract of Pimpinella anisum L. Prevents Dementia by Reducing Oxidative Stress in Neuronal Pathways of Hypermnesic Mice. *Pak. J. Zool.* **2020**, *52*, 1779–1786. [CrossRef]
33. Karimzadeh, F.; Hosseini, M.; Mangeng, D.; Alavi, H.; Hassanzadeh, G.R.; Bayat, M.; Jafarian, M.; Kazemi, H.; Gorji, A. Anticonvulsant and neuroprotective effects of Pimpinella anisum in rat brain. *BMC Complement. Altern. Med.* **2012**, *12*, 76. [CrossRef]
34. Farzaneh, V.; Gominho, J.; Pereira, H.; Carvalho, I.S. Screening of the Antioxidant and Enzyme Inhibition Potentials of Portuguese *Pimpinella anisum* L. Seeds by GC-MS. *Food Anal. Methods* **2018**, *11*, 2645–2656. [CrossRef]
35. Shahamat, Z.; Abbasi-Maleki, S.; Mohammadi Motamed, S. Evaluation of antidepressant-like effects of aqueous and ethanolic extracts of *Pimpinella anisum* fruit in mice. *Avicenna J. Phytomedicine* **2016**, *6*, 322–328.
36. Shobha, R.I.; Rajeshwari, C.U.; Andallu, B. Anti-Peroxidative and Anti-Diabetic Activities of Aniseeds (*Pimpinella anisum* L.) and Identification of Bioactive Compounds. *SSN* **2013**, *1*, 516–527.
37. Erjaee, H.; Rajaian, H.; Nazifi, S.; Chahardahcherik, M. The effect of caraway (*Carum carvi* L.) on the blood antioxidant enzymes and lipid peroxidation in streptozotocin-induced diabetic rats. *Comp. Clin. Pathol.* **2015**, *24*, 1197–1203. [CrossRef]
38. Dadkhah, A.; Fatemi, F. Heart and kidney oxidative stress status in septic rats treated with caraway extracts. *Pharm. Biol.* **2011**, *49*, 679–686. [CrossRef]
39. Sachan, A.R.; Das, D.R.; Kumar, M. Carum carvi—An important medicinal plant. *J. Chem. Pharm. Res.* **2016**, *8*, 529–533.
40. Kooti, W.; Ghasemiboroon, M.; Asadi-Samani, M.; Ahangarpoor, A.; Noori Ahmad Abadi, M.; Afrisham, R.; Dashti, N. The effects of hydro-alcoholic extract of celery on lipid profile of rats fed a high fat diet. *Adv. Environ. Biol.* **2014**, *8*, 325–330.
41. Malik, K.; Ahmad, M.; Zafar, M.; Ullah, R.; Mahmood, H.M.; Parveen, B.; Rashid, N.; Sultana, S.; Shah, S.N.; Lubna. An ethnobotanical study of medicinal plants used to treat skin diseases in northern Pakistan. *BMC Complement. Altern. Med.* **2019**, *19*, 210. [CrossRef]
42. Danciu, C.; Avram, Ş.; Gaje, P.; Pop, G.; Şoica, C.; Craina, M.; Dumitru, C.; Dehelean, C.; Peev, C. An evaluation of three nutraceutical species in the Apiaceae family from the Western part of Romania: Antiproliferative and antiangiogenic potential. *J. Agroaliment. Process. Technol.* **2013**, *19*, 173–179.
43. Sathishkumar, P.; Preethi, J.; Vijayan, R.; Mohd Yusoff, A.R.; Ameen, F.; Suresh, S.; Balagurunathan, R.; Palvannan, T. Anti-acne, anti-dandruff and anti-breast cancer efficacy of green synthesised silver nanoparticles using Coriandrum sativum leaf extract. *J. Photochem. Photobiol. B* **2016**, *163*, 69–76. [CrossRef]
44. Tang, E.L.; Rajarajeswaran, J.; Fung, S.Y.; Kanthimathi, M. Antioxidant activity of Coriandrum sativum and protection against DNA damage and cancer cell migration. *BMC Complement. Altern. Med.* **2013**, *13*, 347. [CrossRef]

45. Sahib, N.G.; Anwar, F.; Gilani, A.-H.; Hamid, A.A.; Saari, N.; Alkharfy, K.M. Coriander (*Coriandrum sativum* L.): A Potential Source of High-Value Components for Functional Foods and Nutraceuticals—A Review. *Phytother. Res.* **2013**, *27*, 1439–1456. [CrossRef]
46. Kim, J.-B.; Kopalli, S.R.; Koppula, S. Cuminum cyminum Linn (Apiaceae) extract attenuates MPTP-induced oxidative stress and behavioral impairments in mouse model of Parkinson's disease. *Trop. J. Pharm. Res.* **2016**, *15*, 765–772. [CrossRef]
47. Masola, B.; Oguntibeju, O.O.; Oyenihi, A.B. Centella asiatica ameliorates diabetes-induced stress in rat tissues via influences on antioxidants and inflammatory cytokines. *Biomed. Pharmacother.* **2018**, *101*, 447–457. [CrossRef]
48. Amjad, S.; Umesalma, S. Protective Effect of Centella asiatica against Aluminium-Induced Neurotoxicity in Cerebral Cortex, Striatum, Hypothalamus and Hippocampus of Rat Brain-Histopathological, and Biochemical Approach. *J. Mol. Biomark. Diagn.* **2015**, *6*, 1–7. [CrossRef]
49. Zofia, N.-Ł.; Martyna, Z.-D.; Aleksandra, Z.; Tomasz, B. Comparison of the Antiaging and Protective Properties of Plants from the Apiaceae Family. *Oxid. Med. Cell. Longev.* **2020**, *2020*, e5307614. [CrossRef] [PubMed]
50. Gooda Sahib, N.; Abdul Hamid, A.; Saari, N.; Abas, F.; Pak Dek, M.S.; Rahim, M. Anti-Pancreatic Lipase and Antioxidant Activity of Selected Tropical Herbs. *Int. J. Food Prop.* **2012**, *15*, 569–578. [CrossRef]
51. Hashim, P.; Sidek, H.; Helan, M.H.M.; Sabery, A.; Palanisamy, U.D.; Ilham, M. Triterpene Composition and Bioactivities of Centella asiatica. *Molecules* **2011**, *16*, 1310–1322. [CrossRef] [PubMed]
52. Barel, A.O.; Paye, M.; Maibach, H.I. *Handbook of Cosmetic Science and Technology*, 4th ed.; CRC Press: Boca Raton, FL, USA, 2014; ISBN 978-1-84214-564-7.
53. de Lima Cherubim, D.J.; Buzanello Martins, C.V.; Oliveira Fariña, L.; da Silva de Lucca, R.A. de Polyphenols as natural antioxidants in cosmetics applications. *J. Cosmet. Dermatol.* **2020**, *19*, 33–37. [CrossRef] [PubMed]
54. Pisoschi, A.M.; Pop, A.; Cimpeanu, C.; Predoi, G. Antioxidant Capacity Determination in Plants and Plant-Derived Products: A Review. *Oxid. Med. Cell. Longev.* **2016**, *2016*, e9130976. [CrossRef] [PubMed]
55. Rahmawati, Y.D.; Aulanni'am, A.; Prasetyawan, S. Effects of Oral and Topical Application of Centella asiatica Extracts on The UVB-Induced Photoaging of Hairless Rats. *J. Pure Appl. Chem. Res.* **2019**, *8*, 7–14. [CrossRef]
56. Finkel, T.; Holbrook, N.J. Oxidants, oxidative stress and the biology of ageing. *Nature* **2000**, *408*, 239–247. [CrossRef]
57. Hamid, A.A.; Aiyelaagbe, O.O.; Usman, L.A.; Ameen, O.M.; Lawal, A. Antioxidants: Its medicinal and pharmacological applications. *Afr. J. Pure Appl. Chem.* **2010**, *4*, 142–151. [CrossRef]
58. Hajlaoui, H.; Arraouadi, S.; Noumi, E.; Aouadi, K.; Adnan, M.; Khan, M.A.; Kadri, A.; Snoussi, M. Antimicrobial, Antioxidant, Anti-Acetylcholinesterase, Antidiabetic, and Pharmacokinetic Properties of *Carum carvi* L. and *Coriandrum sativum* L. Essential Oils Alone and in Combination. *Molecules* **2021**, *26*, 3625. [CrossRef]
59. Abate, L.; Bachheti, A.; Bachheti, R.K.; Husen, A.; Getachew, M.; Pandey, D.P. Potential Role of Forest-Based Plants in Essential Oil Production: An Approach to Cosmetic and Personal Health Care Applications. In *Non-Timber Forest Products: Food, Healthcare and Industrial Applications*; Husen, A., Bachheti, R.K., Bachheti, A., Eds.; Springer International Publishing: Cham, Switzerland, 2021; pp. 1–18. ISBN 978-3-030-73077-2.
60. Brinkhaus, B.; Lindner, M.; Schuppan, D.; Hahn, E.G. Chemical, pharmacological and clinical profile of the East Asian medical plant Centella aslatica. *Phytomedicine* **2000**, *7*, 427–448. [CrossRef]
61. Christensen, L.P.; Brandt, K. Bioactive polyacetylenes in food plants of the Apiaceae family: Occurrence, bioactivity and analysis. *J. Pharm. Biomed. Anal.* **2006**, *41*, 683–693. [CrossRef]
62. Badgujar, S.B.; Patel, V.V.; Bandivdekar, A.H. Foeniculum vulgare Mill: A Review of Its Botany, Phytochemistry, Pharmacology, Contemporary Application, and Toxicology. *BioMed Res. Int.* **2014**, *2014*, 842674. [CrossRef]
63. Sayed-Ahmad, B.; Talou, T.; Saad, Z.; Hijazi, A.; Merah, O. The Apiaceae: Ethnomedicinal family as source for industrial uses. *Ind. Crops Prod.* **2017**, *109*, 661–671. [CrossRef]
64. Vasudevan, M.; Gunnam, K.K.; Parle, M. Antinociceptive and Anti-Inflammatory Properties of *Daucus carota* Seeds Extract. *J. Health Sci.* **2006**, *52*, 598–606. [CrossRef]
65. Begnami, A.F.; Spindola, H.M.; Ruiz, A.L.T.G.; de Carvalho, J.E.; Groppo, F.C.; Rehder, V.L.G. Antinociceptive and anti-edema properties of the ethyl acetate fraction obtained from extracts of *Coriandrum sativum* Linn. leaves. *Biomed. Pharmacother.* **2018**, *103*, 1617–1622. [CrossRef] [PubMed]
66. Chahal, K.K.; Singh, R.; Kumar, A.; Bhardwaj, U. Chemical composition and biological activity of *Coriandrum sativum* L.: A review. *Indian J. Nat. Prod. Resour. IJNPR Former. Nat. Prod. Radiance NPR* **2018**, *8*, 193–203.
67. Majdoub, N.; el-Guendouz, S.; Rezgui, M.; Carlier, J.; Costa, C.; Kaab, L.B.B.; Miguel, M.G. Growth, photosynthetic pigments, phenolic content and biological activities of *Foeniculum vulgare* Mill., *Anethum graveolens* L. and *Pimpinella anisum* L. (Apiaceae) in response to zinc. *Ind. Crops Prod.* **2017**, *109*, 627–636. [CrossRef]
68. Oyenihi, A.B.; Chegou, N.N.; Oguntibeju, O.O.; Masola, B. Centella asiatica enhances hepatic antioxidant status and regulates hepatic inflammatory cytokines in type 2 diabetic rats. *Pharm. Biol.* **2017**, *55*, 1671–1678. [CrossRef]
69. Samojlik, I.; Lakić, N.; Mimica-Dukić, N.; Đaković-Švajcer, K.; Božin, B. Antioxidant and Hepatoprotective Potential of Essential Oils of Coriander (*Coriandrum sativum* L.) and Caraway (*Carum carvi* L.) (Apiaceae). *J. Agric. Food Chem.* **2010**, *58*, 8848–8853. [CrossRef]

70. Kulkarni, S.A.; Nagarajan, S.K.; Ramesh, V.; Palaniyandi, V.; Selvam, S.P.; Madhavan, T. Computational evaluation of major components from plant essential oils as potent inhibitors of SARS-CoV-2 spike protein. *J. Mol. Struct.* **2020**, *1221*, 128823. [CrossRef]
71. Liu, M.; Hu, X.; Wang, X.; Zhang, J.; Peng, X.; Hu, Z.; Liu, Y. Constructing a Core Collection of the Medicinal Plant Angelica biserrata Using Genetic and Metabolic Data. *Front. Plant Sci.* **2020**, *11*, 2099. [CrossRef]
72. Ma, J.; Huang, J.; Hua, S.; Zhang, Y.; Zhang, Y.; Li, T.; Dong, L.; Gao, Q.; Fu, X. The ethnopharmacology, phytochemistry and pharmacology of *Angelica biserrata*—A review. *J. Ethnopharmacol.* **2019**, *231*, 152–169. [CrossRef]
73. Halliwell, B. How to characterize an antioxidant: An update. *Biochem. Soc. Symp.* **1995**, *61*, 73–101. [CrossRef] [PubMed]
74. Przygodzka, M.; Zielińska, D.; Ciesarová, Z.; Kukurová, K.; Zieliński, H. Comparison of methods for evaluation of the antioxidant capacity and phenolic compounds in common spices. *LWT Food Sci. Technol.* **2014**, *58*, 321–326. [CrossRef]
75. Alasalvar, C.; Grigor, J.M.; Zhang, D.; Quantick, P.C.; Shahidi, F. Comparison of Volatiles, Phenolics, Sugars, Antioxidant Vitamins, and Sensory Quality of Different Colored Carrot Varieties. *J. Agric. Food Chem.* **2001**, *49*, 1410–1416. [CrossRef]
76. Liu, D.-K.; Xu, C.-C.; Zhang, L.; Ma, H.; Chen, X.-J.; Sui, Y.-C.; Zhang, H.-Z. Evaluation of bioactive components and antioxidant capacity of four celery (*Apium graveolens* L.) leaves and petioles. *Int. J. Food Prop.* **2020**, *23*, 1097–1109. [CrossRef]
77. Yao, Y.; Sang, W.; Zhou, M.; Ren, G. Phenolic Composition and Antioxidant Activities of 11 Celery Cultivars. *J. Food Sci.* **2010**, *75*, C9–C13. [CrossRef] [PubMed]
78. Embuscado, M.E. Spices and herbs: Natural sources of antioxidants—a mini review. *J. Funct. Foods* **2015**, *18*, 811–819. [CrossRef]
79. Ghasemi, G.; Fattahi, M.; Alirezalu, A.; Ghosta, Y. Antioxidant and antifungal activities of a new chemovar of cumin (*Cuminum cyminum* L.). *Food Sci. Biotechnol.* **2018**, *28*, 669–677. [CrossRef]
80. Rebey, I.B.; Aidi Wannes, W.; Kaab, S.B.; Bourgou, S.; Tounsi, M.S.; Ksouri, R.; Fauconnier, M.L. Bioactive compounds and antioxidant activity of *Pimpinella anisum* L. accessions at different ripening stages. *Sci. Hortic.* **2019**, *246*, 453–461. [CrossRef]
81. Thippeswamy, N.B.; Naidu, K.A. Antioxidant potency of cumin varieties—cumin, black cumin and bitter cumin—on antioxidant systems. *Eur. Food Res. Technol.* **2005**, *220*, 472–476. [CrossRef]
82. Hayat, K.; Abbas, S.; Hussain, S.; Shahzad, S.A.; Tahir, M.U. Effect of microwave and conventional oven heating on phenolic constituents, fatty acids, minerals and antioxidant potential of fennel seed. *Ind. Crops Prod.* **2019**, *140*, 111610. [CrossRef]
83. Gülçın, İ.; Oktay, M.; Kıreçcı, E.; Küfrevıoğlu, Ö.İ. Screening of antioxidant and antimicrobial activities of anise (*Pimpinella anisum* L.) seed extracts. *Food Chem.* **2003**, *83*, 371–382. [CrossRef]
84. Roslon, W.; Wajs-Bonikowska, A.; Geszprych, A.; Osinska, E. Characteristics of Essential Oil from Young Shoots of Garden Angelica (Angelica Archangelica L.). *J. Essent. Oil Bear Plants* **2016**, *19*, 1462–1470. [CrossRef]
85. Haytowitz, D.B.; Wu, X.; Bhagwat, S. *USDA Database for the Flavonoid Content of Selected Foods Release 3.3*; U.S. Department of Agriculture, Agricultural Research Service. Nutrient Data Laboratory: Beltsville, MD, USA, 2018; p. 176.
86. Zainol, M.K.; Abd-Hamid, A.; Yusof, S.; Muse, R. Antioxidative activity and total phenolic compounds of leaf, root and petiole of four accessions of *Centella asiatica* (L.) Urban. *Food Chem.* **2003**, *81*, 575–581. [CrossRef]
87. Xu, D.-P.; Li, Y.; Meng, X.; Zhou, T.; Zhou, Y.; Zheng, J.; Zhang, J.-J.; Li, H.-B. Natural Antioxidants in Foods and Medicinal Plants: Extraction, Assessment and Resources. *Int. J. Mol. Sci.* **2017**, *18*, 96. [CrossRef]
88. Dai, J.; Mumper, R.J. Plant Phenolics: Extraction, Analysis and Their Antioxidant and Anticancer Properties. *Molecules* **2010**, *15*, 7313–7352. [CrossRef]
89. Azmir, J.; Zaidul, I.S.M.; Rahman, M.M.; Sharif, K.M.; Mohamed, A.; Sahena, F.; Jahurul, M.H.A.; Ghafoor, K.; Norulaini, N.A.N.; Omar, A.K.M. Techniques for extraction of bioactive compounds from plant materials: A review. *J. Food Eng.* **2013**, *117*, 426–436. [CrossRef]
90. Altemimi, A.; Lakhssassi, N.; Baharlouei, A.; Watson, D.G.; Lightfoot, D.A. Phytochemicals: Extraction, Isolation, and Identification of Bioactive Compounds from Plant Extracts. *Plants* **2017**, *6*, 42. [CrossRef]
91. Ksouda, G.; Hajji, M.; Sellimi, S.; Merlier, F.; Falcimaigne-Cordin, A.; Nasri, M.; Thomasset, B. A systematic comparison of 25 Tunisian plant species based on oil and phenolic contents, fatty acid composition and antioxidant activity. *Ind. Crops Prod.* **2018**, *123*, 768–778. [CrossRef]
92. Daga, P.; Vaishnav, S.R.; Dalmia, A.; Tumaney, A.W. Extraction, fatty acid profile, phytochemical composition and antioxidant activities of fixed oils from spices belonging to Apiaceae and Lamiaceae family. *J. Food Sci. Technol.* **2021**. [CrossRef]
93. Carocho, M.; Ferreira, I.C.F.R. A review on antioxidants, prooxidants and related controversy: Natural and synthetic compounds, screening and analysis methodologies and future perspectives. *Food Chem. Toxicol.* **2013**, *51*, 15–25. [CrossRef]
94. Christova-Bagdassarian, V.L.; Bagdassarian, K.S.; Stefanova, M. Phenolic Profile, Antioxidant and Antibacterial Activities from the Apiaceae Family (Dry Seeds). *Mintage J. Pharm. Med. Sci.* **2013**, *2*, 26–31.
95. Derouich, M.; Bouhlali, E.D.T.; Hmidani, A.; Bammou, M.; Bourkhis, B.; Sellam, K.; Alem, C. Assessment of total polyphenols, flavonoids and anti-inflammatory potential of three Apiaceae species grown in the Southeast of Morocco. *Sci. Afr.* **2020**, *9*, e00507. [CrossRef]
96. Singh, J.P.; Kaur, A.; Shevkani, K.; Singh, N. Composition, bioactive compounds and antioxidant activity of common Indian fruits and vegetables. *J. Food Sci. Technol.* **2016**, *53*, 4056–4066. [CrossRef] [PubMed]
97. Pittella, F.; Dutra, R.C.; Junior, D.D.; Lopes, M.T.P.; Barbosa, N.R. Antioxidant and cytotoxic activities of *Centella asiatica* (L.) Urb. *Int. J. Mol. Sci.* **2009**, *10*, 3713–3721. [CrossRef]

98. Dragland, S.; Senoo, H.; Wake, K.; Holte, K.; Blomhoff, R. Several Culinary and Medicinal Herbs Are Important Sources of Dietary Antioxidants. *J. Nutr.* **2003**, *133*, 1286–1290. [CrossRef]
99. Ereifej, K.I.; Feng, H.; Rababah, T.M.; Tashtoush, S.H.; Al-U'datt, M.H.; Gammoh, S.; Al-Rabadi, G.J. Effect of Extractant and Temperature on Phenolic Compounds and Antioxidant Activity of Selected Spices. *Food Nutr. Sci.* **2016**, *7*, 362–370. [CrossRef]
100. Karabacak, A.Ö.; Suna, S.; Tamer, C.E.; Çopur, Ö.U. Effects of oven, microwave and vacuum drying on drying characteristics, colour, total phenolic content and antioxidant capacity of celery slices. *Qual. Assur. Saf. Crops Foods* **2018**, *10*, 193–205. [CrossRef]
101. Naeem, A.; Abbas, T.; Ali, T.M.; Hasnain, A. Inactivation of Food Borne Pathogens by Lipid Fractions of Culinary Condiments and Their Nutraceutical Properties. *Microbiol. Res.* **2018**, *9*, 33–38. [CrossRef]
102. Wangensteen, H.; Samuelsen, A.B.; Malterud, K.E. Antioxidant activity in extracts from coriander. *Food Chem.* **2004**, *88*, 293–297. [CrossRef]
103. Huang, D.; Ou, B.; Prior, R.L. The Chemistry behind Antioxidant Capacity Assays. *J. Agric. Food Chem.* **2005**, *53*, 1841–1856. [CrossRef]
104. Apak, R.; Güçlü, K.; Demirata, B.; Özyürek, M.; Çelik, S.E.; Bektaşoğlu, B.; Berker, K.I.; Özyurt, D. Comparative Evaluation of Various Total Antioxidant Capacity Assays Applied to Phenolic Compounds with the CUPRAC Assay. *Molecules* **2007**, *12*, 1496–1547. [CrossRef]
105. Zhong, Y.; Shahidi, F. 12-Methods for the assessment of antioxidant activity in foods. In *Handbook of Antioxidants for Food Preservation*; Shahidi, F., Ed.; Woodhead Publishing Series in Food Science, Technology and Nutrition; Woodhead Publishing: Southston, UK, 2015; pp. 287–333. ISBN 978-1-78242-089-7.
106. Ayeni, E.A.; Abubakar, A.; Ibrahim, G.; Atinga, V.; Muhammad, Z. Phytochemical, nutraceutical and antioxidant studies of the aerial parts of *Daucus carota* L. (Apiaceae). *J. Herbmed Pharmacol.* **2018**, *7*, 68–73. [CrossRef]
107. Shebaby, W.N.; El-Sibai, M.; Smith, K.B.; Karam, M.C.; Mroueh, M.; Daher, C.F. The antioxidant and anticancer effects of wild carrot oil extract. *Phytother. Res. PTR* **2013**, *27*, 737–744. [CrossRef] [PubMed]
108. Schieber, M.; Chandel, N.S. ROS Function in Redox Signaling and Oxidative Stress. *Curr. Biol. CB* **2014**, *24*, R453–R462. [CrossRef] [PubMed]
109. Santos-Sánchez, N.F.; Salas-Coronado, R.; Villanueva-Cañongo, C.; Hernández-Carlos, B. Antioxidant compounds and their antioxidant mechanism. In *Antioxidant Compounds and Their Antioxidant Mechanism*; IntechOpen: London, UK, 2019; Volume 5, pp. 1–28. ISBN 978-1-78923-919-5.
110. Lobo, V.; Patil, A.; Phatak, A.; Chandra, N. Free radicals, antioxidants and functional foods: Impact on human health. *Pharmacogn. Rev.* **2010**, *4*, 118–126. [CrossRef] [PubMed]
111. Brewer, M.S. Natural Antioxidants: Sources, Compounds, Mechanisms of Action, and Potential Applications. *Compr. Rev. Food Sci. Food Saf.* **2011**, *10*, 221–247. [CrossRef]
112. Kiokias, S.; Varzakas, T.; Oreopoulou, V. In Vitro Activity of Vitamins, Flavonoids, and Natural Phenolic Antioxidants Against the Oxidative Deterioration of Oil-Based Systems. *Crit. Rev. Food Sci. Nutr.* **2008**, *48*, 78–93. [CrossRef]
113. Rawel, H.M.; Czajka, D.; Rohn, S.; Kroll, J. Interactions of different phenolic acids and flavonoids with soy proteins. *Int. J. Biol. Macromol.* **2002**, *30*, 137–150. [CrossRef]
114. Škrovánková, S.; Mišurcová, L.; Machů, L. Chapter Three—Antioxidant Activity and Protecting Health Effects of Common Medicinal Plants. In *Advances in Food and Nutrition Research*; Henry, J., Ed.; Academic Press: San Diego, CA, USA, 2012; Volume 67, pp. 75–139.
115. Dayan, N.; Kromidas, L. *Formulating, Packaging, and Marketing of Natural Cosmetic Products*; John Wiley & Sons: Hoboken, NJ, USA, 2011; ISBN 978-1-118-05679-0.
116. Sarkar, R.; Arora, P.; Garg, K.V. Cosmeceuticals for Hyperpigmentation: What is Available? *J. Cutan. Aesthetic Surg.* **2013**, *6*, 4–11. [CrossRef]
117. Tapiero, H.; Townsend, D.M.; Tew, K.D. The role of carotenoids in the prevention of human pathologies. *Biomed. Pharmacother.* **2004**, *58*, 100–110. [CrossRef]
118. Stahl, W.; Sies, H. β-Carotene and other carotenoids in protection from sunlight. *Am. J. Clin. Nutr.* **2012**, *96*, 1179S–1184S. [CrossRef] [PubMed]
119. Sharifi-Rad, J.; Sureda, A.; Tenore, G.C.; Daglia, M.; Sharifi-Rad, M.; Valussi, M.; Tundis, R.; Sharifi-Rad, M.; Loizzo, M.R.; Ademiluyi, A.O.; et al. Biological Activities of Essential Oils: From Plant Chemoecology to Traditional Healing Systems. *Molecules* **2017**, *22*, 70. [CrossRef] [PubMed]
120. Khan, I.A.; Abourashed, E.A. *Leung's Encyclopedia of Common Natural Ingredients: Used in Food, Drugs and Cosmetics*, 3rd ed.; John Wiley & Sons: Hoboken, NJ, USA, 2011; ISBN 978-1-118-21306-3.
121. Elmassry, M.M.; Kormod, L.; Labib, R.M.; Farag, M.A. Metabolome based volatiles mapping of roasted umbelliferous fruits aroma via HS-SPME GC/MS and peroxide levels analyses. *J. Chromatogr. B* **2018**, *1099*, 117–126. [CrossRef]
122. Lagouri, V.; Boskou, D. Screening for antioxidant activity of essential oils obtained from spices. In *Food Flavors: Generation, Analysis and Process Influence*; Charalambous, G., Ed.; Elsevier: Amsterdam, The Netherlands, 1995; Volume 37, pp. 869–879.
123. Singh, R.P.; Gangadharappa, H.V.; Mruthunjaya, K. Cuminum cyminum—A Popular Spice: An Updated Review. *Pharmacogn. J.* **2017**, *9*, 292–301. [CrossRef]
124. Herman, A.; Tambor, K.; Herman, A. Linalool Affects the Antimicrobial Efficacy of Essential Oils. *Curr. Microbiol.* **2016**, *72*, 165–172. [CrossRef] [PubMed]

25. de Groot, A. Linalool Hydroperoxides. *Dermatitis* **2019**, *30*, 243–246. [CrossRef]
26. Morcia, C.; Tumino, G.; Ghizzoni, R.; Terzi, V. Chapter 35—Carvone (*Mentha spicata* L.) Oils. In *Essential Oils in Food Preservation, Flavor and Safety*; Preedy, V.R., Ed.; Academic Press: San Diego, CA, USA, 2016; pp. 309–316, ISBN 978-0-12-416641-7.
27. Nehdia, I.A.; Abutaha, N.; Sbihi, H.M.; Tan, C.P.; Al-Resayes, S.I. Chemical composition, oxidative stability and antiproliferative activity of *Anethum graveolens* (dill) seed hexane extract. *Grasas y Aceites* **2020**, *71*, e374. [CrossRef]
28. Sayed Ahmad, B.; Talou, T.; Saad, Z.; Hijazi, A.; Cerny, M.; Kanaan, H.; Chokr, A.; Merah, O. Fennel oil and by-products seed characterization and their potential applications. *Ind. Crops Prod.* **2018**, *111*, 92–98. [CrossRef]
29. Merah, O.; Sayed-Ahmad, B.; Talou, T.; Saad, Z.; Cerny, M.; Grivot, S.; Evon, P.; Hijazi, A. Biochemical Composition of Cumin Seeds, and Biorefining Study. *Biomolecules* **2020**, *10*, 1054. [CrossRef] [PubMed]
30. Kusumawati, I.; Indrayanto, G. Chapter 15—Natural Antioxidants in Cosmetics. In *Studies in Natural Products Chemistry*; Atta-ur-Rahman, Ed.; Elsevier: Amsterdam, The Netherlands, 2013; Volume 40, pp. 485–505. ISBN 978-0-444-59603-1.
31. Pouillot, A.; Polla, L.L.; Tacchini, P.; Neequaye, A.; Polla, A.; Polla, B. Natural Antioxidants and their Effects on the Skin. In *Formulating, Packaging, and Marketing of Natural Cosmetic Products*; John Wiley & Sons, Ltd: Hoboken, NJ, USA, 2011; pp. 239–257, ISBN 978-1-118-05680-6.
32. Apiaceae. In *Meyler's Side Effects of Drugs*, 16th ed.; Aronson, J.K., Ed.; Elsevier: Oxford, UK, 2016; pp. 651–653, ISBN 978-0-444-53716-4.

MDPI AG
Grosspeteranlage 5
4052 Basel
Switzerland
Tel.: +41 61 683 77 34

Cosmetics Editorial Office
E-mail: cosmetics@mdpi.com
www.mdpi.com/journal/cosmetics

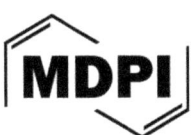

Disclaimer/Publisher's Note: The statements, opinions and data contained in all publications are solely those of the individual author(s) and contributor(s) and not of MDPI and/or the editor(s). MDPI and/or the editor(s) disclaim responsibility for any injury to people or property resulting from any ideas, methods, instructions or products referred to in the content.

www.ingramcontent.com/pod-product-compliance
Lightning Source LLC
LaVergne TN
LVHW070706100526
838202LV00013B/1040